Prevention and treatment of
DIABETIC NEPHROPATHY

TRAVENOL

The European Division of Baxter Travenol Laboratories is privileged to have been able to support the first major inter-disciplinary symposium in Europe on diabetic nephropathy, 'Prevention and Treatment of Diabetic Nephropathy' and to be associated with the publication of these proceedings.

As a manufacturer and supplier of equipment and services for patients suffering from diabetic nephropathy, Baxter Travenol Laboratories believe it is vitally important that industry should be a partner with the health care team in the treatment and welfare of the patient.

As a consequence, 'Prevention and Treatment of Diabetic Nephropathy' was held to investigate both the clinical care and control of diabetes before the patient reaches end-stage renal failure, the treatment of the diabetic with renal failure, and the emerging prospects for prevention.

Travenol is committed to support further developments in the care of the patient with diabetic nephropathy, working in partnership with the medical profession in providing product services and scientific information.

Jean-Pierre Hambursin
Business Manager
Symposium Co-ordinator

Prevention and treatment of
DIABETIC NEPHROPATHY

Proceedings of a European Inter-Disciplinary Symposium
held at the Maison de la Chimie, Paris, France
15-17 April 1983

Edited by

H Keen
M Legrain

1983 MTP PRESS LIMITED
a member of the KLUWER ACADEMIC PUBLISHERS GROUP
BOSTON / THE HAGUE / DORDRECHT / LANCASTER

Published in the UK and Europe by
MTP Press Limited
Falcon House
Lancaster, England

British Library Cataloguing in Publication Data

Prevention and treatment of diabetic nephropathy.
1. Diabetes — Complications — Congresses
I. Keen, H. II. Legrain, M.
616.4′62 RC660

ISBN 0-85200-744-2

Published in the USA by
MTP Press
A division of Kluwer Boston Inc.
190 Old Derby Street
Hingham, MA 02043, USA

Library of Congress Cataloging in Publication Data

European Inter-disciplinary Symposium (1983: Paris, France)
Prevention and treatment of diabetic nephropathy.

Bibliography: p.
Includes index.
1. Diabetic nephropathies—Congresses. I. Keen, H.
II. Legrain, M. III. Title.
RC918.D53E87 1983 616.4′62 83–19605
ISBN 0–85200–744–2

Phototypesetting by Georgia Origination, Liverpool.
Printed by Butler and Tanner Ltd., Frome and London

Contents*

* Corresponding author in *italic* face

Session Two

HYPERGLYCAEMIA AND RENAL RISK
Chairmen: G. Viberti and E. Ritz

Session Three

CLINICAL MANAGEMENT AND PREVENTION OF COMPLICATIONS
Chairmen: J. Mirouze and N. Lameire

List of Speakers

M. Berger
Dusseldorf University
Dusseldorf
W. Germany

H. Brynger
Sahlgrenska Sjukhuset
Göteborg
Sweden

F. Coronel
Universidad Complutense
Madrid
Spain

G. d'Amico
Ospedale S Carlo Borromeo
Milan
Italy

J. M. Dubernard
Hôpital Edouard Herriot
Lyon
France

I. De Leeuw
Academic Hospital Antwerp
Antwerp
Belgium

E. A. Friedman
Downtown Medical Centre
New York
USA

K. H. Gabbay
The Children's Hospital Medical Centre
Boston
USA

C. Jacobs
Centre Pasteur-Vallery-Radot
Paris
France

J. Jervell
Rikshospitalet
Oslo
Norway

T. Kangas
Helsinki Eastern Out-Patient Clinic
Helsinki
Finland

H. Keen
Guy's Hospital
London
United Kingdom

U. Keller
University Hospitalet
Basle
Switzerland

R. Khanna
Toronto Western Hospital
Ontario
Canada

E. Kohner
Hammersmith Hospital and Moorfields Eye Hospital
London
United Kingdom

R. T. Krediet
Academic Medical Centre
Amsterdam
The Netherlands

N. H. Lameire
University Hospital
Gent
Belgium

P. J. Lefèbvre
University of Liege
Liege
Belgium

M. Legrain
Hôpital de la Pitié-Salpétrière
Paris
France

B. Lindholm
Huddinge University Hospital
Sweden

P. V. Mancini
DHSS
London
United Kingdom

C. Mion
Hôpital Saint Charles
Montpellier
France

J. Mirouze
Hôpital Saint-Eloi
Montpellier
France

C. E. Mogensen
Kommunehospitalet
Aarhus
Denmark

V. Parsons
Dulwich Hospital
London
United Kingdom

H.-H. Parving
Herlev Hospital
Copenhagen
Denmark

G. Piccoli
Corso Mon Calieri
Turin
Italy

L. Puertas Vargas
Instituto de Diabetologia CRE
Madrid
Spain

E. Ritz
Ruperto Carola University
Heidelberg
West Germany

J. Rottembourg
Hôpital de la Pitié-Salpétrière
Paris
France

F. L. Shapiro
Hennepin County Medical Center
Minneapolis
USA

G. Slama
Hôtel-Dieu
Paris
France

W. V. Tamborlane
Yale University School of Medicine
New Haven
USA

A. Teuscher
Inselspital
Bern
Switzerland

J. Traeger
Hôpital Edouard Herriot
Lyon
France

R. Van Schilfgaarde
University Hospital
Leiden
Netherlands

G. C. Viberti
Guy's Hospital
London
United Kingdom

A. H. W. Wahba
World Health Organization
Copenhagen
Denmark

J. P. Wauters
Division of Nephrology
University Hospital
Lausanne
Switzerland

Opening remarks

M. LEGRAIN and H. KEEN

Professor Legrain: It is a privilege and a pleasure, and a real honour, to be in a position to welcome to Paris members from the diabetology and the nephrology communities gathered to discuss the *Prevention and Treatment of Diabetic Nephropathy*. For both disciplines the renal lesions of diabetes are of great concern. What is now widely known as the diabetic retinal–renal syndrome represents for the patient a very severe and incapacitating complication.

End-stage renal failure is a major cause of death of juvenile insulin-dependent diabetics, and renal failure is the only growing cause of chronic renal insufficiency requiring replacement therapy - a major financial burden for the community.

The purpose of the Symposium is to offer to diabetic patients better care so far as prevention and treatment are concerned through better collaboration through nephrologists and diabetologists. We can learn a lot from each other if we meet and talk, and all of us are looking forward to closer collaboration between the two disciplines.

The very large experience of the speakers, the chairmen of sessions and the discussants should not only offer a unique opportunity to present to a highly-qualified audience the most recent data on the topic, but also to initiate open and active discussion on all controversial matters. We hope that everybody participating in the Symposium will feel free to express himself in a friendly atmosphere.

Finally, I want to express my warmest thanks to all speakers and session chairmen for coming, and to Travenol Laboratories for initiating and sponsoring the Symposium, and to Messrs Edelman for organizing the meeting in our city.

Professor Keen: Professor Legrain, friends and colleagues. I wish to do little more than to echo the remarks that Professor Legrain has already made. We are co-chairmen of this meeting. In fact, one is a very wakeful chairman and the other is a sleeping chairman.

Professor Legrain has put enormous effort into the organization of these days and it is very much thanks to him that we have the excellent and very exciting programme that lies ahead. So I should like to say thank you to Professor Legrain rather particularly because of that.

Contacts between France and Britain over the diabetic kidney started many years ago. In 1848, Dr Jean-Pierre Pointe paid a visit to Britain, to Guy's Hospital to be precise, from the University of Lyons, and during that visit he met Dr Richard Bright, the father of nephrology. This was at about the time that Richard Bright was describing the heavy proteinuria which could be detected in some patients with diabetes, perhaps taking a first look at the now familiar syndrome of renal failure in the long-term diabetic. It is with this condition that we shall be concerning ourselves primarily over the next days.

Some of the mysteries that confronted Dr Bright have been solved, but many remain unresolved. We hope that the presentations, discussion and informal interactions between the diabetologists and the nephrologists who are here, brought together in this magnificent building in this splendid ambience, will stimulate some new moves forward for the diabetic.

This is a time of change. Only a decade or two ago the diabetic in renal failure was regarded as a poor prospect for the nephrologist; often visually damaged with retinopathy, with widespread arterial disease, perhaps plagued by neuropathy, the diabetic usually came bottom in the priority list for renal support. Now, the diabetic should be much less likely to go blind; timely photocoagulation has substantially reduced the risk of blindness. The diabetic is now eligible for arterial surgery if coronary or peripheral artery disease are causing serious ischaemic disorders; we hope that, with newer approaches to the diabetic diet atherosclerosis will become less common and severe. Improvements in diabetic control should reduce the risk of neuropathy; certainly the tissue damage it may cause can be prevented by good foot care.

So the scene is changing for the diabetic. The earlier fatalistic acceptance of terminal renal failure as the last act in the drama of diabetes is now much less appropriate and less readily justified on the basis of other disabling complications. We must now rethink our positions and take a much more constructive view of the diabetic in renal failure. At the same time we must intensify research into its prevention. That is what we are here for and I hope that this meeting will be the scene of significant progress toward these goals.

May I finish by thanking Messrs Travenol for providing this opportunity not only on behalf of ourselves as a group of doctors meeting to talk about important clinical problems but also on behalf of the diabetic patients themselves who have so much more at stake.

Session One

THE CHANGING SCENE

Chairmen:
M. LEGRAIN and H. KEEN

1
Overview of diabetic nephropathy

E. A. FRIEDMAN

ABSTRACT

In the United States and Western Europe, uraemia complicating diabetic nephropathy has emerged as the single most prevalent cause of renal failure leading to treatment by maintenance haemodialysis or renal transplantation. Coincident vascular damage to other organs particularly the eye prevents rehabilitation in many nephropathic diabetics. By devising a strategy for overall management of each phase of kidney disease, the patient and medical team understand what can be anticipated and accomplished.

The key to optimized therapy is the recognition of the importance of normalizing hypertensive blood pressure while achieving euglycaemia by means of patient self monitoring of blood glucose concentration. The same regimen (consisting of four times daily blood glucose testing coupled with thrice daily injections of insulin) which has proved beneficial to nonazotaemic diabetics has been successfully applied to diabetics in renal failure. Improvement in survival of diabetics treated by haemodialysis and renal transplantation has progressed to the extent that the majority of patients now live for at least 3 years, while an increasing number have been sustained for a decade or longer.

INTRODUCTION

Uraemia is the life limiting complication ending the course of about one half of insulin-dependent diabetics. Glomerular microvasculopathy ultimately causing suppression of glomerular filtration poses the most serious and predictable threat to longevity. Over the past decade, studies of animal models of induced diabetes, coupled with clinical investigation of insulin dependent diabetics, have clarified the natural history of diabetic glomerulopathy. Previous reluctance to sustain life in the uraemic diabetic by peritoneal dialysis, haemodialysis, or renal transplantation has in the United States and parts of Western Europe been supplanted by a growing experience in which life extension, often with substantial rehabilitation, is achievable for many. Once the physician and patient accept the concept that development of uraemia does not necessarily signal inevitable immediate death, a more positive and less desperate attitude permeates longterm diabetic management.

URINARY TRACT INFECTIONS IN DIABETICS

Diabetics have an increased incidence of urinary infections, as well as toxic, neurogenic, and degenerative kidney disorders (Table 1). Bacteruria has been found in increased incidence in diabetics[1]. Bacteria isolated from diabetics with urinary infections are coated with antibody in 43% of samples, suggesting intrarenal rather than bladder infection[2]. The diabetic's greater susceptibility to renal infections has been attributed to a subnormal immune response, detectable by impaired polymorphonuclear leukocyte phagocytosis and chemotaxis, and diminished lymphocyte transformation. Kass, in fact, found bacteruria in 18% of 54 asymptomatic diabetic women and 5% of 37 diabetic men[1]. Other surveys, however, have not confirmed an increased incidence of bacteruria in either diabetic school girls or pregnant diabetics[3]. Repetitive urine cultures in our own unpublished series of diabetic renal transplant recipients revealed no greater incidence of bacteruria than in non-diabetic kidney recipients. There is little doubt, however, that urinary infection, once established, is many times more likely to become seriously complicated in diabetics than in non-diabetics. Treatment of urinary infection in diabetics is

Table 1 Genito-urinary complications of diabetes mellitus

Exacerbation of bacteruria to severe infections
Pyelonephritis
Renal carbuncle
Septicaemia
Enhanced susceptibility to renal toxins
Contrast media-induced nephropathy
Interstitial nephritis (diuretic induced)
Neuropathy of bladder simulating obstruction
Bladder atony (hydronephrosis)
Large artery degenerative syndromes
Nephrosclerosis
Atheromatous embolic disease
Microvasculopathy afflicting glomerulus and retina
Diffuse intracapillary glomerulosclerosis
Nodular intracapillary glomerulosclerosis

not different than that for non-diabetics, though the following principles should be kept in mind:

(1) Normalization of blood glucose concentration probably improves resolution of sepsis. Frequent blood glucose measurements and multiple daily insulin doses will facilitate tight glucose control.

(2) Mechanical obstruction due to ureteric or bladder calculi, tumour, or an enlarged prostate must be corrected to eradicate urinary sepsis.

(3) Avoidance of a bladder catheter will reduce the risk of reinfection. Catheterization should not be performed solely to obtain a urine sample for culture.

(4) Antibiotics and other drugs mainly excreted by the kidney must be administered in lower doses in renal insufficiency.

TOXIC NEPHROPATHY IN DIABETICS

Contrast media studies in azotaemic diabetics, especially in those whose serum creatinine concentration has risen above 3 mg/dl, are risky and ought to be avoided in any circumstance in which the information needed can be developed by other diagnostic means. Both Type I and Type II diabetics may respond to intravenous urography or intravenous or intra-arterial angiographic procedures with the acute onset (hours–2 days) of oliguria and progressive azotaemia. No single contrast material has been identified as more toxic than others. Renal failure has been reported after meglumine iothalamate, meglumine diatrizoate, and sodium diatrazoate given in doses of 36–300 g. The pathogenesis of contrast agent induced nephropathy is incompletely defined. It has been hypothesized that the osmolar load of injected contrast media (about 2000 mosmol/kg H_2O), when added to hyperviscose diabetic plasma in a patient dehydrated by a preparatory cathartic, predisposes to reduced renal perfusion and ischaemic injury. Availability of sonography and radionucleide scans, to discern both renal anatomy and function, permits prudent avoidance of contrast agents in any diabetic whose serum creatinine concentration has reached 3 mg/dl. When angiography must be performed in an azotaemic diabetic, for evaluation of a transient ischaemic attack as an example, normal hydration should be maintained and 25 g of mannitol administered intravenously 1 hour prior to the study to maintain urine flow by an osmotic diuresis.

Our own experience suggests that in the absence of azotaemia or proteinuria, oliguric renal failure does not follow intravenous urography in Type II diabetics. When the creatinine clearance has fallen below 25 ml/min, however, post contrast agent acute renal failure occurs with increasing frequency, afflicting the majority of patients with a clearance of less than

10 ml/min[4]. The course of acute renal failure is variable though in most patients recovery of renal function, heralded by a diuresis, occurs after 3–10 days of oliguria.

Acute renal failure due to drug toxicity, renal ischaemia, or ingestion of or exposure to noxious chemicals may afflict the diabetic at any stage of his illness. Because moderately advanced renal insufficiency (creatinine clearance less than 40 ml/min), though common, may be unrecognized, potentially toxic drugs excreted by the kidneys, such as aminoglycoside antibiotics, must be administered in adjusted (reduced) dosage to avoid excessive accumulation in plasma or tissues. Reference to published tables relating serum levels of drugs to degree of renal insufficiency[5] has minimized the complexity of prescribing an essential yet hazardous drug.

RENAL PAPILLARY NECROSIS

Papillary necrosis in diabetes is usually, though not always, a complication of intrarenal infection. Ischaemic infarction of the renal medulla and papilla may occur in a single papilla without clinical consequence as in sickle cell trait, or may involve multiple papillae leading to destruction of the kidney and obstruction of the ureter by sloughed papillae as seen in analgesic abuse, alcoholism and diabetes. The patient complains of fever, flank pain and dysuria, which may progress to septicaemia and shock. Urine and blood cultures are usually positive for the responsible bacterial or fungal (sometimes both) organism. The urine sediment contains red cells, white cells in clumps, bacteria and renal fragments. Formerly, when radiographic contrast media studies were performed more readily in patients suspected of having papillary necrosis, the extent of renal damage discovered would be surprising. Treatment of papillary necrosis is aimed at removal of any renal tissue fragments causing obstruction and the administration of antibiotics or antifungal drugs.

GLOMERULOSCLEROSIS

Kimmelstiel and Wilson while reviewing *post mortem* findings in the kidneys of seven older age diabetics, recognized nodular intercapillary glomerulosclerosis, a specific lesion present in about half of diabetic kidneys[6,7]. The nodules begin as an increase in mesangial matrix in a glomerular lobule. The growing spherical lesion appears singly or multiply gradually encroaching on still patent capillary loops. The most consistent abnormality in the diabetic glomerulus is diffuse intercapillary glomerulosclerosis, which begins as a thickened glomerular basement membrane, associated with an enlarging mesangium filled with amorphous material that stains with periodic acid–Schiff (PAS).

Mauer and Shvil clarified our understanding of the glomerular mesangium[8], an intercapillary system of cells and matrix through which peripheral branches joined centrally form the axial pole of the glomerulus at the hilum. Within the mesangium, nerve endings, smooth muscle, and angiotensin II receptors have been identified. In diabetic nephropathy, the mesangium enlarges and contains a marked increase in smooth muscle. Mauer *et al.* speculate that some of the functional and haemodynamic aberrations of the diabetic kidney may be attributable to altered mesangial contractibility, which in turn, affects angiotensin and prostaglandin secretion and metabolism[9]. Another recently recognized function of the mesangium is the clearance of macromolecules, which pass through intercellular channels from the periphery of the mesangium to the juxtaglomerular apparatus, and then the distal tubular cells. Diabetic rats have been shown to have impaired clearance of macromolecules[10] which may include products of normal glomerular basement membrane turnover, a defect which could accelerate glomerular injury.

Osterby demonstrated a correlation between the rate of glomerular basement membrane thickening and increased mesangial size after 3½–5 years in Type I diabetics[11]. According to her analysis, the earliest phase in the genesis of diabetic microangiopathy is increased synthesis of glomerular basement membrane[12]. Ultrastructural thickening of the glomerular basement membrane is not present at the time of onset of insulin dependence[13], an important point in the argument tying genesis of microangiopathy to hyperglycaemia, rather than genetic predisposition.

Study of renal biopsies in diabetic nephropathy by immunofluorescence techniques, has detected the presence of plasma proteins, particularly albumin, deposited in a ribbon-like pattern along the tubular basement membrane and Bowman's capsule[14]. The significance of this abnormality, which also occurs in muscle and skin, is obscure.

Kidney size, glomerular diameter, tubular size and glomerular capillary filtration surface area are all significantly (about 130%) increased in diabetes. Similar enlargements have been noted in the streptozotocin induced diabetic rat[15]. Correction of hyperglycaemia by insulin treatment prevents renal and glomerular enlargement in rats. As glomerulosclerosis progresses, the kidneys contract, to the extent that by the time uraemia supervenes, the kidney is smaller than normal (75–125 g) though larger than the end-stage kidneys of interstitial or glomerulonephritis.

FUNCTIONAL CHANGES

Viberti has well summarized the recent literature detailing functional alterations in the diabetic kidney which may be detected before any clinical manifestations of nephropathy are discernable[16]. Proteinuria, mainly consisting of unmodified albumin, is a constant correlate of glomerulosclerosis. Earlier studies which found severe diabetic glomerulosclerosis in autopsy and biopsy kidney specimens in the absence of proteinuria[17,18], are not consistent with our current experience. Depending on the technique employed for protein measurement, proteinuria has been noted in all subjects with diabetes for 6 months–39 years[19], or only after 10 or more years of insulin dependence[20]. Since exercise may induce albuminuria in diabetics with normal basal albumin excretion, the use of exercise as a test for glomerulosclerosis may provide an indication of the degree and rate of progression of nephropathy. Viberti *et al.* have recently observed that serial measurements of urinary β_2-microglobulin excretion provides a reliable estimate of prospective decline in glomerular filtration rate in Type I diabetics[21].

Albumin excretion in newly diagnosed Type I diabetics is a functional abnormality which will revert to normal upon establishment of good glycaemic control with insulin treatment. Only scanty information is on hand to explain what determines the onset and degree of proteinuria in long duration diabetic nephropathy. Contradictory results have been reported in comparative biochemical analyses of glomerular basement membranes from normal and diabetic patients. Measurements of apparent glomerular pore radius by fractional clearances of dextran polymers of molecular radii of 20–40 ° indicate a size of 54–55 ° in short duration Type I diabetics, which is similar to the pore size in non-diabetics[22]. Haemodynamic factors, and alteration in electrical charge of glomerular cells and membranes, effect glomerular permselectivity of macromolecules. Albuminuria in diabetes therefore reflects more than a thickened glomerular basement membrane, and results from factors other than increased membrane pore size. Whatever the mechanism for increased permeability of glomerular capillaries, of which albumin is the most readily noted, there follows an accumulation of large macromolecules, immune globulins, and non-immune circulating aggregates within the glomerular wall and mesangium[23]. These plasma constituents are thought to serve as a stimulus to mesangial matrix production, leading to diffuse and nodular intercapillary glomerulosclerosis.

NATURAL HISTORY OF NEPHROPATHY

Careful longterm observation of Type I diabetics for more than 20 years has permitted construction of a typical course for the clinical expression of progressively severe glomerulosclerosis. The often less clear onset, and older age at onset, of Type II diabetics however, has until now blurred their follow-up study. In Type I diabetes, proteinuria is usually first noted in routine urine samples after 10–15 years of insulin dependence. By the 20th year of insulin treatment, about one half of patients have continuous proteinuria[24]. That fixed proteniuria is an ominous sign is apparent from the survival curves of a 1961 study in which only 28% of diabetics could anticipate a life expectancy of 10 years after onset of proteinuria[25]. Mogensen calculated that diabetics who had a normal glomerular filtration rate (GFR) at the onset of proteniuria, would lose GFR at the rate of 11 ml/min^{-1}y^{-1}. The interval between appearance of proteinuria and an elevation of serum creatinine concentration is about 1 year, though there is a wide variability with some patients evincing proteinuria without azotaemia for 5 or more years[26].

Other than fluid retention, there are few clinical consequences of the early stages of nephrotic syndrome due to glomerulosclerosis, though urinary protein losses may reach 10–30 g/day. Its onset can be so insidious that the patient is unsure of its presence until a weight gain of approximately 7 kg and a change in belt or shoe size has occurred. The assumption that massive (greater than 4 g/24 h) proteinuria in a diabetic is a consequence of glomerulosclerosis is supported by the nearly universal presence of diabetic retinopathy. In these instances where the fundi are benign, or the findings unusual (red cell casts in the urinary sediment, for example), a percutaneous renal biopsy should be performed to clarify the renal diagnosis. Once azotaemia occurs, after a mean of 17.3 years of diabetes in the study by Rutherford *et al,* subsequent decline in renal function is exponential, lasting a mean of 3 years[27]. Jones *et al* found that deterioration in renal function varies considerably from one diabetic to another, but its rate is constant in individuals[28]. For each patient followed by Jones *et al*, there was a linear relation between the months which elapse from the time at which serum creatinine reaches 2.3 mg/dl and the inverse (reciprocal) of the serum creatinine level. Of 9 patients whose course was plotted starting at a serum creatinine of 2.3 mg/dl, 7 reached end-stage uraemia in 5–43 months but 2 others had only minimal decline after 35 and 47 months, respectively. More recently, Viberti *et al. (vide supra)* have suggested that a simplified prospective plot of the patient's course could be obtained by repetitive measurements of urinary β_2-microglobulin[21].

Clinical manifestations

There are no clinical signs or symptoms of progressive glomerulosclerosis prior to the development of nephrotic range proteinuria. The first 13–18 or more years of glomerulosclerosis constitute the silent phase of diabetic nephropathy. Nephrotic diabetics differ from other nephrotic patients mainly in the profundity of their illness. The fluid overloaded diabetic with prior marginal cardiac compensation and wide excursions in plasma glucose concentration, lacks resilience and is distracted and enervated by multiple annoying problems. Each day may bring another new complication, be it breakdown of a foot ulcer, or a fresh vitreous haemorrhage, blocking restoration of reasonable (functional) health. Insulin dependent diabetics may experience frequent and profound hypoglycaemic episodes as renal function is lost and renal catabolism of exogenous insulin (normally about one third of insulin is metabolized by the kidney) diminishes. With further reduction in GFR to below 10 ml/min, uraemic signs including anaemia, acidosis, lethargy,

Table 2 Clinical expression of diabetic nephropathy

Stage	*Creatinine clearance*	*Strategy*
Silent	Normal – super normal	Maintain euglycaemia Control hypertension Consult ophthalmologist
Early proteinuria	30 ml/min – normal	As in silent stage, search for typical features and other renal diseases Inform patient
Late proteinuria (nephrotic)	20–29 ml/min	Plot 1/creatinine *vs* time Consider dialysis access Inventory kidney donors Review eye status Emphasize hypertensive regimen Assess cardiac status
Azotaemia	5–19 ml/min	Review alternative uraemia therapies Review eye status Create dialysis access Treatment if symptomatic
Renal death	5 ml/min	Uraemia therapy

nausea, and uncontrollable hypertension dictate the end of conservative care and signal the need for dialysis or renal transplantation. Table 2 gives the signs of renal insufficiency as a correlate of residual GFR. Lacking an overall plan, the azotaemic diabetic faces fragmented, often contradictory approaches to correcting organ or systemic disease. Successful rehabilitation of uraemic diabetics by dialysis or renal transplantation requires a team approach, in which a single physician, identifiable as the patient's doctor, follows through in integrating the needed services of ophthalmologist and nephrologist. Patients have proven remarkably able to tolerate long complicated uraemia therapy regimens so long as there remains a chance of a successful outcome. We believe a policy of full disclosure of available options, including the statistical chances of success for each, has been helpful. Delegation of a portion of responsibility to the patient, as in finger stick glucose monitoring or home haemodialysis, promotes a feeling of accomplishment and maintains self esteem.

PRE-END-STAGE URAEMIA THERAPY

Management of renal insufficiency in the diabetic just beginning an exponential decline in GFR, requires co-ordination of specialty consultants with the nephrologist, perforce, as captain of the team consisting of opthalmologist, podiatrist, vascular surgeon and psychiatrist. Depending on local circumstances, and patient preference, the co-ordinating physician might equally well be an endocrinologist or general internist, so long as patient and physician understand what is intended. Lacking overall direction, the patient may be subjected to unneeded repetitive studies, delay in urgently required treatment (such as panretinal photocoagulation) and avoidable anxiety.

Renal–retinal syndrome

Type I diabetics facing imminent uraemia must also cope with impending loss of vision due to progressive retinopathy. The prevalance of retinopathy in newly diagnosed uraemic diabetics exceeds 95%, half of whom are blind, or have reduced visual acuity. Reports of the course of uraemia therapy in the mid 1970s detailed what at first appeared to be an inevitable high incidence (50%) of blindness[29], in what has been termed a renal–retinal syndrome[30]. Appreciation of the importance of control of hypertension, and improved regulation of blood glucose concentration, has sharply reduced the rate of visual decline in haemodialysed and renal transplanted diabetics[31,32].

Hypertension

Hypertensive diabetics suffer an accelerated risk of stroke, coronary artery disease, congestive heart failure, peripheral vascular disease, retinopathy and loss of renal function[33]. Reduction of elevated blood pressure will reduce proteinuria[34] and slow the rate of declining GFR[35] in nephropathic diabetics. Christlieb reviewed the mechanism(s) for an increased rate of hypertension in diabetics without evidence of nephropathy, and suggested that hyperglycaemia induced expanded blood volume might be responsible[36]. Most hypertensive diabetics without renal disease have normal plasma renin activity (PRA). In nephropathic diabetics with proteinuria of 2 g or more daily, both plasma renin activity and plasma aldosterone concentration are significantly reduced, characterizing a 'low-renin hypertension'[37]. Defects identified in low-renin hypertensive diabetics include: decreased sympathetic activity altering stimulation of renin release[38]; defective synthesis of renin as prorenin[39]; hyalinization of afferent arterioles inhibiting passage of renin from juxtaglomerular cells into the lumen[40]; and expanded intravascular volume. Arteriolar hyalinization is a component of diabetic vasculopathy, and also contributes to hypertension by raising peripheral vascular resistance. An additional factor responsible for hypertension is an increased cardiac output as a compensation (tachycardia) to the anaemia of renal insufficiency. In this light, hypoaldosteronism (promoting natriuresis and plasma volume fall), and low-renin activity (decreased circulating angiotensin II and lowered peripheral vascular resistance), can be viewed as compensatory mechanisms to counteract hypertension.

Hypertension should be reduced to a standing blood pressure of about 120/80 mmHg employing diuretic and vasodilator drugs. In severe hypertension (diastolic pressure above 120 mmHg), potent additional drugs, including captopril and minoxidil, are effective. The keystone to hypertensive management in azotaemic diabetics is a sufficient dosage of diuretics. As GFR declines to about 25% of normal, chlorthiazide and hydrochlorthiazide become ineffective, and must be replaced by a loop diuretic such as furosemide. To effect diuresis at creatinine clearances as low as 10–20 ml/min may require total doses as high as 480 mg of furosemide daily. Adding metalazone, a long acting thiazide retaining activity in renal insufficiency, in daily doses of 5–20 mg, often promotes diuresis in resistant cases. Bi-nephrectomy for control of intractable hypertension has not been required in our programme in over 5 years. Diabetics may develop unusual or particularly severe complications of antihypertensive drugs, including worsened hyperglycaemia from diuretics; muted or altered signs and symptoms of hypoglycaemia from β-blockers; and intensified fluid retention from sympathetic inhibitors and vasodilators. An important signal indicating the limit of conservative management is persistent hypertension, poorly responsive to maximal doses of diuretics and other antihypertensive drugs.

Creatinine clearance below 20 ml/min

The necessity for impending dialytic therapy or a kidney transplant ought not to come as a surprise, but rather be an anticipated event. Timing of initiation of uraemia therapy has been advocated 'early' (creatinine clearance of 10–25 ml/min) or later, though all would agree that a creatinine clearance of less than 5 ml/min is an absolute indication for switching from conservative to more aggressive treatment. Urgent indications for dialytic treatment or a kidney transplant, in patients whose serum creatinine has reached 8 mg/dl, are: development of uraemic bleeding due to gastritis or colitis; pericarditis; convulsions; and most typically in diabetics, a non-specific deterioration characterized by weight loss, worsening hypertension and lethargy. Lacking either prospective or retrospective studies of the ideal time to start dialysis, it is reasonable to select that point in a patient's course at which further deterioration, especially of visual acuity, and the cardiovascular system, appears inevitable. Proper anticipatory planning should prepare for smooth initiation of uraemia therapy, in which an informed patient has selected the most appropriate course. Young Type I diabetics must thoroughly consider the feasibility of a kidney transplant, reflecting on potential intrafamilial donors.

END-STAGE URAEMIA

Haemodialysis

In the early 1970s, annual mortality for Type I diabetics on maintenance haemodialysis exceeded 60%, while progression of vision loss resulted in blindness for half of the survivors[41]. However, by the latter half of the 1970s appreciation of the importance of control of hypertension and intravascular volume overload improved survival, to the extent that half of the patients now live for at least 3 years[42]. A typical haemodialysis regimen requires 3 weekly treatments, each of 4–7 hours duration. Death is most often due to myocardial infarction, or failure, followed in frequency by sepsis, stroke, and withdrawal from treatment[43]. Of haemodialysis survivors, only about one in four can be termed rehabilitated, contrasted with about three in four non-diabetics who achieve gainful employment or return to work or school responsibilities[44]. Admittedly, quantification of life quality is imprecise and highly subjective. Yet our experience indicates that even blind diabetics, hemiparetic after a stroke, may opt to begin or continue haemodialysis, subjectively deriving benefit from the life that is extended. On the other hand, observation of the minority who work, raise families and lead vigorous lives, precludes a prediction of a poor outcome *a priori* for any diabetic about to begin a dialysis. Haemodialysis, when performed at home by the patient (not a family member), provides a sense of accomplishment and self control conducive to rehabilitation.

Peritoneal dialysis

Intermittent peritoneal dialysis via a surgically implanted silastic catheter has been utilized for Type I diabetics, yielding a 1 year survival as high as 52%. Others, however, have achieved less satisfactory results with as few as 22% surviving for 2 years[45]. Continuous Ambulatory Peritoneal Dialysis (CAPD), however, has yielded much more encouraging results in uraemic Type I diabetics; the treatment requires the patient to perform four dialysate exchanges daily. In the initial Toronto experience, survival of CAPD-treated patients exceeded 80% at 1 year[45]. Advantages of CAPD over haemodialysis include rapid training (under a week), absence of a machine and minimal cardiac stress. Initial clinical trials in diabetics suggest that when insulin is added to the dialysate daily blood glucose excursions are blunted, yielding control superior to that effected during haemodialysis or intermittent peritoneal dialysis[46,47]. It must be emphasized that the longterm utility of CAPD for diabetics is unknown.

Haemofiltration

Haemofiltration is a technique in which blood circulated extracorporeally is placed under pressure against a semipermeable membrane, producing an ultrafiltrate containing water and nitrogenous wastes. Prior to its reinfusion, the contracted plasma is re-expanded with a balanced salt solution. Treatment by haemofiltration performed thrice weekly for 3–6 h has proven successful for ureamic diabetics[48] though very few patients have been reported to date. Whether haemofiltration will be preferable to haemodialysis is a question answerable by prospective trials now in progress.

Kidney transplantation

Mainly pioneered and perfected by Najarian and his associates, kidney transplantation for diabetics is the uraemia therapy most likely to promote true re-

Table 3 Self monitored blood glucose during uraemia therapy

Pt Age	*Rx*	*Daily Glucose Pre* (mg/dl)	*Daily Glucose* Post* (mg/dl)	*Glycohaemoglobin Pre* (%)	*Glycohaemoglobin*† *Post* (%)
35	Transplant	181–350	100–180	—	—
48	Transplant	31–152	100–180	9.0	7.0
37	Transplant	96–314	80–80	9.3	6.8
51	Transplant	280–612	120–120	7.9	7.0
41	Transplant	96–224	110–120	10.5	9.7
54	Haemodialysis	160–375	80–180	12.9	8.1
54	Haemodialysis	78–162	80–120	9.1	6.8
44	Haemodialysis	192–495	150–180	10.8	9.4

* Using Chemstrip
† Lowest value achieved during first 6 months of self monitoring

habilitation. Immunosuppression is accomplished with the same regimen employed in non-diabetics, most often a combination of azathioprine, anti-thymocyte (lymphocyte) globulin and prednisone. Survival after cadaveric kidney transplantation is about 50% at 3 years, but exceeds 65% at 3 years in intrafamilial grafting[49]. Subsequent survival of those reaching 3 years is very good, with 73% still functioning 7 years later[50]. In their most enthusiastic comments to date, the Najarian's Minnesota surgical team concludes that 'Diabetics are no longer at high risk for graft loss or patient death in relationship to nondiabetics, at least in the first 2 years after transplantation'[51]. The introduction of cyclosporine may allow for improved kidney graft survival in diabetics as well as combined kidney and pancreas allografting[52]. Diabetic kidney transplant recipients can experience true rehabilitation providing that usable vision was present at the time of engrafting, and that a serum creatinine level below 3 mg/dl is maintained. According to the only longitudinal study to date, about 4 of 5 recipients will have sustained or improved vision 3 years post kidney transplantation[53].

Recognizing that CAPD is incompletely evaluated, and that there may be enhanced survival, and reduced morbidity, in uraemic diabetics subjected to tight glucose regulation, the relative merits of available treatments are compared in Table 3. Intrafamilial kidney transplantation is advised as the preferred therapy for Type I diabetics below age 45 y. Additional investigation is required to determine the appropriate extent of study to exclude sibling donors liable to near term development of diabetes. Until this information is in hand, there is some uneasiness in accepting a diabetic's siblings and children as organ donors.

GLUCOSE REGULATION IN URAEMIC DIABETICS

Substantial evidence[54] supports the rationale for striving towards continuous euglycaemia in non-uraemic diabetics. Wide swings between hyperglycaemia and hypoglycaemia are no more desirable in uraemic diabetics than in those diabetics who retain normal renal function. Indeed, it is probable that one important factor responsible for earlier reports of inferior survival in diabetics treated by haemodialysis and kidney transplantation, was poor diabetic regulation. The technique of self monitoring of blood glucose concentration as a guide to fractional insulin doses throughout the day has markedly improved glucose regulation in non-azotaemic insulin dependent diabetics[55]. To explore its applicability to patients undergoing uraemia therapy, we conducted a pilot study in five renal transplant recipients and three haemodialysis patients[56]. We achieved improved glucose control documented by a reduction in mean glycosylated haemoglobin concentration (Table 3). The level of glycosylated haemoglobin appears to be a reliable indicator of glucose control in treated uraemic patients[57], though in the common assay, carbamylated haemoglobin, an

Table 4 Factors determining choice of uraemia therapy for the diabetic

Treatment	*Advantages*	*Disadvantages*
Renal transplantation	Cures uraemia for duration of graft function Stabilizes retinopathy Permits long intervals (months) away from treatment facility Reverses neuropathy Best rehabilitation Longterm survival (> 15 years in some cadaveric graft recipients)	Steroids complicate glucose control Risk of infectious complication High mortality in cadaveric graft recipients Risk of developing diabetes in familial donors Poor survival of secondary grafts Not applicable to elderly or patients with cardiovascular instability Glomerulosclerosis can recur Lower limb loss in > 15% at 2 years
Peritoneal dialysis	Avoids major surgery Minimizes burden on cardiovascular system Facilitates glucose regulation when insulin is added to dialysate Adaptable to home care (intermittent peritoneal dialysis or continuous ambulatory peritoneal dialysis (CAPD) in selected patients First year CAPD survival excellent (> 90% in one report)	Recurrent peritonitis High mortality Retinopathy may progress Limited longterm success
Haemodialysis	Avoids major surgery Permits care by experienced staff Available in most countries	Poor rehabilitation Retinopathy may progress Mortality equivalent to that for cadaveric graft recipients Inexorable 'failure to thrive' syndrome in about 25% of patients

Table 5 1984 preferred therapy for uraemic diabetic

Age range (years)	*Renal Transplant*	*Peritoneal Dialysis*	*Haemodialysis*
18–44	+ +	*	+
45–65	Selected patients	+	+
Over 65 (or presence of intractable heart failure)	–	+	+

+ + strongly recommended, especially if family donor available
+ recommended
– not recommended
* Insufficient experience is on hand to advise either intermittent peritoneal dialysis or CAPD over a renal transplant as definitive therapy for the longterm management of young Type I diabetics who may be rehabilitated by a renal transplant

abnormal metabolite caused by high blood urea concentration, may be misidentified as glycosylated haemoglobin[58]. Self monitored patients can apply their experience to blood glucose regulation after kidney transplantation, including the usually difficult to control interval after administration of large steroid doses to reverse rejection episodes.

It may be anticipated that introduction of self glucose monitoring to longterm transplant management will prove salutary in three ways:

(1) All of the subjective benefits of euglycaemia observed in tightly controlled nonazotaemic diabetics, will be extended to kidney recipients.
(2) Euglycaemia will protect the renal transplant from morphologic and functional components of diabetic nephropathy attributable to hyperglycaemia.
(3) Post transplant confusion in distinguishing between rejection and pseudorejection[59] (a spurious rise in serum creatinine attributed to hyperglycaemia) will be avoided.

Happily for those conducting trials of tight control, there do not seem to be any negative consequences of careful glucose regulation after kidney transplantation. The author's analysis of available uraemia therapy for the diabetic and advice over which choice to select are given in Tables 4 and 5.

References

1. Kass, E.H. (1956). Asymptomatic infections of the urinary tract. *Trans. Assoc. Am. Physicians,* **69,** 56
2. Forland, M., Thomas, V. and Shelokov, A. (1977). Urinary tract infections in patients with diabetes mellitus. Studies on antibody coating of bacteria. *JAMA,* **238,** 1924
3. Kunin, C.M., Southall, I. and Paguin, A.J. (1960). Epidemiology of urinary tract infection: pilot study of 3057 school children. *N. Engl. J. Med.,* **263,** 817
4. Harkonen, S. and Kjellstrand, C.M. (1977). Exacerbation of diabetic renal failure following intravenous pyelography. *Am. J. Med.,* **63,** 939
5. Bennet, W.M., Muther, R.S., Parker, R.A., Feig, P., Morrison, G., Golpere, T.A. and Singer, I. (1980). Drug therapy in renal failure: Dosing guidelines for adults. Part I: Antimicrobial agents, analgesics. Part II: Sedatives, hypnotics, and tranquilizers; cardiovascular, antihypertensive, and diuretic agents; miscellaneous agents. *Ann. Intern. Med.,* **93,** 62
6. Kimmelstiel, P. and Wilson, C. (1936). Intercapillary lesions in glomeruli of kidney. *Am. J. Pathol.,* **12,** 83
7. Gellman, D.D., Pirani, C.C., Soothill, J.F., Muehreke, R.C. and Kark, R.M. (1959). Diabetic nephropathy; a clinical and pathologic study based on renal biopsies. *Medicine,* **38,** 321
8. Mauer, S.M. and Shvil, Y. (1979). The glomerular mesangium. In Black, Sir D. and Jones, N.F. (eds.). *Renal Disease.* pp. 93–106 (Oxford: Blackwell Sci. Publ.)
9 Mauer, S.M., Steffes, M.W. and Brown, D.M. (1981). The kidney in diabetes. *Am. J. Med.,* **70,** 603
10. Mauer, S.M., Steffes, M.W., Chern, M. and Brown, D.M. (1979). Mesangial uptake and processing of macromolecules in rats with diabetes mellitus. *Lab. Invest.,* **41,** 401
11. Osterby, R. (1975). Early phases in the development of diabetic glomerulopathy. *Acta Med. Scand.,* (Suppl) **1,** 574
12. Foglia, V.G., Manccini, Re, and Cardeza, A.F. (1950). Glomerular lesions in the diabetic rat. *Arch. Pathol. Lab. Med.,* **50,** 75

13. Ireland, J. T. (1970). Diagnostic criteria in the assessment of glomerular capillary basement membrane lesions in newly diagnosed juvenile diabetics. In Camerini-Davalos, R. A. and Cole, H. S. (eds.). *Early Diabetes.* p. 273. (New York: Academic Press)
14. Burkholder, P. M. (1974). Renal disease associated with diabetes mellitus. In Burkholder, P. M. (ed.). *Atlas of Human Glomerular Pathology.* p. 325. (Hagerstown, Md: Harper and Row)
15. Rasch, R. (1979). Prevention of diabetic glomerulopathy in streptozotocin diabetic rats by insulin treatment. Kidney size and glomerular volume. *Diabetologia,* **16,** 125
16. Viberti, G. C. (1979). Early functional and morphological changes in diabetic nephropathy. *Clin. Nephrol.,* **12,** 47
17. Hatch, F. E., Watt, M. F., Kramer, N. C., Parrish, A. E. and Howe, J. S. (1961). Diabetic glomerulosclerosis: a long-term follow-up study based on renal biopsies. *Am. J. Med.,* **31,** 216
18. Thomsen, A. C. (1965). The kidney in diabetes mellituus. (Copenhagen: Munksgaard Press)
19. Mogensen, C. E. (1976). Renal function changes in diabetes. *Diabetes,* **25,** 872
20. Viberti, G. C. (1979). Effect of control of blood glucose on urinary excretion of albumin and β_2-microglobulin in insulin-dependent diabetes. *N. Engl. J. Med.,* **300,** 368
21. Viberti, G. C., Bilous, R. W., MacKintosh, D. and Keen, H. (1983). Monitoring glomerular function in diabetic nephropathy. A prospective study. *Am. J. Med.,* **74,** 256
22. Mogensen, C. E. (1971). Kidney function and glomerular permeability to macromolecules in early juvenile diabetes. *Scand. J. Clin. Lab. Invest.,* **28,** 79
23. Mauer, S. M., Fish, A. J., Day, N. K. and Michael, A. F. (1974). The glomerular mesangium. II. Quantitative studies of mesangial function in nephrotoxic nephritis in rats. *J. Clin. Invest.,* **53,** 431
24. Knowles, H. C. Jr. (1974). Magnitude of the renal failure problem in diabetic patients. *Kidney Int.,* **4,** (Suppl 1), 52
25. Caird, R. I. (1961). Survival of diabetics with proteinuria. *Diabetes,* **10,** 178
26. Mogensen, C. E. (1976). Renal function changes in diabetes. *Diabetes,* **25,** 872
27. Rutherford, W. E., Blondin, J., Miller, J. P., Greenwalt, A. S. and Vavra, J D. (1977). Chronic progressive renal disease: rate of change of serum creatinine concentration. *Kidney Int.,* **11,** 62
28. Jones, R. H., Mackay, J. D., Hayakawa, H. and Parsons, V. (1979). Progression of diabetic nephropathy. *Lancet,* **1,** 1105
29. Chazan, B. I., Rees, S. B., Balodimos, M. C., Younger, D. and Ferguson, D. B. (1969). Dialysis in diabetics. *JAMA,* **209,** 2026
30. Friedman, E. A. (1980). Diabetic renal–retinal syndrome. The prognosis improves. *Arch. Intern. Med.,* **140,** 1149
31. Ramsay, R. C., Cantrill, H. L., Knobloch, W. H., Goetz, F. C., Sutherland, D. E. R. and Najarian, J. S. (1983). Visual parameters in diabetic patients following renal transplantation. *Diabet. Nephr.,* **2,** 26
32. Ramsay, R. C., Cantrill, H. L., Knobloch, W. H., Shapiro, F. L., Comty, C. M. and Kjellstrand, C. M. (1983). Visual parameters in diabetic patients on chronic dialysis. *Diabet. Nephr.,* **2,** 30
33. Kannel, W. B., Hjortland, M. and Castelli, W. P. (1974). Role of diabetes in congestive heart failure: The Framingham Study. *Am. J. Cardiol.,* **34,** 29
34. Mogensen, C. E., Christensen, C. K., Christensen, N. J., Gundersen, H. J. G., Jacobssen, E. K., Pedersen, E. B. and Vittinghus, E. (1981). Renal protein handling in normal hypertensive and diabetic man. *Contr. Nephrol.,* **24,** 139
35. Mogensen, C. E. (1980). Antihypertensive treatment inhibiting the progression of diabetic nephropathy. *Acta Endocr. Copenh.,* **94** (Suppl. 238) 103
36. Christlieb, A. P. (1973). Diabetes and hypertensive vascular disease. *Am. J. Cardiol.,* **32,** 592
37. Christlieb, A. R., Kaldany, A. and D'Elia, J. A. (1976). Plasma renin activity and hypertension in diabetes mellitus. *Diabetes,* **25,** 969
38. Christensen, N. J. (1972). Plasma catecholamines in long-term diabetics with and without neuropathy and in hypophysectomized subjects. *J. Clin. Invest.,* **51,** 779
39. Day, R. P., Leutscher, J. A. and Gonzales, C. M. (1975). Occurrence of big renin in human plasma, amniotic fluid, and kidney extracts. *J. Clin. Endocrinol. Metab.,* **40,** 1078

40. Schindler, A. M. and Sommers, S. C. (1966). Diabetic sclerosis of the renal juxtaglomerular apparatus. *Lab. Invest.,* **15,** 877
41. Leonard, A., Comty, C. and Raij, L. (1973). The natural history of regularly dialyzed diabetics. *Trans. Am. Soc. Artif. Intern. Organs,* **19,** 282
42. Comty, C. M., Kjellsen, D. and Shapiro, F. L. (1976). A reassessment of the prognosis of diabetic patients treated by chronic hemodialysis. *Trans. Am. Soc. Artif. Intern. Organs,* **22,** 404
43. Goldstein, D. A. and Massry, S. G. (1978). Diabetic nephropathy - clinical course and effect of hemodialysis. *Nephron,* **20,** 286
44. Gutman, R. A., Stead, W. W. and Robinson, R. R. (1981). Physical activity and employment status of patients on maintenance dialysis. *N. Engl. J. Med.,* **304,** 309
45. Katirtzoglou, A., Izatt, S., Oreopoulos, D. G., Dombros, N., Blair, G. R., Chisholm, L., Meema, H. E., Ogilvie, R., Vas, S., Leibel, B. and McCreedy, W. (1980). Chronic peritoneal dialysis in diabetics with end-stage renal failure. In Friedman, E. A. and L'Esperance, F. A. Jr. (eds.). *Diabetic Renal-Retinal Syndrome.* p. 317 (New York: Grune & Stratton)
46. Flynn, C. T., (1980). Diabetic control by CAPD. In Friedman, E. A. and L'Esperance, F. A. Jr. (eds.). *Diabetic Renal-Retinal Syndrome.* p. 435 (New York: Grune & Stratton)
47. Khanna, A. P., Leibel, R., Pierratos, A. *et al.* (1982). Continuous ambulatory peritoneal dialysis in diabetics with end-stage renal disease. *N. Engl. J. Med.,* **306,** 625
48. Shaldon, S. (1981). Progress from haemodialysis. *Nephron,* **27,** 2
49. Kjellstrand, C. M., Goetz, F. C. and Najarian, J. S. (1980). Transplantation and dialysis in diabetic patients: An update. In Friedman, E. A., L'Esperance, F. A. Jr. (eds.). *Diabetic Renal-Retinal Syndrome.* p. 345 (New York: Grune & Stratton)
50. Sutherland, D. E. R., Fryd, D. S., Simmons, R. L., Kjellstrand, C. M., Ramsay, R. C., Goetz, F. C., Mauer, S. M. and Najarian, J. S. (1980). Long-term diabetic renal transplants. In Friedman, E. A. and L'Esperance, F. A. Jr. (eds.). *Diabetic Renal-Retinal Syndrome.* p. 353 (New York: Grune & Stratton)
51. Sutherland, D. E. R., Morrow, C. E., Fryd, D. S., Ferguson, R., Simmons, R. L. and Najarian, J. S. (1982). Improved patient and primary renal allograft survival in uremic diabetic recipients. *Transplantation,* **34,** 319
52. Calne, R. Y., White, D. J. G., Evans, D. B., Thiru, S., Henderson, R. G., Hamilton, D. V., Rolles, K., McMaster, P., Duffy, T. J., MacDougall, B. R. D. and Williams, R. (1981). Cyclosporin A in cadaveric organ transplantation. *Br. Med. J.,* **282,** 934
53. L'Esperance, F. A., James, W. A., Friedman, E. A., Feinroth, M. V. and Mondschein, L. G. (1982). Long term retention of vision following vitrectomy in diabetic patients. In Friedman, E. A. and L'Esperance, F. A. (eds.). *Diabetic Renal-Retinal Syndrome - Prevention and Management* p. 277 (New York: Grune & Stratton)
54. Jackson, R. L., Esterly, J. A., Guthrie, R. A., Hewett, J. E. and Waiches, H. B. (1982). Capillary basement membrane changes in adolescents with type I diabetes. *JAMA,* **248,** 2143
55. Peterson, C. M., Forhan, S. E. and Jones, R. L. (1980). Self management: An approach to patients with insulin-dependent diabetes mellitus. *Diabetes Care,* **3,** 82
56. Levitz, C. S., Hirsch, S., Ross, J. M., Butt, K. M. H. and Friedman, E. A. (1980). Lack of blood glucose control in hemodialyzed and renal transplantation diabetics. *Trans. Am. Soc. Artif. Intern. Organs,* **26,** 362
57. Zawada, E. T. Jr., Virji, A. and Gomez, E. (1980). Glycosylated hemoglobin test in diabetic and non-diabetic hemodialysis patients. *Dialys. Transpl.,* **9,** 360
58. Fluckiger, R., Harmon, W., Meier, W., Loo, S. and Gabbay, K. H. (1981). Hemoglobin carbamylation in uremia. *N. Engl. J. Med.,* **304,** 823
59. Matas, A. J., Simmons, R. L., Kjellstrand, C. M. and Najarian, J. S. (1977). Pseudo-rejection: Factors mimicking rejection in renal allograft recipients. *Ann. Surg.,* **186,** 51

2
The changing scene in the treatment of diabetic patients with terminal uraemia in Europe

C. JACOBS, F. P. BRUNNER, H. BRYNGER, S. CHALLAH, P. KRAMER, N. H. SELWOOD, A. J. WING

INTRODUCTION

Ten years ago, the diabetic patient with end-stage renal failure (ESRF) was practically doomed to death in almost any country in Europe, regardless of his/her age or type of diabetes. Routine exclusion of diabetics with terminal uraemia from methods of treatment of ESRF was deemed justified, not only by the overall dearth in treatment facilities which prevailed almost everywhere in Europe, but also by the overt scepticism that was broadcast by the early pioneers in the field about the anticipated poor outcome from the application of maintenance haemodialysis to this group of patients[1].

At the end of 1981, however, more than 5000 diabetics were listed on the file of the European Dialysis and Transplantation Registry (EDTA)[2]. Diabetes accounts for the sole cause of terminal uraemia that provides year by year an increasing number of new patients accepted all over Europe for Renal Replacement Therapy (RRT). This complete reversal of the situation is the result of a combination of factors, among which can be mentioned: (1) the wide spread of treatment facilities over the last decade in most of the European countries, (2) the considerable advances made in the medical management of diabetic patients with ESRF, and also (3) the increasing pressure exerted by the patients and diabetologists or nephrologists, who gradually took up the challenge of accepting for RRT patients with systemic diseases, whose former systematic exclusion from the various modes of treatment of terminal uraemia became less and less warranted.

This paper describes the 'changing scene' thus observed in Europe regarding the treatment of terminal uraemia in diabetic patients, over the period 1973–1981, reviewing the number and distribution of diabetics in various European countries, the evolution in techniques of treatment and the results currently being achieved.

METHODS

Data were collected by the EDTA registry through individual patient questionnaires, which were returned annually by the medical staff in charge of the patients treated with maintenance dialysis methods or renal transplantation. In 1981, patient questionnaires were returned by 85% of all Centres whose addresses were known in 32 countries. Over 130 000 patient records were held on the Registry Computer files, and close to 81 000 patients were recorded alive on December 31st, 1981[2]. All over the years the EDTA individual patient questionnaire included questions on patient's age, sex, primary renal disease, successive sequences of treatment of ESRF, source and data of kidney transplant and the date and causes of death. However, no distinction was made among patients with diabetic nephropathy between those with type I (juvenile, insulin-dependent) and type II (non-insulin-requiring) diabetes.

RESULTS

Number and distribution of diabetics taken on Renal Replacement Therapy in Europe

Whilst the total number of patients on the Registry rose five fold over 8 years, a 20-fold increase was recorded in diabetics. They were only 245 in December, 1973[3]. Eight years later close to 5200 had been reported to the Registry of whom 2661 were alive at the end of December, 1981. The proportion of patients alive on all modes of treatment who were diabetic rose from 1.2% in 1973 to 1.9% in 1976[4] and reached 3.4% in 1981[2]. The proportion of new patients who were diabetic increased steadily over the years. The 124 patients who started some form of treatment in 1973 represented 1.8% of the new patients who had been accepted for RRT during that year. In 1981, the 1182 diabetics accounted for 7.4% of patients newly taken onto treatment in Europe. This percentage was however much smaller than that reported from the United States, where diabetics are claimed to account for about 25% of new patients taken onto RRT in recent years[5].

The proportion of diabetics aged less than 40 years at the start of RRT dropped from 40% in the small group of patients accepted in 1973 to 27% in 1981. The percentage of patients in the 40–60 year age group remained stable over the years, around 45%, whereas the proportion of diabetics older than 60 years jumped from 16% in 1976 to 27% in 1981. These changes in age distribution are roughly similar to the ones observed in the large group of non-

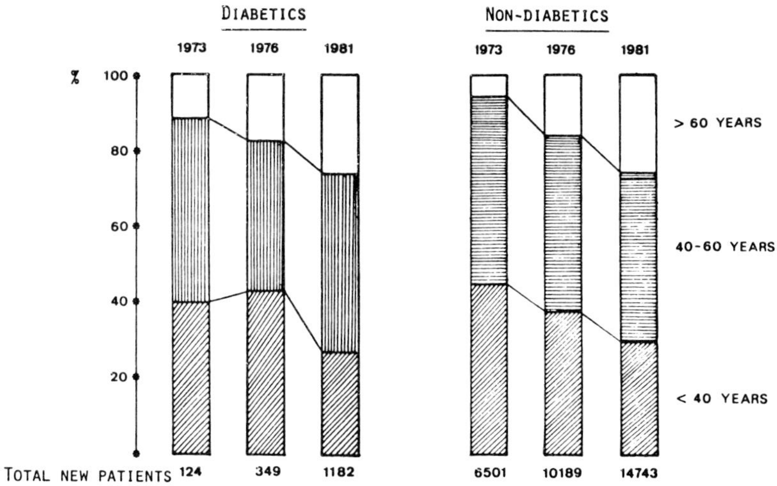

Figure 1 Age distribution of diabetic and non-diabetic patients at start of renal replacement therapy

diabetic patients (Figure 1). They also suggest an increasing preponderance of type II (non-insulin-requiring) diabetics among the patients taken onto RRT in recent years.

The geographical pattern of diabetics on treatment for ESRF varies between European countries. These differences must be accounted for by epidemiological factors and selection policies which are often, although not exclusively, determined by the availability of treatment facilities. To illustrate these differences, we have thus picked out:

The Scandinavian countries: (Denmark, Norway, Sweden and Finland) where all modes of treatment of ESRF have been widely available for a long time, and in which the proportion of patients with renal failure due to diabetes could be shown as particularly high[2]. The yearly percentage of diabetics taken onto RRT in Scandinavia rose from 4% of all new patients accepted for dailysis and renal transplantation in 1976 to 9% in 1979 and to 18.8% in 1981.

The Western Continental European countries: (Belgium, France, Federal Republic of Germany, Netherlands and Switzerland) in which there is currently no real dearth in treatment facilities, and where no stringent selection according to age or primary renal disease has had to be made in recent years. Diabetics accounted, however, for only 7.9% of all new patients accepted for treatment in these countries in 1981.

The Southern European countries: (Italy, Spain and Greece) in which epidemiological data on diabetes appear somewhat less firmly established than in the Northern European countries, but where a widespread availability of treatment facilities should currently permit a wide acceptance of diabetics. This situation is in sharp contrast to,

The United Kingdom and Ireland, where the growth in number of uraemic patients accepted for treatment has been restricted by economic rationing, which still predominates over medical needs. In the Southern European countries as well as in the United Kingdom, diabetics accounted for 5% of the uraemic patients who started RRT in 1981. However, this rather low proportion compared to the other Western European countries represented a threefold increase over the years 1976–1981.

Evolutive trends in the modes of treatment

The rapid spread of continuous peritoneal ambulatory dialysis (CAPD) greatly influenced the initial mode of treatment chosen for diabetics with terminal uraemia[6]. CAPD was unknown in Europe in 1976, at which time 19% of the diabetics taken on treatment were started on intermittent peritoneal dialysis (IPD). Five years later, 20% of new diabetics started treatment on CAPD. IPD has, however, not been completely abandoned, still being performed as initial mode of treatment in 15% of the new diabetics in 1981. Peritoneal dialysis techniques were thus used in more than one third of the new diabetics in 1981.

There are wide differences in the choice of initial mode of therapy for diabetics with terminal renal failure in the various European countries. In Scandinavia, the proportion of patients first treated with haemodialysis remained stable, at 45% to 47% over a 5 year period (1976–1981), whilst the percentage of diabetics who received a transplant without prior dialysis declined from 22% to 8%. Forty-four per cent of the diabetics who commenced treatment in 1981 started on CAPD (23%) or IPD (21%). Haemodialysis was by far the most popular initial mode of treatment in the five Western Continental countries considered in this study. The proportion of patients starting RRT on CAPD rocketed from 1% to 18% in 2 years (1979–1981). In the United Kingdom, nearly 80% of new diabetics in 1981 were treated initially with CAPD (44%) or IPD (35%). These figures demonstrate that most of the diabetics with ESRF in the United Kingdom owe their survival to the fact that peritoneal dialysis techniques can be performed at home. In the Southern European countries, there was a steady increase in the proportion of new diabetics for whom peritoneal dialysis methods were initially chosen (40% of the 238 new diabetics accepted for treatment in 1981), but in contrast to other European countries, IPD remained more popular than CAPD in these countries in 1981.

At the close of 1981, 60% of the 2401 diabetics alive with RRT in Europe, and whose mode of treatment was known with certainty, were treated with hospital haemodialysis, whereas only 3.2% performed haemodialysis in their own homes. Almost as many patients were alive with functioning transplants (16%) as with CAPD (18%). Over the preceding 5 years the proportion of

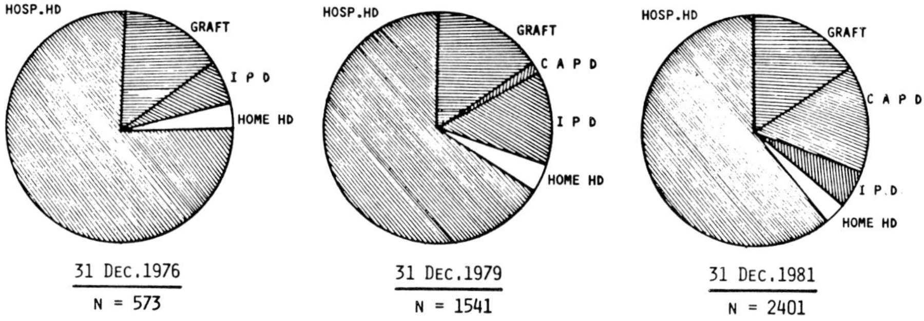

Figure 2 Evolution of modes of treatment in diabetics with terminal uraemia in Europe (1976–1981)

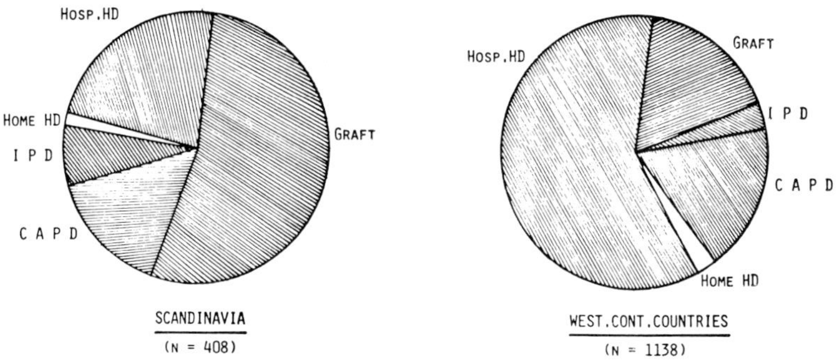

Figure 3 Modes of treatment of terminal renal failure in diabetics alive in Scandinavia ($n = 408$) and in five Western European Continental countries ($n = 1138$) on December 31st, 1981

patients treated by hospital haemodialysis fell by 15%. There was no significant change in the respective role of home haemodialysis and renal transplantation. CAPD dramatically overtook IPD in the last 2 years (Figure 2).

The very high proportion of diabetics alive in Scandinavia at the end of 1981 with functioning grafts demonstrate that most of the patients initially taken on haemodialysis or peritoneal dialysis are eventually transplanted. This appears as the consequence of an active transplantation programme together with a high acceptance rate of 'young' diabetics (aged less than 40 years) in the Scandinavian countries[2]. In the Western European Continental countries only 17% of the diabetics alive at the end of 1981 had functioning transplants (Figure 3). In the UK, the same all-out 'extra-Center' treatment policy was applied for diabetics as it was for all other uraemic patients. Nearly 50% of diabetics were treated with PD techniques and renal transplantation also had an important role (Figure 4). In contrast, hospital haemodialysis was the overwhelming method of treatment used for diabetics in the Southern European countries (Figure 4). The percentage of patients treated with CAPD and IPD

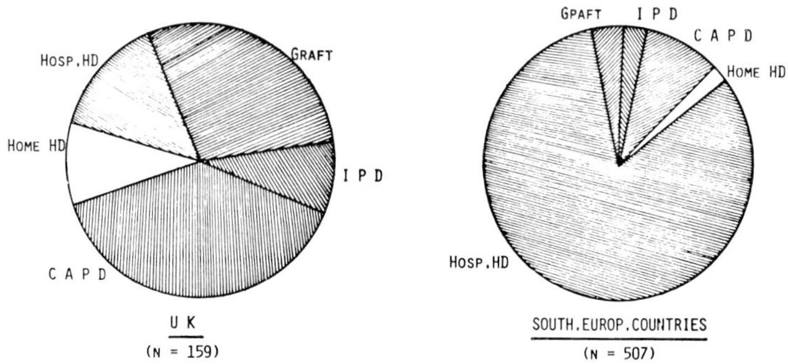

Figure 4 Modes of treatment of terminal renal failure in diabetics alive in the United Kingdom ($n = 159$) and in three Southern European countries ($n = 507$) on December 31st, 1981

looks small in contrast to the 40% of patients who started on peritoneal dialysis in 1981. This discrepancy illustrates the lag between a change in choice of initial therapy and its impact on the distribution of all living patients, especially when the proportion on PD may be eroded by a high drop-out rate.

Survival of diabetics on Renal Replacement treatments

The survival of diabetics on RRT has tended to improve in recent years, at least in the group of patients aged less than 40 years at start of treatment. The actuarial survival rate at 2 years rose from 43% for patients starting treatment

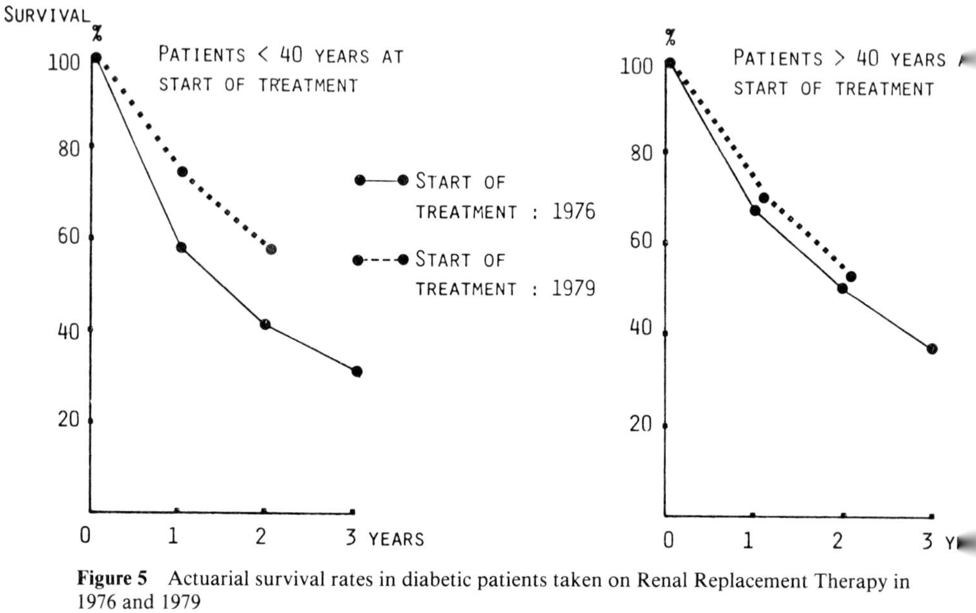

Figure 5 Actuarial survival rates in diabetic patients taken on Renal Replacement Therapy in 1976 and 1979

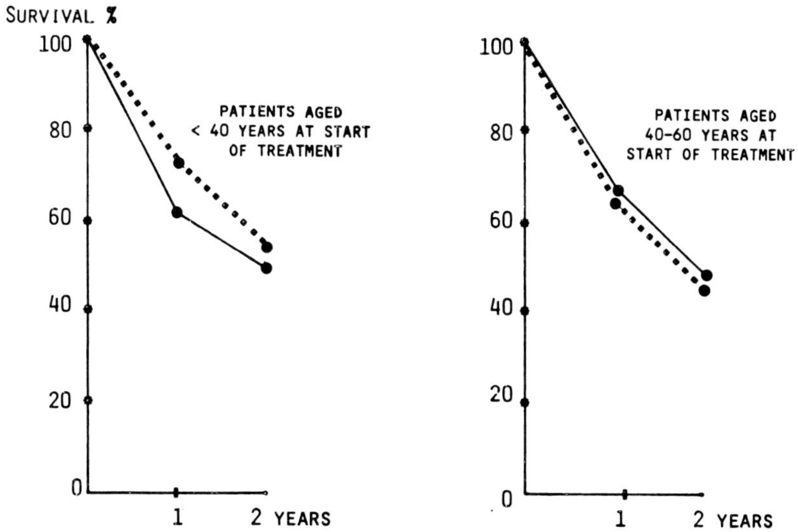

Figure 6 Actuarial survival rates in diabetics who started haemodialysis (•—•) or CAPD (•---•) after January 1st, 1979

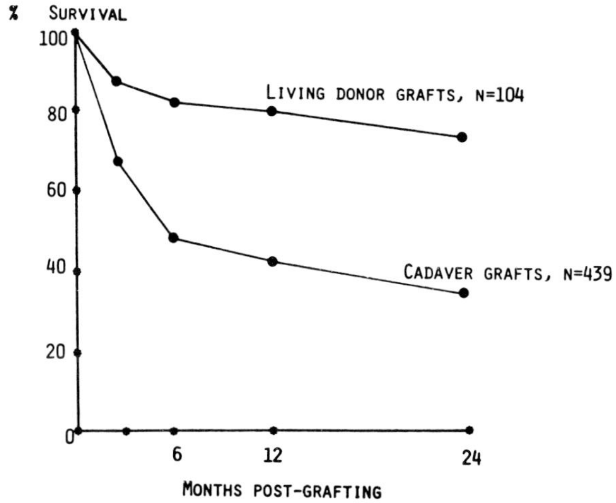

Figure 7 Living donor and cadaver donor graft survival rates in diabetic recipients aged <40 years at time of grafting

in 1976 to 59% for those starting in 1979 (Figure 5). This latter figure, which is in accordance with the results currently being achieved in large series of patients treated by experienced groups in the United States, is still about 20% lower than the survival rate of the whole treated population aged 35–44 years[7]. There is no such favourable trend in diabetics aged over 40 years, whose survival at 2 years is stuck at a steady 51%, that is about 20% less than in the whole treated population aged 45–65 years.

The analysis of survival rates, according to the mode of therapy, recorded in diabetics who commenced treatment after January 1st, 1979 shows that among the under 40 year olds, the 643 diabetics who started on CAPD had a 10% better survival at 1 year than the 1098 starting on haemodialysis. This advantage is not maintained over time, and survival turns out to be the same at 2 years. In the older patients, aged 40–60 years, CAPD and haemodialysis yielded similar results at 1 and 2 years (Figure 6).

As for the 104 patients aged less than 40 years who benefited from a living donor transplant, the actuarial graft survival rates (Figure 7) were 80% at 1 year and 73% at 2 years. The 439 cadaver grafts did not do so well, with only 42% surviving at 1 year and 35% at 2 years, a result approximately 20% lower than in the non-diabetic transplant recipients[8]. The much better results achieved in living donor graft diabetic recipients is well in accordance with those obtained in a large American series[9].

Causes of death

The distribution of causes of death in diabetics treated exclusively with haemodialysis remained consistent over a 5 year period (Figure 8). Cardiac causes (myocardial infarction, heart failure, hyper- or hypokalaemia and fluid overload) accounted for a steady 40% of all deaths. There was a 5% decline in the proportion of fatal cerebro-vascular accidents in 1981 compared to 1976. Although infections accounted for 10% of deaths occurring in diabetics on RRT, this proportion is no higher than in non-diabetic patients[4]. On peritoneal dialysis, the proportion of deaths due to infections steadily diminished, and in 1981 it was quite similar to that recorded on haemodialysis (Figure 9). Cardiac and cerebro-vascular causes of death were similar in 1979 and in 1981, accounting for 55–58% of deaths. These data suggest that poor control of blood pressure and fluid balance probably represent a more vital threat to

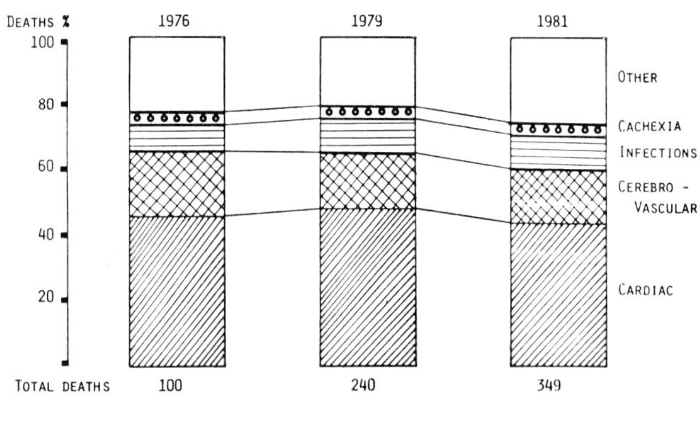

Figure 8 Causes of death in diabetics treated exclusively by haemodialysis (Hospital + Home)

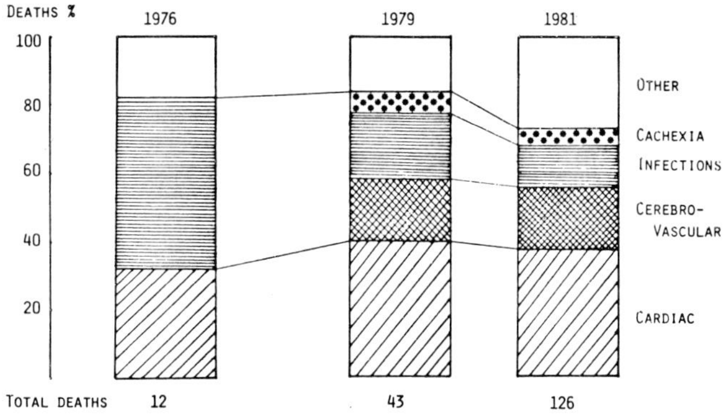

Figure 9 Causes of death in diabetics treated exclusively by peritoneal dialysis (CAPD + IPD)

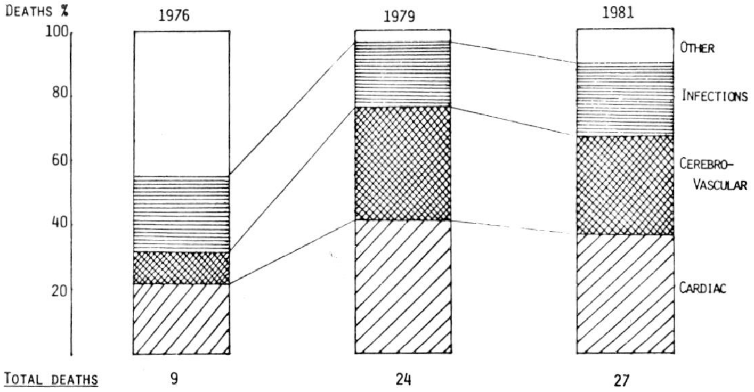

Figure 10 Causes of death in diabetics with first cadaver transplant

diabetics treated with CAPD than do infectious complications. Cachexia accounted for 5% of the deaths recorded in diabetics undergoing peritoneal dialysis, a proportion that is quite similar to the one observed in haemodialysis patients, whereas no death could be attributed to this cause among the grafted patients. In the small group of patients who died after first cadaver transplant, more deaths were due to cerebro-vascular accidents than to infectious causes, which is all the more remarkable in view of the younger age of transplant recipients (Figure 10).

SUMMARY AND CONCLUSIONS

More than 5000 diabetics with terminal uraemia had been accepted for renal replacement therapy in Europe by the end of December, 1981. 2661 were alive, and accounted for 3.4% of all patients on treatment. 7.4% of all patients who started some form of RRT in Europe in 1981 were diabetic. Three to four times as many diabetics were taken onto treatment in recent years in the Scandinavian countries as in the United Kingdom or in Italy.

Peritoneal dialysis, mainly CAPD, gained wide acceptance for uraemic diabetics all over Europe. At the end of 1981, 63% of the diabetics alive in Europe were treated with haemodialysis (of whom only 3.2% performed this procedure in their homes), 15% with CAPD, 6% with IPD. 16% of the live diabetics had a functioning kidney graft. Survival improved in recent years for diabetics aged less than 40 years at the start of treatment, but was still about 20% lower than in non-diabetics of the same age group. Haemodialysis and CAPD yielded similar survival rates at 2 years. Living donor kidney transplantation had a rather good outcome with a 73% graft survival at 2 years, whereas cadaver graft survival remained poor, being only 35% at 2 years.

Deaths in diabetics on RRT were mostly of cardiac and cerebro-vascular origin, irrespective of the mode of treatment. Infectious causes of death were no more frequent in patients treated with CAPD than in those who underwent haemodialysis.

Although further progress in survival and quality of life remains to be made, the results currently being achieved completely invalidate the ominous predictions that had been stated a decade ago about the anticipated grim outcome from the application of dialysis to diabetics with terminal uraemia. The analysis of causes of death recorded in these patients suggests that an efficient management of metabolic and vascular complications of diabetes prior to the stage of terminal uraemia is of utmost importance to reduce the differences in survival rates that still exist between diabetics and the other patients who undergo renal replacement therapy for end-stage renal failure.

ACKNOWLEDGEMENTS

We gratefully acknowledge the work of doctors and staff who completed the questionnaires for the EDTA Registry, and also thank Miss Elizabeth Goupy for skilful assistance in preparing the manuscript.

The work of the EDTA Registry is supported by the Council of the Association, and grants from Governments of many European countries, and from several commercial companies who are acknowledged in the reports published annually in the Proceedings of the EDTA.

References

1. Ghavanian, M., Gutch, C. F., Kopp, K. F. and Kolff, W. J. (1972). The sad truth about haemodialysis in diabetic nephropathy. *JAMA*, **222**, 1386
2. Kramer, P., Broyer, M., Brunner, F. P., Brynger, H., Donckerwolcke, R. A., Jacobs, C., Selwood, N. H. and Wing, A. J. (1982). Combined report on regular dialysis and transplantation in Europe, XII, 1981. *Proc. Eur. Dial. Transplant. Assoc.*, **19**, 4

3. Parsons, F.M., Brunner, F.P., Burck, H.C., Gräser, W., Gurland, H.J., Härlen, H., Schärer, K. and Spies, G.W. (1974). Combined report on regular dialysis and transplantation in Europe, IV, 1973. *Proc. Eur. Dial. Transplant. Assoc.*, **11**, 3
4. Jacobs, C., Brunner, F.P., Chantler, C., Donckerwolcke, R.A., Gurland, H.J., Hathway, R.A., Selwood, N.H. and Wing, A.J. (1977). Combined report on regular dialysis and transplantation in Europe, VII, 1976. *Proc. Eur. Dial. Transplant. Assoc.*, **14**, 3
5. Friedman, E.A. (1982). Diabetic nephropathy. Strategies in prevention and management. *Kidney Int.*, **21**, 780
6. Rottembourg, J., El Shahat, Y., Agrafiotis, A., Thuillier, Y., de Groc, F., Jacobs, C. and Legrain, M. (1983). Continuous ambulatory peritoneal dialysis in insulin dependent diabetic patients: a 40 month experience. *Kidney Int.*, **23**, 40
7. Kjellstrand, C.M., Whitley, K., Comty, C.M. and Shapiro, F.L. (1983). Dialysis in patients with diabetes mellitus. Editorial Review. *Diab. Nephr.*, **2**, 5
8. Jacobs, C., Broyer, M., Brunner, F.P., Brynger, H., Donckerwolcke, R.A., Kramer, P., Selwood, N.H., Wing, A.J. and Blake, Ph. (1981). Combined report on regular dialysis and transplantation in Europe, XI, 1980. *Proc. Eur. Dial. Transplant. Assoc.*, **18**, 3
9. Najarian, J.S., Sutherland, D.E.R., Simmons, R.L., Howard, R.J., Kjellstrand, C.M., Ramsay, R.C., Goetz, F.C., Fryd, D.S. and Sommer, B.G. (1979). Ten year experience with renal transplantation in juvenile onset diabetics. *Ann. Surg.*, **190**, 487

3.1
An overview of the health economics of diabetic nephropathy

A. H. W. WAHBA

INTRODUCTION

Nephropathy in diabetic patients is a relatively serious clinical, ethical and economic problem in the community, indicated by the progress of the disease itself and its sequelae as well as its two alternative therapeutic measures, dialysis and transplantation.

Diabetic vascular disease (microangiopathy) affects the kidneys at the microscopic level. It generally takes about 10 years before the first symptoms of nephropathy appear. Effective diabetes control, early diagnosis and therapy of any renal impairment in infection may postpone the onset of irreparable damage. The number of diabetic patients enrolled in dialysis and/or kidney transplants in European countries varies from 8 to 12 per million inhabitants per year. In industrialized countries in general, an incidence rate of 20 new cases of juvenile diabetes per million population per year may be estimated, and approximately half of them will develop a severe nephropathy.

Whenever the management of such patients is envisaged, the economic aspects of both the continuing therapy of the underlying disease, i.e. diabetes, and the urgent replacement of the kidney function have to be considered in the context of the more or less simple diabetological principles and the more complex nephropathy therapy policies and priorities. Diabetic nephropathy is one disease in the group of conditions in need of dialysis, and transplantation and national authorities have to deal with all of them '*en bloc*'.

A close collaboration, dialogue and comprehensive approach between the treating diabetologist, the consulting nephrologist and/or surgeon and the patient, as well as the latter's family are essential for the full understanding of all the implications.

A comprehensive evaluation of the alternatives available should therefore be performed at the *micro* level, while another one considering national needs and means will be done at the *macro* level. The results of different assessment studies cannot be adopted as such under the various prevailing national, regional and local settings. But general guidelines developed nationally and internationally, provide a useful framework, as long as they are adapted according to the local real needs and available resources.

An economic assessment alone of nephropathy treatment will never provide decision makers with the total and comprehensive picture. Technical aspects (safety to patients and operators, ergonomics, accuracy and precision), clinical aspects (relevance, timing and site), quality of life aspects (work, recreation, pain, worry, communication, sleep, dependency on others, excretion and sexual activity) and of course the cost-effectiveness aspects must all be included.

The present paper will concentrate on the economic aspects of nephropathy in general, with special reference to the disease as a complication of diabetes.

GENERAL APPROACHES TO AN ECONOMIC ANALYSIS

It appears that relatively many economic evaluations have been undertaken in the field of kidney dialysis or transplantation. The impact on the actual management of end-stage renal failure is different according to the prevailing policy decisions, available technological conditions, financial and reimbursement regulations. The role of national pressure groups, patient and community associations, the media as well as the professional and industrial lobbies should also be considered. Another problem which affects the calculation of socio-economic costs of diabetes is that this disease, and its various complications including deaths, may be classified under different headings, and that many costs and production losses are assigned to other denominators. This may lead to a final underestimation of the real and total economic consequences.

Any major diagnostic, therapeutic or rehabilitative programme can be evaluated on the micro-economic and the macro-economic levels, the ultimate goal being to find an answer to the question: is it 'worth' doing something?

Clinicians seek answers to the following questions: Is diagnosis made more precise? Is patient outcome improved? Are adverse side effects or incidental risks to patients reduced? At this 'micro' level, 'worth' is judged essentially in terms of the beneficial and harmful effects on the patients.

By contrast, policymakers and planners face questions of a different sort: Are there net health benefits to the large number of eligible patients from the use of a particular technology? How and where should this technology be provided? What are the alternatives? At this 'macro' level, 'worth' is judged in terms of a wider set of advantages and disadvantages; their very diversity raises questions of how to measure them and how to judge their value to different types of person (e.g. patients, patients' families, potential patients and the public at large; the young and the old; those in employment and the unemployed, the retired; men and women).

Cost analysis

In a cost analysis end results are not considered, i.e. there is no analysis of cost per life year gained. The analysis simply attempts to estimate the cost per dialysis or annual costs or per transplant.

The usefulness of cost analyses *per se* is somewhat limited. They may be useful when trying to estimate the cost side in a cost-effectiveness study, provided that a clear cost concept has been employed. Most often the perspective of the hospital is taken – and in some instances no distinction is made between real costs and expenditures. A comparison of costs of both types of treatment generally demonstrates a considerable difference in favour of transplantation. This type of analysis is then used at national levels to recommend that transplantation activities ought to be expanded.

In any case, cost studies represent only one aspect of the evaluation process, but are still useful in the holistic approach to dialysis and transplant.

In Table 1 costs of hospital dialysis as reported in 6 studies are shown.

Interpretation of these figures is difficult as it is often not known how capital

Table 1 Costs of hospital dialysis

Author	*Year of estimate*	*Country*	*Annual Cost**	
Annual total cost per patient				
Klarman *et al* (1968)	1968	USA	$14 000	(11 000)
Pearson *et al* (1976)	1972	USA	$14–25 000	(9–16 500)
Douglas (1973)	1972	USA	$20–30 000	(13–20 000)
Schippers and Kalff (1976)	1973	Netherl.	$26 000	(16 000)
Stewart *et al* (1973)	1973	Australia	$A7400	(6000)
Buxton and West (1975a)	1972	UK	£5600	(8800)

* $US except where stated; 1975 sterling equivalent in brackets (from Parkin[3])

Table 2 Costs of home dialysis

Author	*Year of estimate*	*Country*	*Capital cost**		*Maintenance*†*	
Klarman *et al* (1968)	1968	USA	—		$5000	(4000)
Pearson *et al* (1976)	1972	USA	—		$5600	(3700)
Rae *et al* (1972)	1972	Canada	$Can8750	(5700)	$Can5854	(3800)
Douglas (1973)	1973	USA	—		$4–6000	(2500–4000)
Stewart *et al* (1973)	1973	Australia	$A6000	(4800)	$A2600	(2100)
Hull (1976)	1975	USA	—		$15600	(7600)
Kerr (1967)	1967	UK	£3500	(7600)	£1150	(2500)

* $US except where stated; 1975 sterling equivalent in brackets (from Parkin[3])
† includes equipment, home adaptation and 'training'

costs (premises, machines and salaries of staff) have been calculated on a patient per year basis. There is a general agreement that treatment at home is undoubtedly less expensive than treatment in hospital, in addition to having other advantages. Costs are easier to estimate than those of hospital care, since a price for equipment and home adaptation is relatively easy to obtain. The only problem is in estimating part of the cost of the 'back-up' hospital unit to each home dialysis patient, since all patients and a family member require initial training in a hospital unit, and some will require subsequent readmission for complications. Some estimates of capital costs and maintenance in home dialysis are shown in Table 2.

Survival in hospital (about 65% at 3 years) is poorer than that at home (81% at 3 years), although this largely reflects selection of patients rather than intrinsic differences. Likewise, the degree of rehabilitation achieved by patients is considerably better for home dialysis than hospital care, and almost as good as that of transplant patients.

The calculation of the cost of a renal transplant is even more of a problem, and since there are very few units which are devoted entirely to this activity, separating the cost of a transplant patient from hospital running costs is extremely difficult. In Table 3 some studies on the costs of renal transplantation are shown. The actual values by themselves mean little, but comparing them with dialysis costs it is clear that a transplant operation probably costs less than dialysis for 1 year in hospital.

Table 3 Costs of a renal transplant

Author	*Year of estimate*	*Country*	*Cost of operation**		*Cost of follow-up**	
Klarman *et al* (1968)	1968	USA	$13 000	(10 000)	—	
Kountz (1969)	1969	USA	$10 000	(7500)	—	
Douglas (1973)	1972	USA	$13–16 000	(8500–10 500)	—	
Schippers and Kalff (1976)	1973	Netherl.	$18 000	(11 300)	$3200	(2000)
Stewart *et al* (1973)	1973	Australia	$A7100	(7100)	$A800	(700)

* $US except where stated; 1975 sterling equivalent in brackets (from Parkin[1])

It must also be noted that after the high initial cost of the transplant operation and the necessary postoperative care, costs become relatively small, drugs and outpatient attendances, but mortality is quite high, 40% at 3 years, and a further 20% of grafts fail necessitating a return to dialysis care. Even allowing for this, however, cost per life-year is lowest for this form of treatment, as well as offering the most satisfactory quality of life.

Cost–benefit analysis (CBA)

There is an enormous potential expenditure on treatment for chronic renal failure. Therefore, the implicit question arises about the proportion of national health services budgets that should be spent on such treatment. In industry decisions on courses of action are determined on the basis of the return on the money invested. In health care an alternative approach, based on similar principles, is cost–benefit analysis.

According to Weisbrod's concept the monetary losses which accrue as a result of morbidity and mortality are:

(1) Indirect Costs
The loss of economic production due to premature death of a member of the production force
Temporary and/or intermittent losses of economic production due to sickness
Decreased production efficiency due to disease induced debility

(2) Direct Costs
The economic costs of diagnosis, treatment, rehabilitation and capital investment in health care facilities

These items are the cost to society rather than to individuals or their families. Measurement of the indirect costs can be done in various ways. The 'human capital' approach, which considers a human person as human capital for production, has been most frequently used. There are, however, other approaches to valuing a life, including explicit statements of value by individuals. Another major category of indirect costs, which is difficult to quantify, is that of pain and suffering of the individual and the burden of illness on the family.

In the case of a cost–benefit analysis of a contemplated treatment programme, the indirect costs, when they can be obviated, may then become benefits, namely, 'saved costs'. The size of these savings depend mainly on the efficacy of the treatment thus preventing costly sequelae. Some of the direct costs may become benefits too, for instance in connection with a national well-coordinated programme, where all sorts of unnecessary expenditures and duplications can be eliminated.

For a properly organized cost–benefit study some *epidemiological* information must be provided: (1) incidence and/or prevalence of diabetic nephropathy, (2) number of cases discovered and/or treated, (3) treatment or diagnostic techniques actually, or potentially available, (4) cure rate and survival period for the various treatment modalities/techniques, and, ideally, (5) some indication of the 'quality of life' (patient's own feelings, rehabilitation and social function) after treatment.

Some workers have envisaged studying all costs and benefits through a *cohort analysis*, by relating costs and benefits to the present and future history of a cohort. Usually a cohort of 1000 persons is studied for say 20–30 years. The cohort must be characterized in terms of sex, age, potential earnings and morbidity and mortality patterns, as this will enable the results of the analysis to be translated into equivalent economic terms. Studies of this sort are based on a series of assumptions and extrapolations, such as survival after defined

Table 4 Percentage survival of patients

	5 years	*10 years*
Hospital haemodialysis	53.2	35.6
Home haemodialysis	74.0	55.6
1st live donor graft	71.2	60.0
1st cadaver graft	58.1	44.2

From *Proc. EDTA* 1980, Table XVII

periods and rehabilitation, in terms of ability to work and maintain either the totality or a part of the earnings.

An example of survival periods is given in Table 4.

The benefit–cost ratios are calculated by forming a fraction of discounted benefits and costs. If the ratio is greater than 1, then benefits exceed costs, and the investment is 'profitable', provided that no other relevant alternatives with greater ratios exist. Put differently, given limited resources, it is possible to rank-order the various available therapeutic and/or rehabilitative measures according to their benefit–cost ratios.

From studies on both sides of the Atlantic, and in spite of differences in assumptions, time and place, it appears that the costs of dialysis clearly outweigh benefits. In these terms and by an improved quality of life for those in whom it is successful, kidney transplantation has been justified. This should not imply that kidney transplantation is, in fact, highly successful. The survival of the grafted kidney (as opposed to the patient) is of the order of 50% in the first year. These figures relate to cadaver grafts from unrelated donors. Kidney transplants from live related donors do considerably better (80% still functioning at 1 year) but there has been some reluctance on the part of doctors and relatives in most countries, except the USA, to use kidneys from this source. It has been noted that patient and graft survival rates have improved little since the late 1960s, but it must also be remembered that the present 1 year survival rates for dialysis are near 90%.

For those who survive with a functioning kidney for over 1 year after transplantation the outlook is relatively good. However, they still have to contend with the longterm effects of immune suppression and drug toxicity which includes higher incidence rates of cancer and cataracts, changes in appearance due to steroids and infection hazards. While the survival of those with terminal renal failure has been markedly improved since the advent of longterm dialysis, transplantation does not seem to have added to this.

While some weighing of benefit against cost goes on in many fields of medical decision making, and although many doctors reject such a notion as somehow unethical, it is probably better to be as explicit as possible about the basis of decisions, rather than relying upon subjective value-judgements.

The cost-effectiveness approach (CEA)

As most health care services expected to examine the alternatives in a comprehensive integrated dialysis/transplantation programme, the costs and effects of the treatment appears to be the most rational approach in an economic evaluation.

The broad format for a cost-effectiveness analysis is simple:

Effectiveness is measured by a change in some index of health (i.e. quality-adjusted life-expectancy).

Cost is measured by the net value of the changes in resource availability occasioned by the technology under appraisal.

The key difference between CEA and CBA is the valuation of all the benefits/outcomes of a health practice. Ideally, in CBA all outcomes/benefits are valued in money terms, including loss of life, quality of life and other intangibles. CEA serves to place priorities on alternative treatments, but without requiring that the dollar value of life and health be assessed.

The typical CEA situations can be envisaged, both involving two or more treatments: (1) given or assumed that the alternatives under consideration have the same clinical effectiveness, which procedure is the least costly, i.e. in this situation cost differences between two alternatives are important, (2) outcomes are not the same, either with respect to type of outcome or level of outcome. Assuming that outcomes vary with respect to level, (e.g. life expectancy or 'quality of life'), one might attempt to cost the units of outcome, for instance cost per life year gained, and then compare the alternatives this way. It is this latter version of CEA which has been used in studies of dialysis and transplantation.

CEA can be conducted from (1) a sectoral perspective, i.e. the health care sector or even narrower, a hospital or a community, and (2) a broad societal perspective. The general results emerging from various cost-effectiveness studies are that for dialysis, home dialysis systematically is cheaper than hospital dialysis. Comparing dialysis and transplantation, it appears that transplantation is the cheaper alternative. It is to be noted, however, that in the case of cadaveric transplantation the difference between home dialysis and transplantation is negligible. In the latest American studies only the live related donor transplant is better than dialysis.

A computer simulation model for the investigation of the end-stage renal disease systems of care was developed, and has shown its usefulness in determining cost-effectiveness. The analysis of the simulation also showed that live related donor transplantation was the least costly and had the greatest survival time, while centre haemodialysis had the poorest cost-effectiveness.

CONCLUSIONS

The relative merits of dialysis and transplantation for the management of diabetic nephropathy have been the subject for a scientific, administrative and public debate. One important aspect of this debate being the economic aspects.

The present judgment is that transplantation from a living donor, ideally an HLA-identical sibling, offers the best chance for decent life. Fortunately, haemodialysis and peritoneal dialysis offer acceptable alternatives for survival, if transplantation is not possible.

Trials of alternative methods of therapy which may inhibit the progression of diabetic nephropathy such early and improved diabetes control as anti-hypertensive treatment should be more widely investigated.

Methods for reducing dialysis costs should be envisaged.
Research is necessary so that a truly direct attack on the underlying lesion of diabetic glomerulosclerosis can be initiated.

Technical, clinical, epidemiological, socio-ethical and economic aspects are essential for the appropriate assessment of both dialysis and transplantation. Very few – if any – evaluative issues can be satisfactorily resolved by using only one single parameter. In the most apparently clinical of all questions of evaluation – is the patient's health improved? – economic notions of welfare and utility are essential in the measurement of health status. Conversely, in the most apparently economic of all questions of evaluation – is the benefit greater than the cost? – clinical and epidemiological understanding of the links between what is done and what happens to patients is essential.

This interactive and symbiotic relationship between the disciplines should be reflected in research and development, education and training, health planning and management and clinical practice.

EPILOGUE

It may be difficult to invent something new, but we can improve and master something already known.

References

1. Goetz, F.C. and Kjellstrand, C.-M. (1979). The treatment of diabetic kidney disease. *Diabetologia,* **17,** 267
2. Gurland, H.J. *et al.* (1976). Combined report on regular dialysis and transplantation in Europe, VI, 1975. *Proc. Eur. Dial. Transplant Assoc.,* **13,** 3
3. Parkin, D.M. (1978). Chronic renal failure: the economics of treatment. *Community Health,* **9,** 134
4. Pedersen, K.M. (1983). Economic Evaluation of Dialysis, Wolfsberg Symposium. In *Symposium on the Economic and Medical Evaluation of Health Care Technologies,* April 13–16, Wolfsberg (in press)
5. Roberts, S.D. *et al.* (1980). Cost-effective care of End-Stage Renal Disease: A Billion Dollar Question. *Ann. Intern. Med.,* **92,** 243
6. *Symposium on the Economic and Medical Evaluation of Health Care Technologies,* 13–16 April 1982, Wolfsberg (in press)

3.2
Diabetic nephropathy in the UK – health economics

P. V. MANCINI

ABSTRACT

The economic view of disease is discussed in terms of the monetary and non-monetary burdens it imposes on society and the individual. The burden of diabetes is set in the context of estimates of the burden of all diseases in the UK.

Diabetic nephropathy is shown to impose chiefly non-monetary costs on individuals and their families, but also incurs direct monetary costs of treatment, most dramatically when end-stage renal failure is reached. It is argued that the indirect monetary costs from morbidity are attributable not to clinical nephropathy but to other, earlier, complications of diabetes.

The system of resource allocation in the UK and the reluctance on the part of doctors to treat diabetics for renal failure are discussed. Modes of therapy and the role of economics are considered.

Estimates of the costs of treatment for end-stage renal failure (ESRF) are presented on the basis of a survey of hospitals undertaken by the Department of Health and Social Security (DHSS) in 1981, and the cost–effectiveness of therapy for diabetics considered.

Finally, the paper discusses the possibility of preventing clinical nephropathy, and the economic aspects of prevention.

INTRODUCTION – THE ECONOMIC VIEW OF DISEASE

Any disease puts a burden on the person who suffers from it, and on the society of which he is a member. It is possible to categorize the burden, or cost, in two ways: monetary and non-monetary. Monetary costs do not imply an expenditure or cash payment, but mean that the costs, which may be lost time, or lost production, can be quantified and valued in money terms. Other costs, such as pain and suffering, which are not easily quantifiable and very difficult to value, are referred to as non-monetary costs: attempts have been made to put values on what are at present non-monetary items such as loss of life for its own sake, but these are controversial.

The monetary costs, which by definition are more readily calculable, comprise the effect on society's resources, in terms of the production of goods and services. The *direct* monetary cost of disease is the value of resources used in treating it; the *indirect* monetary costs of disease relate to changes in the production of goods and services, leisure (non-working) time, and any use of other resources (e.g. transport) by the patient and his family or friends, as a result of the patient's morbidity or premature death. Various attempts have been made to estimate the costs of disease[1,2]. The early work by Black and Pole[2] showed that in 1972–3 Diabetes Mellitus in the UK accounted for 0.87% of total in-patient days, compared with 31.31% for Psychoses and Neuroses (ICD Nos 290–309); and only 0.81% of estimated life-years lost compared with 21.51% for Hypertension (ICD Nos 400–404).

Most of the studies of this type have naturally concentrated on the monetary costs. What they reveal, at first sight, is the relative unimportance, in terms of direct costs, of diabetes, at a national level. But this is not to deny the tremendous importance of such disease to the individual and to the doctors who treat him.

DIABETIC NEPHROPATHY

Clinical diabetic nephropathy is a spectacular, distressing, and late-manifesting complication of diabetes. One of the problems of the 'burdens of disease' approach is of course the need for categorization. The figures quoted earlier for diabetes would probably not include life-years lost nor in-patient days attributable to end-stage renal failure associated with diabetes.

Diabetic nephropathy certainly imposes costs in terms of pain, suffering, etc, and in direct monetary terms (costs of treatment, if treated), but it is difficult to attribute much in the way of lost output to diabetic kidney disease, since diabetes has many other complications which develop before the appearance of clinical nephropathy. By the time a person has reached end-stage renal failure, he has probably undergone at least one other serious complication, chiefly blindness from retinopathy. Kjellstrand *et al*[3] suggest that 21 years after the onset of diabetes is the average time for a patient to develop end-stage renal failure. By this time about one third of patients already have severe visual problems.

Any indirect monetary costs arising from morbidity are, therefore, probably attributable to other complications of diabetes which occur before overt clinical nephropathy, especially renal failure, develops.

IMPLICATIONS IN THE UNITED KINGDOM

Since the indirect monetary costs of diabetic kidney disease may be trivial, economic interest centres on the direct costs of treatment of end-stage renal failure occasioned by diabetes, and the non-monetary costs of morbidity and premature mortality (i.e. the value of pain and suffering).

Professor Stewart Cameron of Guy's Hospital[4] quoting Fuller[5] states that at least 500 diabetics in the UK reach end-stage renal failure each year. EDTA estimates that in 1981 only 80 diabetics were accepted for treatment (5.5% of the intake that year)[6]. This low rate of acceptance for treatment, while reflecting the UK's generally low acceptance rate, is also a legacy from the early days of renal therapy for diabetics, when their prognosis was especially poor. Historically, many renal units have been unwilling to start diabetics on dialysis because of the prospect of difficult haemodialysis, difficult and diminishing vascular access, and because of the possibility of intervening death from cardiovascular disease.

Part of the reason for the relatively low acceptance rate for renal replacement therapy (RRT) generally in the UK is that the DHSS does not usually allocate funds for particular services except on an experimental and limited basis. Instead, it allocates National Health Service (NHS) funds on a geographical basis to regional health authorities, which in turn allocate to district health authorities. In practice, money is allocated to hospitals, which may or may not have a renal unit. In allocating funds the authorities have to consider the needs of many competing specialties, and the policies of the Department, with regard to particular client groups.

However, UK nephrologists ask that the Department should take on a central role and take the funding of renal services out of what they consider the lottery of the geographical system, arguing that RRTs are proven effective techniques of a different nature from the more mundane activities of the NHS. However, as will be shown later there are other equally important activities which are more cost-effective in saving life.

Even if the Department did undertake such a central responsibility for this one specialty, it is by no means certain that doctors would be willing to treat all patients with end-stage renal failure, nor that all such patients would wish to be treated. Diabetics seem to do badly on many doctors' acceptance criteria[7], especially those diabetics who have already developed blindness.

TREATMENT MODES FOR DIABETICS

In the UK, haemodialysis has not generally been offered to diabetics in renal failure: transplantation has been considered the more successful therapy, if any. But now, Continuous Ambulatory Peritoneal Dialysis (CAPD), which does not require repeated access to the vascular system, seems to be a technique particularly suited to the diabetic patient, not least because of the possibility of introducing insulin (though in increased quantity[8]) into the peritoneal dialysate. Not only might CAPD act as a technique in its own right, but it might also offer the chance of maintained survival until transplantation is possible.

THE ROLE OF ECONOMICS

The classical model of cost–benefit analysis has a very simple decision rule – undertake those activities whose benefits exceed their costs (and, conversely, do not undertake those activities whose costs exceed their benefits). This rule, simple though it sounds, begs many questions – the estimation of benefits, the estimation of costs and the estimation of the net benefits of alternative uses of resources.

Estimating benefits of therapy depends ultimately on medical evidence, as to whether one mode is better than another in terms of clinical outcome for a particular (type of) patient. Even this is not clearcut, since patients are *selected* for particular modes of therapy whose outcomes of treatment are thereby affected[3,9,10]. As Glass[9] points out, randomized controlled trials are not easily practicable in this area. The benefits of a health care activity, in this case renal replacement therapy, can be conceived of in terms of avoided costs (or the 'burden' discussed earlier). To 'justify', in the cost–benefit sense, the treatment of patients with end-stage renal failure, one has to show that the benefits outweigh the costs. Since it is difficult to value the benefits of therapy, *viz* increased survival (of a variable quality), one has to look at the costs of therapy and consider what is the implied value of 'life'.

THE COSTS OF RENAL REPLACEMENT THERAPY (RRT)

Because of the lack of comparable cost data in the UK, the DHSS undertook a study in three renal units in 1981, to determine the basic costs of dialysis and transplantation and the costs of complications. The data on complications only relate to the experiences of 48 renal patients, whereas the basic cost data are based on the activity of the whole of each renal unit. Of the 48 patients who were studied in detail, it is interesting to note that only one, who had a successful transplant, was a diabetic. It is probable, in view of the figures quoted by Cameron[4] (above) that the cost figures calculated relate almost exclusively to non-diabetic patients. Accordingly, since diabetics probably experience more complications than the non-diabetic patient, the cost figures ought to be regarded as *minimum* estimates of treating diabetic end-stage renal failure.

Table 1 shows the annual basic costs of dialysis in three UK hospitals. These costs relate only to the performance of dialysis sessions and do not include the

Table 1 Basic annual costs of dialysis

	£, Nov 1981 prices
Hospital haemodialysis	9500–11 000
Home haemodialysis	6500–7 000
CAPD	5400–6 200

1. Figures exclude cost of in-patient admissions, out-patient attendances, drugs, tests, etc.
2. Apart from haemodialysis machines, home conversion costs, and minor CAPD equipment, they are current costs (machines etc are annuitized at 5% p.a.)
3. Training costs are extra in first year

Table 2 Estimated annual total costs of dialysis

	£, Nov 1981 prices
Hospital haemodialysis	11 200–13 650
Home haemodialysis	7100–8 700
CAPD	7550–9 800

1. Figures include costs of out-patient attendances, drugs, etc and in-patient admissions for complications
2. Complications data based on experiences of 48 patients (one diabetic)
3. Figures to be regarded as minimum estimates of treatment costs for diabetics
4. CAPD data on complications based on very few patients, and early experience of technique (people commencing RRT in 1978)

Table 3 Costs of first transplants

	£, Nov 1981 Prices
SUCCESSFUL	
First Year	5000–5700
Annual Maintenance	1400–1650
UNSUCCESSFUL	
First Year Cost (Survivors)	8500–13 500

3 year cadaver graft survival = 53%

costs of in-patient admissions, out-patient attendances, drugs or tests. The range of costs encountered reflects not only differences in technique but, for example, different prices paid for dialysate. For hospital haemodialysis the basic costs range from £9500 to £11 000, for home haemodialysis the basic costs are between £6500 and £7000, and for CAPD between £5400 and £6200. Of course complications which result in admissions, together with regular out-patient attendances, push the basic cost up. These full costs are shown in Table 2.

For hospital haemodialysis, the range of costs is £11 200–£13 650; for home haemodialysis £7100–£8700; and for CAPD £7550–£9800. For diabetic patients home haemodialysis is probably not an option – they will probably have to be dialysed in hospital or by CAPD. As has been alluded to earlier, transplantation is often regarded as the preferred option for diabetics (and non-diabetics).

Our estimates[11], presented in Table 3, suggest that a successful transplant costs between £5000 and £5700, with annual maintenance costs of about £1500. These figures do not include any estimates for costs, in the case of diabetics, of such problems as amputations.

However, UK data[12] suggest a 3 year cadaver graft survival of only 53%, and for *diabetics* in the USA[9] the equivalent cadaver graft survival is about 40%. Only a small proportion of diabetics, as also non-diabetics, are lucky enough to have identical live-related donors, which is a factor in improving success[13].

It is still too early to quote the longterm survival of CAPD patients – it is known that after a couple of years on CAPD many patients cannot continue on that mode, and have to revert to haemodialysis. However, the respite offered by CAPD to diabetics may be long enough to permit the opportunity of transplantation[13] and an improved prognosis if the graft fails.

COST-EFFECTIVENESS ANALYSIS

Non-economists confuse cost-benefit and cost-effectiveness analysis. The latter is a more limited, and some might argue more useful, technique. Cost-effectiveness analysis assumes, or does not question, that a given outcome, such as prolongation of life, is desirable. Assuming that a particular patient were treatable equally by haemodialysis, CAPD or transplantation, what would cost-effectiveness tell us? In non-diabetics it would show that hospital haemodialysis was much more expensive per life year added than was home haemodialysis; home haemodialysis was probably as cost-effective as CAPD, and successful transplantation the most cost-effective. In the case of diabetics, however, there would be the increased risk of amputations[3]. These statements about relative cost-effectiveness measured in terms of added life-years are intuitively and anecdotally plausible, but they do raise the important issue of patient selection – not all patients can have a successful transplant, not all can dialyse at home (particularly diabetics).

In circumstances such as these, economic analysis is chiefly directed to the question: what must be the minimum value placed on life (in practice a 'life year') in order to justify an annual expenditure of the order of £10 000?

Clearly, since in the case of diabetic nephropathy, the benefit from treating the disease is chiefly non-monetary, a decision to treat a patient by dialysis implies acceptance of a value of life of at least £10 000 p.a. This figure is several times higher than the cost per life-year estimated for Bone Marrow Transplantation (BMT) for acute myeloid leukaemia[14], £750–£1500. This is not to suggest that resources ought to be taken away from renal failure, but that in considering any expansion, if the NHS had to choose where to inject its new money, other life-saving interventions might come higher in the priority list than dialysis. This comparison brings home, of course, the fact that kidney transplantation is more cost-effective than dialysis, and only a little less cost-effective than BMT.

PREVENTION

End-stage renal failure occurs relatively late in the natural history of diabetes. The warning signs of changes in morphology and in kidney function happen long before the clinically critical decline of function which necessitates renal replacement therapy.

If the critical point of clinical nephropathy could be delayed by improved diabetic control[15] or other means, the costs of renal failure in non-monetary and direct monetary terms could be delayed or avoided all together. Unanswered questions are whether this prevention is possible[16] and, if so, whether it is cost-effective. A preventive measure is of course an investment whose benefits may not accrue for several years – e.g. an intervention to halt the course of nephropathy may have to occur 15 or so years before overt clinical nephropathy develops. In such circumstances, economists would advocate using a discount factor to give more weight to immediate effects, and progressively less weight to the more distant ones. However, since it is unlikely that the costs of prevention would be anything like the costs of treating end-stage renal failure in diabetics, and may indeed only relate to improved diabetic control, prevention would not only confer a net benefit in monetary terms but also in terms of the avoided non-monetary burden imposed by clinical nephropathy.

ACKNOWLEDGEMENTS

I am grateful to Alan Angilley and Andrew Burchell for helpful comments.

DISCLAIMER

Any views expressed are those of the author alone, and ought not to be ascribed to the Department of Health and Social Security.

References

1. Rice, D.P. (1966). Estimating the cost of illness. *Health Economics Series,* **No. 6,** US Public Health Service
2. Black, D.A. and Pole, J.D. (1975). Priorities in biomedical research: Indices of burden. *Br. J. Prev. Soc. Med.,* **29,** 222
3. Kjellstrand, C.M., Whitley, K., Comty, C.M. and Shapiro, F.L. (1983). Dialysis in patients with diabetes mellitus: editorial review. *Diab. Nephr.,* **2,** 5
4. Cameron, J.S. (1983). The management of diabetic renal failure in the United Kingdom: editorial. *Diab. Nephr.* **2,** 1
5. Fuller, J. Personal communication
6. Jacobs, C. *et al* (1983). The first five thousand diabetics treated by dialysis and transplantation in Europe. *Diab. Nephr.,* **2,** 13
7. Parsons, V. and Lock, P. (1980). Current issues in medical ethics: Triage and the patient in renal failure. *J. Med. Ethics,* **6,** 173
8. Kjellstrand, C.M. (1977). Dialysis in diabetics. In Friedman, E.A. (ed.). *Strategy in Renal Failure,* pp. 345–391 (New York: Wiley)
9. Glass, N.R., Miller, D.T., Sollinger, H.W. and Belzer, F.O. (1983). Transplantation is the treatment of choice for diabetic nephropathy. *Diab. Nephr.,* **2,** No. 1
10. Berger, P.S., Alpert, P.E. and Longnecker, R.E. (1983). Dialysis therapy for diabetics. *Diab. Nephr.* **2,** 24
11. Mancini, P.V. and Davis, M.J.S. (1982). The costs of renal replacement therapy. DHSS (unpublished)
12. UK Transplant Service, 1972–82. Anniversary Report, p. 46
13. Amair, P., Khanna, R., Leibel, B. *et al* (1982). Continuous ambulatory peritoneal dialysis in diabetics with end-stage renal disease. *N. Engl. J. Med.,* **306,** 11
14. Black, D. (1982). (Chairman). *Report of Working Group on Bone Marrow Transplantation.* (London: HMSO)
15. Brenner, B.M., Hostetter, T.H. and Humes, H.D. (1978). Dietary protein intake and the progressive nature of kidney disease. *N. Engl. J. Med.,* **298,** 826
16. Viberti, G.C., Bilous, R.W., Mackintosh, D., *et al* (1983). Longterm correction of hyperglycaemia and progression of renal failure in insulin dependent diabetes. *Br. Med. J.,* **286,** 598

Open Discussion

Professor Legrain: If I can add one little fact to Mr Mancini's data on transplantation, on the extra costs of diabetic transplant cases. In La Pitié Hospital the average duration of hospitalization time in the first year following transplantation is 25 days for the non-diabetic and 55 for the diabetic; which gives some measure of the extra costs.

Professor Keen: We have had a wide-ranging first look at the problem of diabetic nephropathy, and an entry into the difficult question of cost-benefit analysis, difficult to me, and I suspect difficult to most doctors. As physicians, we do not primarily concern ourselves with costs but try to concern ourselves primarily with benefits. With some forms of treatment it is we who are saying yes while those who administer us who are saying no. In a sense there is almost inevitably an adversarial relationship between the doctor and the health economist, which may be deflected into a competitive relationship between doctors for scarce resources. I do not apologize for it, but I understand that it must always be difficult for the health economist to argue his case with a group of practising doctors.

Professor Friedman also ranged widely over the problem of diabetic nephropathy from the point of view of the nephrologist and he has a comment on health economics.

Professor Friedman: Professor Wahba and Mr Mancini made me exceptionally uncomfortable with their scholarly presentations and illustrate the danger of having economists look at a part of the problem without understanding the whole. They could hardly be expected to understand the whole problem without close clinical collaborators.

In one of his slides, Professor Wahba made recommendation as to the desirability of shifting patients from one treatment to another; more transplantation, more home haemodialysis. But the data are not available to support that contention. As a specific example, the two year death rate in England from kidney transplantation in diabetics as reported from the King's College Hospital in December 1982 in *Br. Med. J.* was 40%. 60% of the grafts had ceased to function in two years. Under those circumstances, would anyone really wish to advocate more kidney transplantation? Further, the evidence that haemodialysis in the home or CAPD is less or more expensive is unavailable, because no study to my knowledge has been done with age-matched patients of equivalent severity.

Lacking these data, health administrators can hardly advocate anything other than the funding of research to get more information.

Mr Mancini claimed to talk about the facts of life. What are the facts? That it is more cost-effective to lose a destroyer in the Falkland Islands than to deny – for that same amount of money – two years of health care for Britain's diabetics? There are no facts. There are contentions.

As scholars concerned with a mutual problem we ought to sit down with each other and suffer and think and reason, but not come in with recommendations without the facts to support them. I say this in friendship and collegiality.

Professor Keen: That is a splendid polemic. I suspect, too, that Professor Friedman would spend much more than the equivalent of five battleships, given the opportunity. Unfortunately somebody has to call a halt, on some economic or political basis. In some way the resources of a nation have to be divided amongst all those who make calls upon them. There is a housing call, there is an educational call, and there is a health call.

As doctors we cannot make those decisions, but we should shout as loudly as we can for the things we need. Nevertheless, resources are not unlimited.

Mr Mancini: Professor Keen has made my point. That is the fact of life I was speaking about. Resources are limited and people do choose. In the United Kingdom, decisions on the high-level funding between government spending departments are taken at cabinet level. The Department of Health gets its vote of money, and we try to do the best with it we can. The same with the Regional and District Health Authorities when they get their share.

It would be very nice to sell a few destroyers – if we could get anything for them – and give the funds to renal patients, but it does not work like that, unfortunately.

Professor Wahba: I should like to clear up a misunderstanding. I did not advocate nor make any recommendations. These were simple alternatives and possibilities but not recommendations. We cannot make any recommendations on these subjects.

There are two kinds of health economist. One kind has an executive position and is forced to apply cuts and is paid to do so. Then there is the health economist who works on a different level, who helps the clinician to work more effectively and more efficiently and tries to provide him with alternatives. He is only an adviser and has no sort of authoritative power.

Mr Mancini: I am the latter kind of economist. I have no power. I only make recommendations.

Dr H J Goldsmith (UK): The results of transplantation have improved in the last two years. We do not yet know how much of it is due to blood transfusion and how much is due to cyclosporin A. But if we use cyclosporin A, then at present prices there will in the future be very little to choose between the cost of a transplant and the cost of, say, home dialysis or CAPD.

My other point is quite a separate one. Civilized nations accept that it is wrong to kill people because they are of no use to society. Thus in our mental hospitals we have a very large number of patients, more probably than the number of renal patients, even if we managed to treat them all. The cost of looking after such a patient is equivalent to the cost of treating a patient on haemodialysis in hospital.

Dr E Kohner (UK): Why is it that so many of Professor Friedman's patients who go on haemodialysis are blind? Usually retinopathy presents quite a long time before there is any significant renal failure. In the United States there is an ophthalmologist on every street corner and they are grossly underworked. I wonder why they do not photocoagulate more patients, in good time and adequately.

Incidentally, 1600 was the number of photocoagulation burns mentioned. We find 2000–6000 much more common. Very few patients can be adequately treated with 1600 burns. That may be one of the reasons why the patients are blind. Or is it that the patients are not seen regularly by a doctor? Or is it that the interns do not look at the eyes, or if they do they do not know what they see?

Professor Friedman: Most of the patients in the United States who have visual loss when they are seen by the nephrologist have visual loss because of either non-management or mismanagement of their retinopathy on the way towards renal failure. The *Journal of the American Medical Association* reported an interesting study in 1982 performed by retinal specialist ophthalmologists who had a panel of diabetic patients with proliferative retinopathy examined by house staff, general physicians, opthalmologists who were not specialists in diabetes and ophthalmologists who were specialists in diabetes. Forty per cent of the ophthalmologists who were not specialists in diabetes missed proliferative retinopathy. There are other studies like this making the same point. Even though we spend a great deal of money in the USA on health care, it is far from optimal. We have undernourished, hypertensive, untreated patients, and diabetics who go blind. The statistics that I gave are from the Scandia Transplant Report of the 97% with retinopathy, 50% who had lost vision at the time of transplantation. They were not my own data. Ours are worse. If we had Dr Kohner on our team, or on every street corner, I feel sure we would have fewer blind patients and I would be delighted to have her suggest the proper number of photocoagulative burns to administer.

Professor Legrain: There is something I do not understand. Professor

Friedman seems to have major problems with eyes, but he seems to have solved the problem of the feet. How does he do it? No more amputations?

Professor Friedman: The reason is that the fate of the foot is totally in my hands. The fate of the eye is predetermined by the time that the patient has come to me.

There is another interesting experiment on this point. Davidson at Emery University and Grady Memorial Hospital in Atlanta began a diabetic foot awareness control programme; not uraemic diabetics, all diabetics. Within one year, the amputation rate was reduced by 50% just by simple care. Dr Khanna, who will speak in a later session, is associated with Professor Oreopoulos. When I visited Professor Oreopoulos he agreed to the importance of a podiatrist in the renal failure team. He established a foot care programme amongst his patients, and though I do not know the results specifically, he told me his amputation rate is going way down.

If those in this audience go back to their own institutions and control blood pressure - listen to what Mogensen says, and control blood sugar - listen to what Keen, Parving and others say, and get a podiatrist to look after the feet, their patients will hold their renal function longer and the amputation rate will go down. If Professor Keen and Legrain achieve nothing else in this conference than to make participants aware of those points, that will keep a lot of European feet moving for a long time.

Professor M Leski (Switzerland): Professor Jacobs presented data on the transplant success rate in diabetics, but he gave no information on patient survival following graft failure. Would it be possible to have some information?

Professor Jacobs: We covered this at the EDTA Conference in Paris two years ago, but I shall recall it now.

There is something even worse for a diabetic than having to undergo haemodialysis under bad conditions or having CAPD and performing it badly, and that is to have a failed transplant. In the European experience as well as our individual experience, it is clear that when a transplant has failed, the survival of the patient is greatly threatened, and the survival of the diabetic with a failed transplant is in the general European experience very bad. Three years ago the one year survival in diabetics when a transplant had failed was only 20%.

I should welcome advice, but this is my personal feeling and it comes out everywhere that the diabetic with the failed transplant has a very poor survival.

Professor Friedman: It used to be that any patient with a failed transplant had a very poor survival, because of the large doses of immunosuppressive drugs that were used as the transplant was failing. The data that Professor Jacobs showed were up to 1981. Things have got very much better. Professor Roy Calne's demonstration of the use of cyclosporin has revolutionized cadaveric graft and patient survival. It is not 50% at one year and 45% at two years any longer. It can be as high as 90% at one year and 88% at two years.

The December 1982 Paper by Sutherland, Najarian and associates in *Transplantation*, and the March 1983 Paper by the same group in *Transplantation Proceedings*, which grew out of their presentation at the Brighton meeting a year earlier, concludes with the statement that there is no longer for the first two years an excess mortality in cadaveric kidney transplants in diabetics as compared to non-diabetics. Furthermore, Professor Thomas Starzl at Denver now regularly makes the statement that the use of living related donor kidneys in his opinion is obsolete – his word: not unethical, as he has been misquoted, but obsolete. And the reason it is obsolete is that the results of cadaveric transplants have improved so much as to compare with the live donor.

Professor J Simoes (Portugal): Are the 20–25% of diabetic patients in the United States patients with 5 mg% creatinine, or are they end-stage failure patients by other criteria?

Professor Friedman: I do not know. The figure that I quoted is not even subdivided into type 1 and type 2. It is just all diabetics. Our records are not as good as EDTA.

Professor Simoes: But with more than 5 mg%? Just with that indication?

Professor Friedman: I wish not to mislead anyone to think that I knew the creatinine levels. It is just new patients accepted on dialysis, one in four nationwide.

Professor Simones: We were told they should be accepted with 5 mg%. This is the reason for the question.

Professor Friedman: I said that uraemia therapy for the diabetic is often necessary at 5 mg%, and in fact most of my patients begin between 4.5 and 8 mg%.

Professor Simoes: This could be very important because of the different incidence in diabetic nephropathy in the United States and diabetic nephropathy in Europe.

Professor Friedman: It would only be of importance for one year – if we started early. What has happened year by year is that the proportion has risen even higher than 25%.

Professor Simoes: I agree.

Secondly, I do not think the figures from the EDTA Registry give a completely accurate picture of the incidence of nephropathy and of end-stage renal failure of nephropathy in Europe, although they are well-known figures. Why was Portugal not included? We are a very healthy country but we have left our Spanish friends just in front of the Atlantic.

Had anyone wanted to know the results in Portugal they could have asked for them.

Professor Jacobs: In building up a presentation for a meeting one has to make a choice. I made the choice which I have shown. Furthermore, I have had the honour and pleasure of being invited to Portugal three years ago, and I discussed the situation with my Portuguese colleagues. As far as I know, the Portuguese dialysis and transplant programme was just starting at that time. So I took the decision to discuss countries for which I, or the EDTA Registry at least, have had information spanning several years.

Professor Simoes: But the information should be fully factual.

Session Two

HYPERGLYCAEMIA AND RENAL RISK

Chairmen:
G. VIBERTI and E. RITZ

4

Early changes in kidney function, blood pressure and the stages in diabetic nephropathy

C. E. MOGENSEN, C. K. CHRISTENSEN, H. BECK NIELSEN and E. VITTINGHUS

INTRODUCTION

Systematic studies over the last decade have revealed that multiple changes are already present in the kidney at the time of clinical diagnosis of diabetes mellitus[1-6]. These early changes in renal function and structure in diabetes may well set the stage for the late diabetic nephropathy and its devastating consequences[7,8]. Therefore, much more detailed investigations of the early changes are pertinent.

Generally, we now have a much more active approach to the problems related to the patient with manifest diabetic nephropathy or incipient nephropathy. The changing scene in diabetic nephropathy during the 1970s and the early 1980s can be summarized as follows:

(1) The prognosis for uraemic diabetics entering end-stage renal failure programmes has continued to improve[9].

(2) Two studies have now documented the beneficial effect of anti-hypertensive treatment in diabetic nephropathy by considerably postponing uraemia[10-14]. This topic is dealt with specifically elsewhere in this volume.

(3) Supercontrol of metabolism is another avenue for exploration, with respect to the prevention of future decline in kidney function[15-17]. Much more work needs to be done in this area.

(4) It is indeed encouraging that more research is now being performed all

over the world to combat diabetic nephropathy[9,18]. On the other hand, only amounts corresponding to a minute fraction of the cost of treatment of end-stage renal failure are allocated, at present, for research into renal disease in diabetes[19]

A number of survey articles on the topic have appeared during the last few years[3-6,8,13,20-23]. This paper will not deal with the morphological lesion in diabetic renal disease, but relevant papers have recently been published elsewhere[24,90-92].

METHODS

The methods used for the study of early changes in diabetes from the functional point of view are listed in Table 1. Measuring protein excretion by sensitive methods has proved to be one of the most important advances[6,22,25-28]. Provocative tests, such as the physical exercise test reveals very early changes in the kidney of diabetic patients[15,29-36] Naturally, the classical measurements of kidney function, e.g. glomerular filtration rate (GFR) and renal plasma flow (RPF), by very exact techniques are quite indispensible for the study of renal involvement in diabetes[1,37-40], also with respect to progression studies[13,41-44]. The use of serum creatine and creatinine clearance has its limitation[10,44-46]. By defining the exact rate of progression, it is now possible to study the effect of any form of intervention. Indeed, progression rate in diabetic nephropathy seems to be a very well-defined linear parameter[13,42-44].

Table 1 Methods for the study of early renal changes in kidney function

Protein excretion
Albumin by RIA, or other sensitive methods
IgG by RIA, or other sensitive methods
β_2-microglobulin by RIA
Provocative test
Physical exercise
GFR
Inulin or ^{125}I-iothalamate clearance (constant infusion with urine collection)
EDTA clearance (single-short method)
RPF
PAH or ^{131}I-hippuran clearance
Progression studies
Define rate of progression

Also, acute effects of blood pressure changes, administration of glucose, amino acids, drugs, and hormones etc. can be studied by these methods[22,27,40,47-64].

THE CONCEPT OF MICROALBUMINURIA

This paper will survey a number of studies on renal involvement in diabetes, with 'microalbuminuria' as a key parameter. Microalbuminuria is defined as increased albumin excretion without clinical proteinuria. (Table 2 and Figure 1.) To the left on Figure 1 is shown the excretion rate in young normal males in strict baseline condition after drinking water for 2 hours (200 ml/15 min)[64]. The mean excretion rate is 5.0 μg/min ± 1.8 SD. To the right is shown albumin concentration (μg/ml) in Albustix trace-positive and Albustix positive diabetics. Provided that the urine flow is 1 ml/min, the values correspond. It can be seen that abnormal excretion rate exists over a wide range, and also when the Albustix test is negative. This illustrates that early phases of renal disease can only be detected by sensitive assays for protein or albumin excretion. Therefore, such methods are quite indispensible for the detection of early phases of renal disease, including the incipient diabetic nephropathy.

Table 2 Increased urinary albumin excretion but *not* clinical proteinuria (microalbuminuria)

Type I-diabetes
(1) Newly diagnosed diabetes
(2) During poor metabolic regulation
(3) During daily life activities – physical exercise
(4) Control of diabetes
(5) Non-diabetic renal or systemic disease
(6) Early phases of diabetic nephropathy (incipient nephropathy)

Type II-diabetes
(7) What is the predictive value of microalbuminuria

Microalbuminuria is a rather crude expression, since it has multiple aetiologies[22,27], also in diabetes. It is found in newly diagnosed diabetes and during poor metabolic control. It may be found during daily life activities, such as physical exercise, more commonly in diabetics than in non-diabetics.

Microalbuminuria is dependent upon control of diabetes, e.g. 'poor-control-related'-microalbuminuria is reversible during optimal conventional treatment or insulin pump treatment.

Microalbuminuria may also be found in non-diabetic renal or systemic disease, coexisting with diabetes, although diagnostic problems often arise in this special situation. Urinary tract infection is a possibility. Essential hypertension, known to increase microalbuminuria during poor blood pressure control[22,48,65–67], may in some instances coexist with diabetes. However, no specific marker is yet available to differentiate essential hypertension from increased pressure due to diabetic nephropathy or renal changes in diabetes.

Importantly, gradually increasing microalbuminuria is the hallmark of the

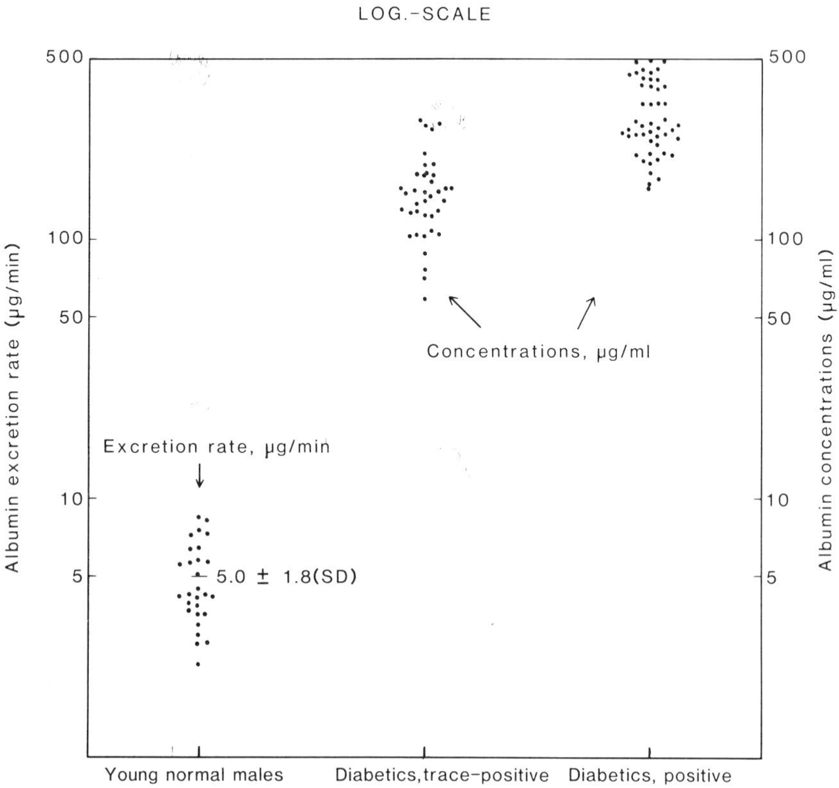

Figure 1 Albumin excretion rate in 28 young normal men, and in 38 diabetics with trace-positive Albustix, and in 48 diabetics with positive Albustix (morning urines)

early phase of diabetic nephropathy, also termed *incipient diabetic nephropathy*. Optimal standard diabetes control as well as strict baseline resting condition during urine collection should be ensured – as well as multiple collections.

Type II diabetes has been somewhat neglected in studies of kidney function over the last decade, but more interest in the non-insulin dependent diabetes is now evident. This paper will also deal with some data on the predictive value of microalbuminuria, specifically in type II diabetes[68,69].

Microalbuminuria, renal function and size at clinical diagnosis of diabetes

Abnormalities have been documented at the clinical onset of diabetes[54,68,70]. Figure 2 shows urinary albumin excretion in newly diagnosed type I diabetes (insulin-dependent diabetes mellitus) before and after standard insulin treatment, both in the erect position during the day and in the recumbent position during the night. The hatched area indicates mean values for normals ± one standard deviation. It is clear that there is a much narrower

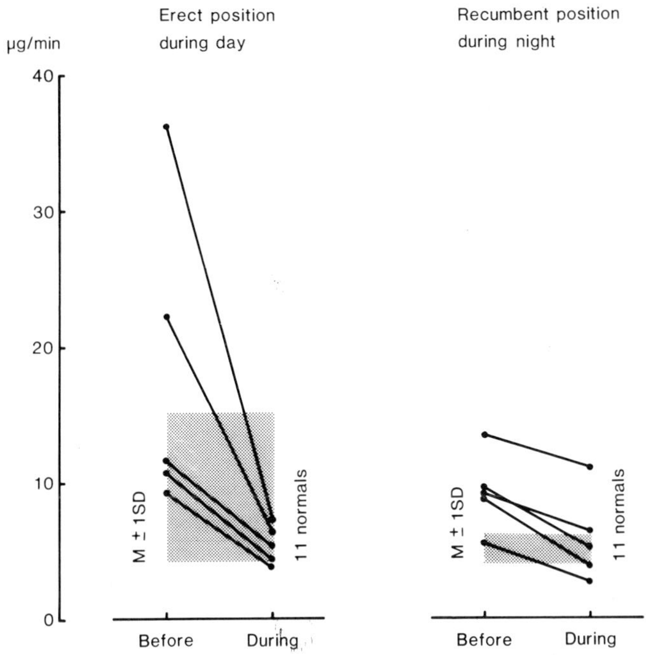

Figure 2 Urinary albumin excretion in newly diagnosed type I diabetics before and during insulin treatment

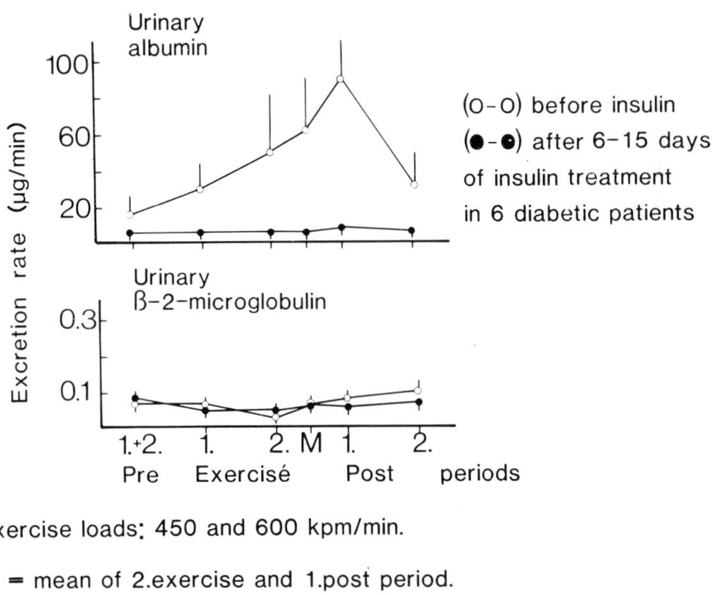

Figure 3 Urinary albumin excretion in urinary β_2-microglobulin excretion before and after insulin treatment in newly diagnosed insulin-dependent diabetic patients. Exercise tests

range for albumin excretion in the recumbent position for normals. Therefore, baseline resting conditions are preferable in comparison to 24 hour periods when studying renal involvement in diabetes. It is evident that there is a clear-cut fall in urinary albumin excretion during insulin treatment in both situations. There seems to be a tendency to higher values in diabetics during the day time, and this may be explained by the provocative effect of physical exercise on protein excretion in diabetes. Figure 3 shows urinary albumin excretion before and during exercise, on light (450 kpm/min for 20 min) and moderate (600 kpm/min for 20 min) exercise. The elevated baseline values in the untreated situation are further increased after physical exercise. After insulin treatment the values are totally normalized.

The increase in albumin excretion is clearly of glomerular origin, because urinary β_2-microglubulin excretion is quite normal also during physical exercise. The mechanism behind the exercise induced microalbuminuria in the untreated situation may well be an increased pressure in the glomerulus, permitting albumin to escape through the glomerular wall[36,61,71,72].

Excretion rate is normalized after a few weeks of insulin treatment. However, during standard control, on our ordinary insulin regime, an exercise-induced rise in albumin excretion is found again after a few years of diabetes in

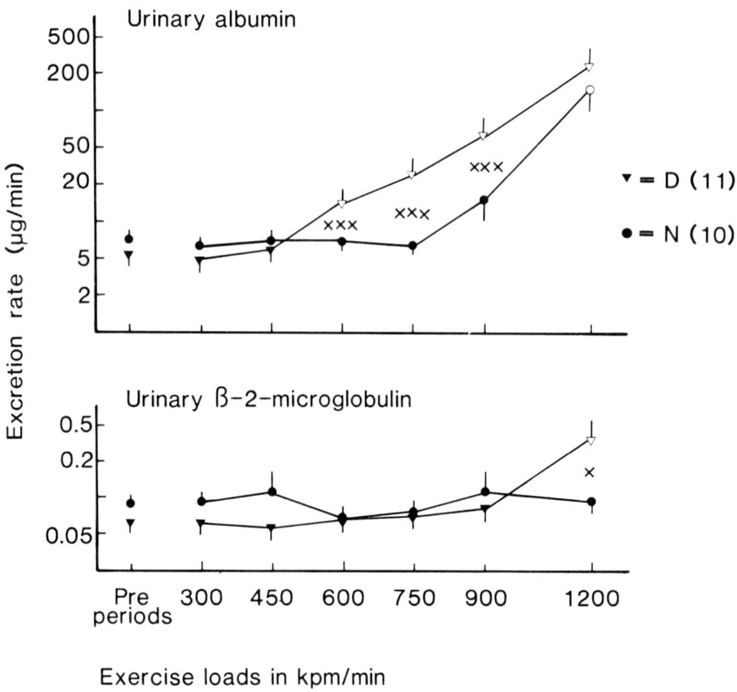

Figure 4 Urinary albumin excretion and β_2-microglobulin excretion during graded exercise in young male insulin treated diabetic patients and comparable controls

most patients at work loads not causing an increase in normals, as shown in Figure 4. Values are most often normal in baseline situations in ordinary good clinical control[70,73,74], where GFR is still high.

GFR is also significantly increased in newly diagnosed diabetes and becomes normal or nearly normal after insulin treatment[53,75]. RPF is found to be normal or slightly increased, but is depressed when expressed per gram kidney weight[4,76]. (Table 3.)

Table 3 Renal plasma flow calculated per gram kidney weight

Group	*Mean* ($ml\,min^{-1}\,g^{-1}$) ± SD	*Statistical significance of difference from normal values* (2p)
Normal subjects ($n=12$)	1.713 ± 0.229	—
Newly diagnosed diabetics ($n=6$)	1.470 ± 0.143	3.2%
Patient with diabetes duration of 1–12 years ($n=12$)	1.547 ± 0.172	5.6%
All diabetics considered together ($n=18$)	1.521 ± 0.163	1.2%

Table 4 Metabolic control and renal function in insulin-dependent diabetics (Reference 61)

	Poor control	*Good control*
Albumin excretion	↑ (+125%)*	n
β_2-micro- excretion	↑ (+123%)	n
Ratio	n.s. (+32%)	n
^{51}Cr-EDTA (GFR)	↑ (+21%)	n

* Changes primarily of glomerular origin
n.s. not significant
n = normal

After experimentally induced poor control, albumin excretion is increased (Table 4). There is also a small increase in urinary β_2-microglobulin excretion in the situation of very bad control. However, the ratio albumin : β_2 is not increased, indicating that the changes are predominantly of glomerular origin. GFR is also increased in this situation. During good control, complete or partial normalization takes place, underlining the important role of good metabolic control for normalization of these parameters[61]. Renal size is increased in early diabetes. The weight of the kidney, as measured from urograms, is significantly increased, both in newly diagnosed diabetes and after a few years of diabetes, in fact renal size is usually increased to the same extent as GFR. Thus GFR per gram kidney weight is not increased in diabetic patients[52,77–79].

Renal function after years of diabetes

During standard control in non-proteinuric patients, GFR is elevated, independent of the actual plasma glucose level[39,80–82].

During standard control renal plasma flow measured by labelled hippuran clearance may be normal or slightly increased. Some studies, including our own, revealed a higher mean value, but not a statistically significant difference[4,76]. In other studies a slightly different result with somewhat higher differences between normals and diabetics were found, the increase being statistically significant[4]. Thus it can be concluded that renal plasma flow is in the normal range or slightly elevated in early diabetes, but not to the same extent as GFR.

Table 3 shows data on renal plasma flow per gram kidney weight and, as mentioned, depressed values are found. Thus it is difficult to imagine that the increased GFR is a simple consequence of elevated plasma or blood flow to the kidney.

Intensified conventional treatment and insulin pump treatment, effect on microalbuminuria

In two short-term studies insulin pump treatment has been shown to normalize an exercise-induced increase in albumin excretion[15,17]. However, there are only a few controlled studies being performed.

Figure 5 shows the effect on 24 hour urinary albumin excretion of intensified conventional insulin treatment and insulin pump treatment. The data are from the study by Beck Nielsen *et al.* (in preparation). The intensified conventional regime consisted of the following measures: more education on diabetes, more control visits at the clinic and home monitoring of blood glucose. The patients in the two groups had a mean DD of 9.4 years $\pm$ 6.0 *vs.* 10.7 $\pm$ 5.6 SD, were aged 29.8 $\pm$ 7.9 *vs.* 28.8 $\pm$ 7.1 and had no, or very few signs, of microvascular disease. Both groups have been followed for 6 months so far and the study continues. There is a fall in all patients with elevated values (above the normal range of 22 mg/24 hours) irrespective of the treatment modality. Such elevations before treatment cannot be considered as stage III changes, i.e. not incipient diabetic nephropathy (see Table 5), since they are readily reversible with intensified control. It appeared that one patient, who increased to an abnormal value, did not respond well to the pump treatment, due to difficulties in handling the pump. No significant change in mean glucose concentration and HbA_{cI} was seen in this single patient.

For the material as a whole there was a highly significant fall in both mean blood glucose and HbA_{cI}, considerably more so for the pump treated group than for the conventionally intensified treated group.

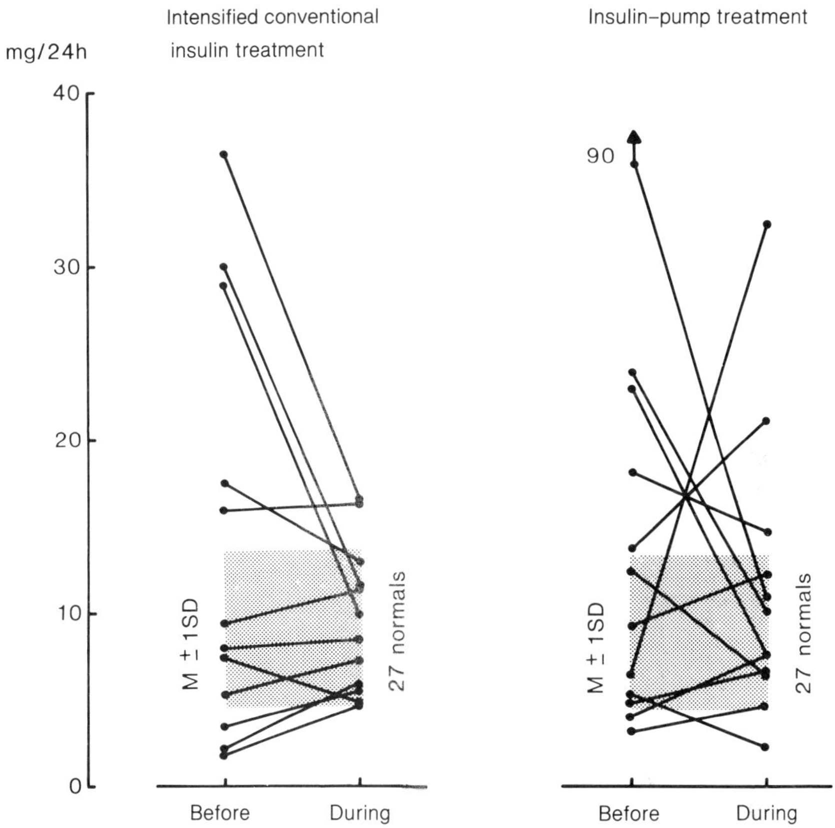

Figure 5 Urinary albumin excretion (24 hour urine collection) before and during intensified conventional insulin treatment (left) and insulin-pump treatment (right). Duration of treatment 6 months

INCIPIENT DIABETIC NEPHROPATHY

Seen from the point of early intervention in diabetic nephropathy, the most interesting stage is the early phase of clinical nephropathy or the incipient diabetic nephropathy[23,31,42,83-85]. We are dealing with the transition phase between normal excretion of albumin and clinical proteinuria, which means an excretion rate above ~15 μg/min in albumin excretion in the baseline resting situation. On the other hand, clinical proteinuria is not present. This stage III (Table 5) is seen in patients with a diabetes duration of 10–15 years. We have studied seven young male patients over a number of years, and looked at the

Table 5 Stages in diabetic nephropathy

Stage	*Proposed term*	*DD*	*Morphological change or lesion*	*Microalbuminuria*	*GFR*	*RPF*	*Blood pressure*	*Renal vascular resistance*
I	Early hyperfunction-hypertrophy stage	0–2 y	Increase in glomerular and kidney size	May be present, but reversible	↑↑↑	n or ↑	n	n
II	Renal-lesion-without-clinical-signs-stage	2–50 y	GBM: thickened MR: augmented	At poor control At exercise Otherwise usually not	↑↑	n or ↑	n	n
III	Incipient nephropathy	~10–15 y	Probably more advanced changes	Increasing microalbuminuria	Still high	Starts to decline	Diastolic pressure increases	↑
IV	Clinical nephropathy (30–40%)	~15–20 y	Glomerulosclerosis	Already developed into clinical proteinuria ($>0.5\,g/24\,h$)	Declining*	Declining	Elevated	↑↑
V	End-stage renal failure	~25–30 y	Glomerular closure	Declining proteinuria	Very low	Very low	Elevated	?

GMB: Glomerular basement membrane
MR: Mesangial regions
* Antihypertensive treatment reduces rate of progression by 50–60%
n = normal

development of renal abnormalities in this very decisive stage of renal disease in diabetes.

Data on albumin excretion are shown in Figure 6. By definition excretion is elevated in this phase, a transition phase between the normal values found in patients in good control in the preceding phase II, but below the values of clinical proteinuria, phase IV. Definition of these stages in diabetic nephropathy is given in Table 5.

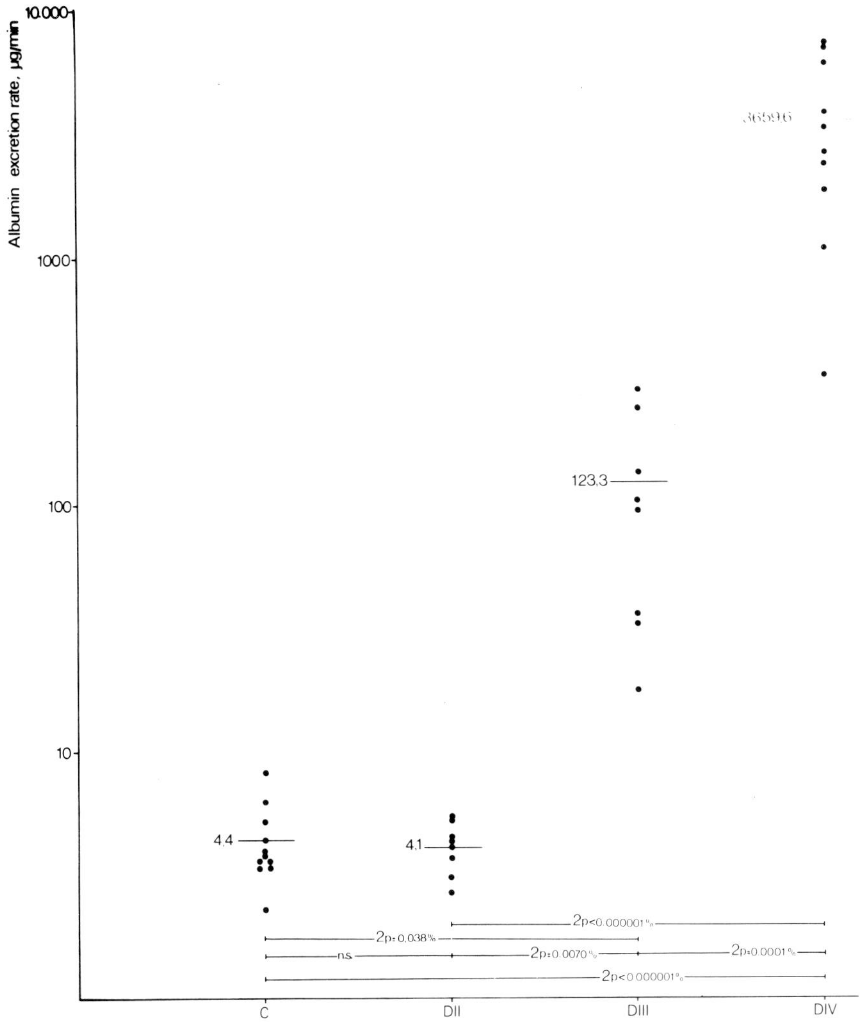

Figure 6 Urinary albumin excretion. Baseline values in yo g normal subjects (C), insulin-treated diabetic patients (D_{II}), patients with incipient diabetic nephropathy (D_{III}), patients with overt diabetic nephropathy (D_{IV}) (see also Table 5 for stages)

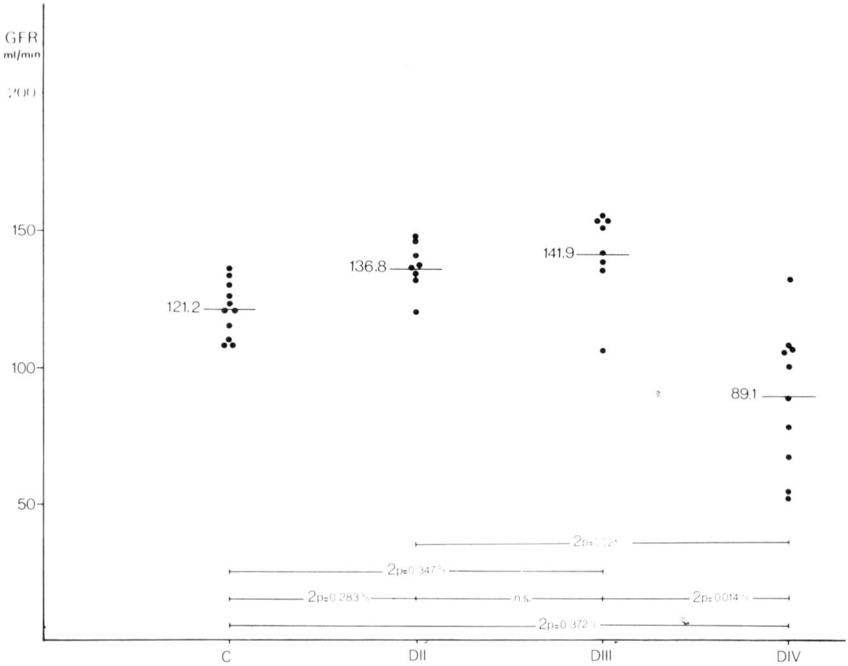

Figure 7 GFR baseline values in young normal subjects (C), insulin-treated diabetic patients (D_{II}), patients with incipient diabetic nephropathy (D_{III}), patients with overt diabetic nephropathy (D_{IV})

Figure 7 shows data on GFR in patients with incipient nephropathy as well as in the stages indicated above. GFR is significantly increased in this group, which means that we still have supranormal renal function in these patients. Diabetic patients with normal baseline albumin excretion of course also exhibit high GFR in comparison to normal subjects. On the other hand, GFR decreases in patients with overt diabetic nephropathy. The important point appears to be that GFR is very well preserved in patients with incipient nephropathy.

Data on mean arterial blood pressure values are shown in Figure 8. A very significant increase in mean blood pressure (diastolic + $\frac{1}{3}$ pulse pressure) is found already in incipient diabetic nephropathy, compared to the normal values in patients with normal albumin excretion (stage II). Still higher mean blood pressure values are of course found in overt diabetic nephropathy, so here again we see the transition phase between patients with normal baseline albumin and overt nephropathy, the incipient nephropathy. This increase in blood pressure may well be of importance in initiating the decline in renal function to be expected later in these patients.

Renal plasma flow starts to decline in these patients and furthermore, there is a marked increase in renal vascular resistance[83] (Table 5).

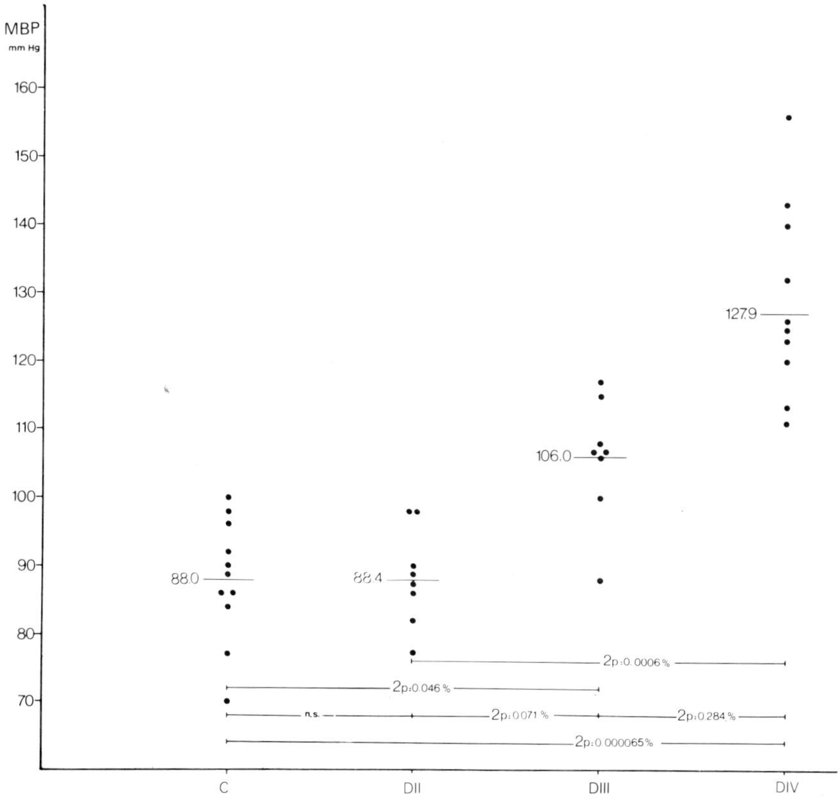

Figure 8 Mean arterial blood pressure (diastolic + $\frac{1}{3}$ pulse pressure). Baseline in young normal subjects (C), insulin-treated diabetic patients (D_{II}), patients with incipient diabetic nephropathy (D_{III}), patients with overt diabetic nephropathy (D_{IV})

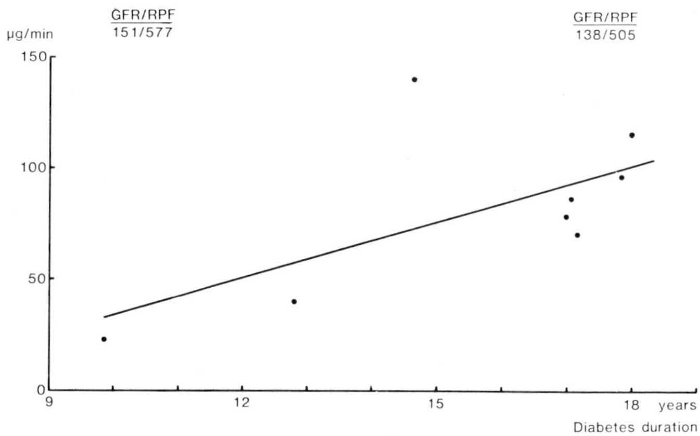

Figure 9 Urinary albumin excretion in the development of incipient diabetic nephropathy, from diabetes duration of 10–18 years. GFR and RPF indicated above

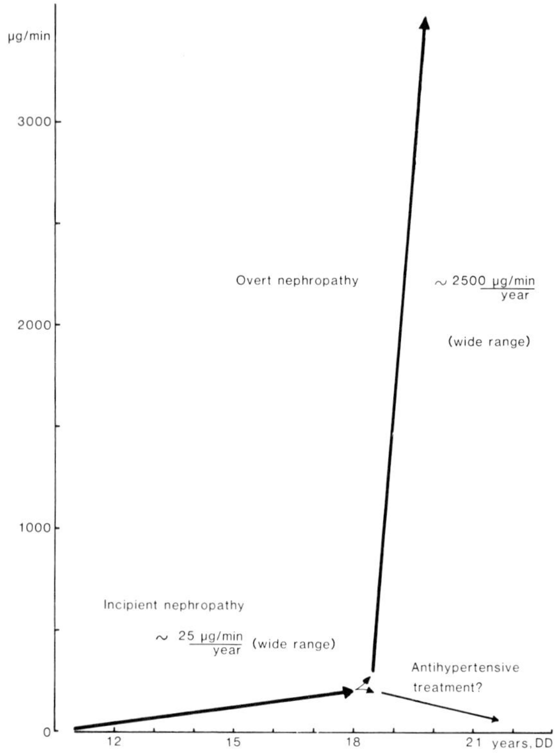

Figure 10 Outline of urinary albumin excretion in the development of incipient and overt diabetic nephropathy. Will antihypertensive treatment reverse the abnormality in the incipient phase of nephropathy?

Development of kidney disease has been followed in these patients, and an example of the course in patients with diabetes duration of 11–18 years is shown in Figure 9. A slow increase in urinary albumin excretion is found over the years. The increase rate in albumin excretion is considerably less pronounced than in overt nephropathy[42,83,86].

There is great variability in the increase rate of microalbuminuria, some patients exhibit rapid increase, some show a non-progressive pattern. Also here blood pressure seems to be of importance.

A significant correlation is found between increase rate in albuminuria ($\mu g\ min^{-1}\ year^{-1}$) and diastolic pressure, suggesting that high blood pressure is of significance for this early development of renal damage, as outlined in Figure 10. The hypothetical effect of early antihypertensive treatment is illustrated in the figure.

At present we are undertaking a trial in order to establish whether antihypertensive treatment is able to revert or arrest microalbuminuria in this early phase of diabetic nephropathy. As antihypertensive treatment, cardioselective β-blockers are being used, so far without notable side-effects. The preliminary results indicate that patients showing a good reduction in mean baseline blood pressure during treatment also exhibited a fall in baseline albumin excretion.

In essential hypertension marked changes in albumin excretion are a prominent finding, even in Albustix-negative patients[48,65]. Changes are reversed by effective treatment of hypertension[48,66,67].

Exercise-induced changes in albumin excretion and blood pressure in incipient diabetic nephropathy

Generally, baseline blood pressure and 24 hour urine collection are used in evaluating patients, also in diabetics. We have been interested in seeing the effect of daily life activities on blood pressure and albumin excretion, also in patients with incipient nephropathy, and have started investigations on the

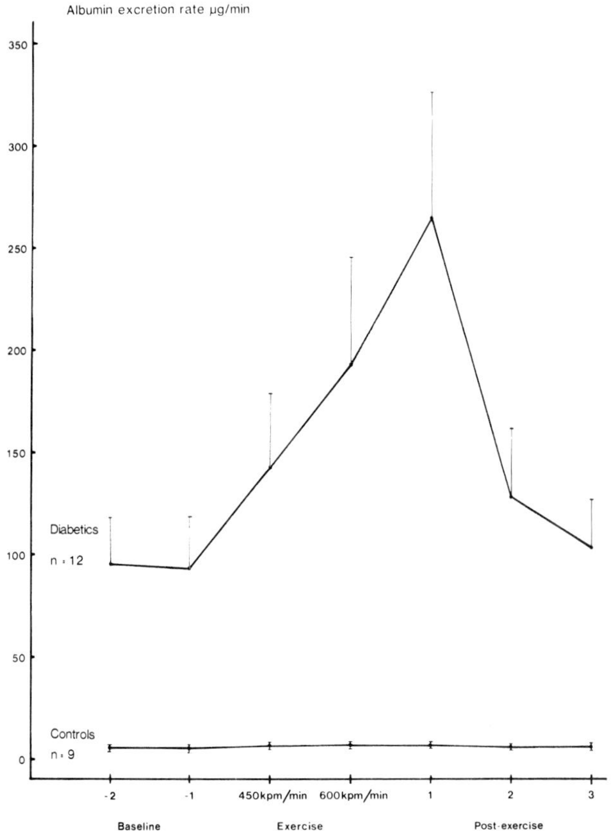

Figure 11 Urinary albumin excretion in incipient diabetic nephropathy before, during and after exercise (450 kpm/min for 20 min, followed by 600 kpm/min for 20 min). Values are given as mean ± 1SD

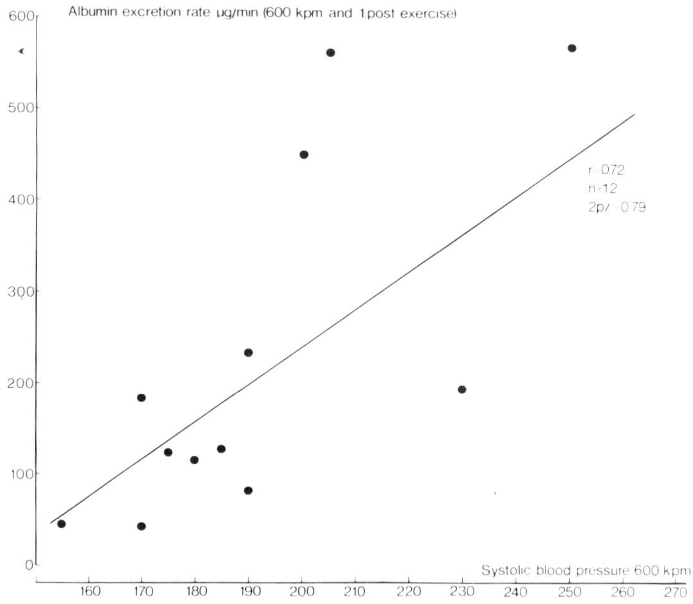

Figure 12 Data from exercise experiments. Urinary albumin excretion plotted against systolic pressure, recorded at the work-load of 600 kpm/min

effect of physical exercise. The exercise test was performed starting with two baseline periods without exercise then two exercise periods with light and moderate exercise, followed by three post-exercise periods (Figure 11). A very marked increase in urinary albumin excretion is seen during these levels of physical exercise, which is quite normal for daily life activities. Blood pressure is also abnormally increased during exercise in these diabetic patients with early diabetic nephropathy. Thus the slightly elevated baseline blood pressure is still more increased during exercise. Indeed, a correlation between increase in albumin excretion, and increase in systolic blood pressure could be documented in these patients (Figure 12). In diabetics with very marked increases in systolic pressure, exercise also induced the highest increases in albumin excretion. One might wonder whether such high increases in blood pressure during daily life, sometimes increases of 100 mmHg or more in systemic pressure, followed by an increase in microalbuminuria or albuminuria, would appear to be damaging to the diabetic kidney.

OVERT DIABETIC NEPHROPATHY (STAGE IV)

Established diabetic nephropathy is primarily characterized by permanent proteinuria (>0.5 g/24 h). Why is it that decline in GFR always continues when proteinuria is present? The diabetic alterations in metabolism have

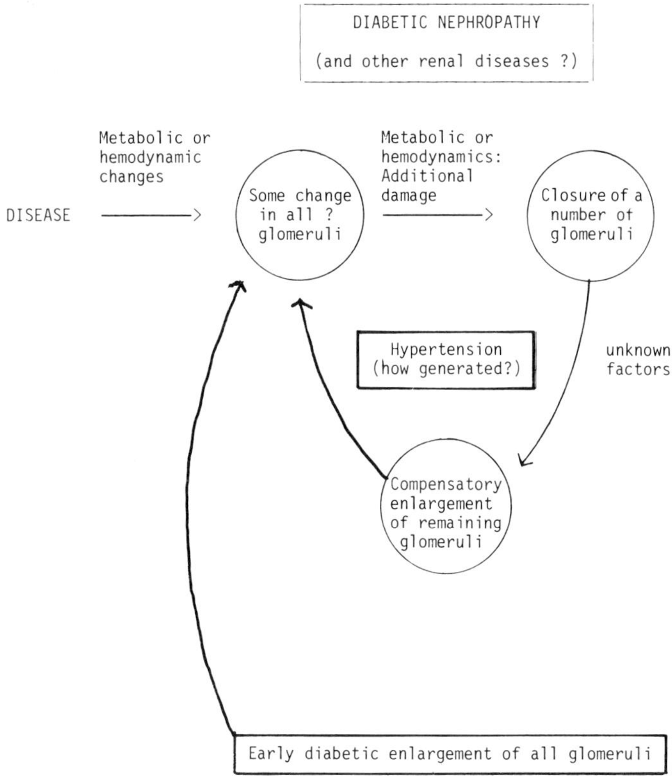

Figure 13 The hypothetical positive feed-back loop promoting decline in renal function

marked influence on the glomerulus[24]. When diabetes is present, metabolic and possibly haemodynamic changes induce damage in all glomeruli. Additional damage, again due to metabolic and haemodynamic factors, later cause closure of a number of glomeruli, perhaps after 12–16 years of diabetes. Thereafter, extra compensatory enlargement of remaining glomeruli takes place. This process may again induce additional damage to all remaining glomeruli, thus generating a positive feedback loop, promoting loss of renal function. A sketch of this development is shown in Figure 13.

Such a process, albeit hypothetical, may be common for a number of renal diseases[87], but in the case of diabetes there is a special situation, since in the early phase of diabetes, enlargement of all glomeruli is already seen. Therefore, this self-perpetuating process may be more easily established in diabetic patients. Increased GFR alone, without renal lesions, is less likely to provoke renal damage and probably a combination of metabolic induced and haemodynamic induced abnormalities is required. Hypertension is well recognized as a prominent finding in this condition with proteinuria, and hypertension may

Table 6 Summary of studies on progression of overt nephropathy (Reference 42)

Patients:	10 young male patients (<40 y) with constant proteinuria
Methods:	GFR (^{125}I-iothalamate-clearance) measured several times over a 2–5 y period
Results:	Fairly linear fall in GFR in all patients (mean fall rate 1.2 ml min^{-1} month^{-1}) Rapid fall in GFR associated to high diastolic pressure (Wide range of pressures: 85–120 mmHg)
Perspective:	Will antihypertensive treatment *slow progression of nephropathy* and reduce proteinuria?

play a decisive role in the development of both incipient and overt diabetic nephropathy.

In a study of diabetic nephropathy (Table 6), performed some years ago on proteinuric patients, a fairly linear fall in GFR was established in most diabetic patients[42]. A rapid fall was associated with a higher diastolic pressure, the study being characterized by a rather wide pressure range, which may be important in comparison with somewhat different results obtained in other studies[43]. The perspective that emerged was of course: will antihypertensive treatment slow the progression of nephropathy and reduce proteinuria? An antihypertensive trial was started in a number of patients, and blood pressure could be reduced on conventional 'triple therapy', however, not quite normalized as indicated in Figure 14. After several weeks of treatment albumin

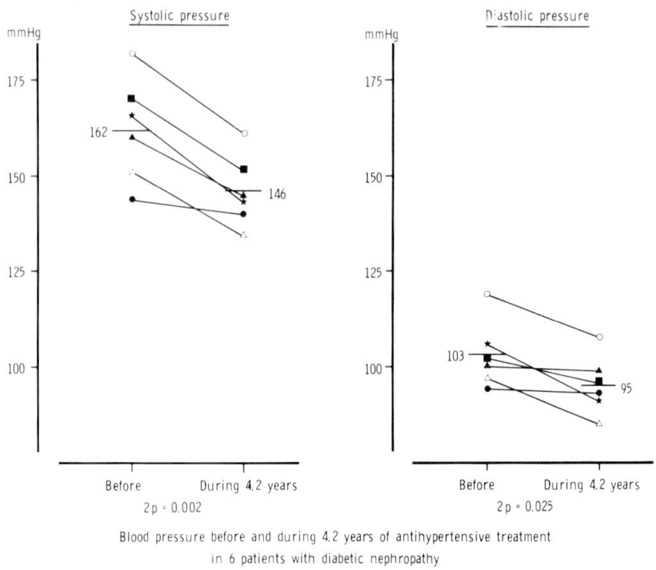

Figure 14 Blood pressure before and during longterm antihypertensive treatment in patients with diabetic nephropathy

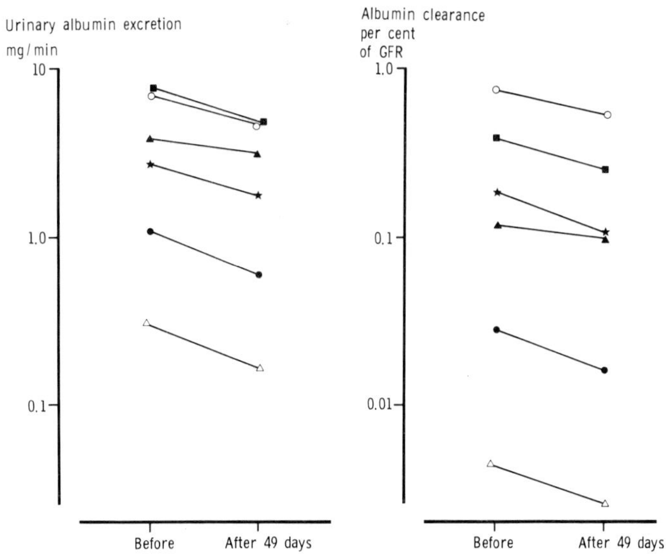

Figure 15 Urinary albumin excretion before and during short-term antihypertensive treatment in patients with diabetic nephropathy. To the left urinary albumin excretion rate. To the right albumin clearance as a per cent of GFR

excretion was significantly decreased (Figure 15). Figure 16a shows an example of the longterm effect on GFR and albumin clearance of treatment in an individual patient. The fall in GFR before and during treatment is characterized by linearity, and there is a marked alteration in the slope after antihypertensive treatment. Also, the increase in albumin clearance is virtually halted during treatment as shown in Figure 16b.

In all patients there was a significant reduction in the rate of decrease of GFR, and the increase in albumin clearance was arrested (Figure 17a,b). Thus antihypertensive treatment postpones uraemia by many years[10–12,41,88], as recently also shown by Parving[13,14]. However, it should be emphasized that nephropathy is not arrested, only postponed. Earlier intervention in incipient diabetic nephropathy may indeed prevent the decline in kidney function.

Longterm correction of hyperglycaemia in diabetic nephropathy does not seem to slow progression, although there was a tendency in this direction[89]. Antihypertensive treatment was started in a number of the patients during the study, after correction of hyperglycaemia.

MICROALBUMINURIA IN TYPE II DIABETES

The aim of this study was to define the predictive value of microalbuminuria in type II diabetes, both for clinical proteinuria and with respect to mortality[69]. In

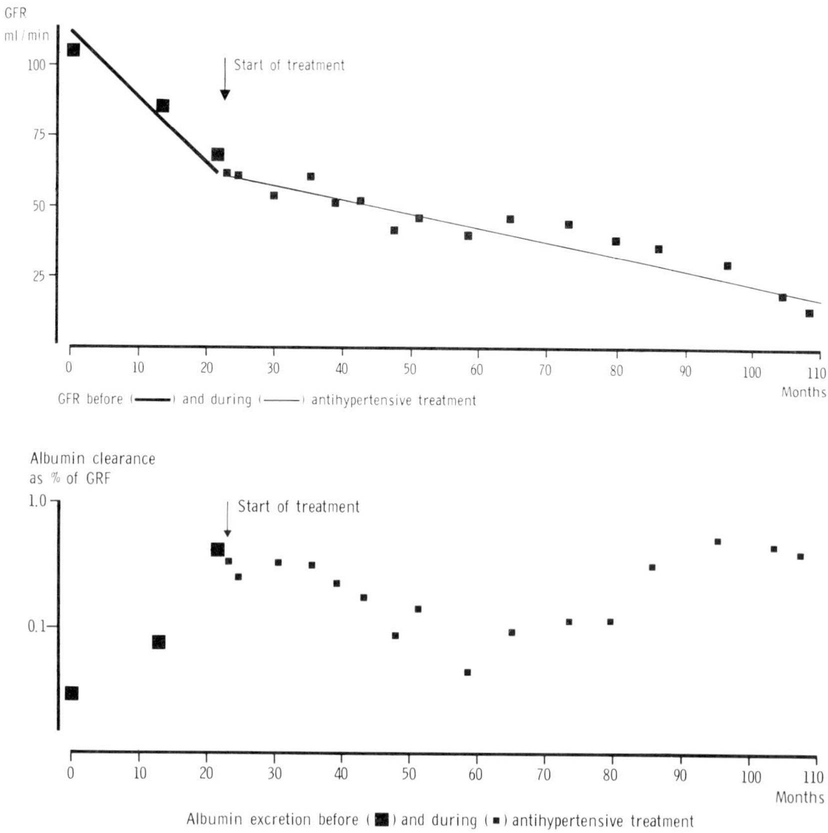

Figure 16a + b GFR and albumin clearance as a per cent of GFR before and during antihypertensive treatment in diabetic patients followed for 110 months

type II diabetes the situation is more complex than in type I diabetes. In these patients it is difficult to know whether the increase in albumin concentration is due to poor metabolic control or other factors. Some patients may be in the phase of incipient diabetic nephropathy. Albumin excretion may also be increased due to non-diabetic renal or systemic disease, such as cardiovascular disease, urinary tract infection and hypertension, often found in elderly patients.

During 1973 the albumin concentration was determined in all morning urines from patients attending our clinic.

Microalbuminuria was defined as the range between 30 and 140 μg/ml in accordance with the study by Viberti[85]. Two groups with lower concentrations, below 15 and 16–30 μg/ml, and one group with a higher concentration, more than 140 μg/ml, served as controls. Patients were aged 50–75 years, and all had their diabetes diagnosed after the age of 45.

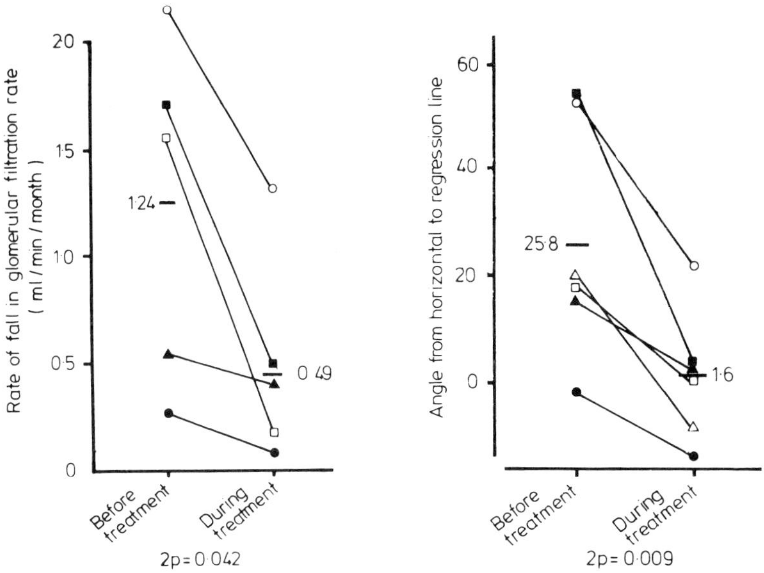

Figure 17a + b Rate of fall in glomerular filtration rate and progression in proteinuria before and during antihypertensive treatment in diabetic nephropathy. Progression of proteinuria expressed as angle from horizontal to regression line

Identical values for groups with respect to age, duration of diabetes, plasma glucose, blood pressure and weight were ensured.

Microalbuminuria was associated with a significant increase in the development of clinical proteinuria. A small proportion of patients with a low albumin concentration developed proteinuria in comparison with a rather large number of patients in the microalbuminuria range.

In all groups a significant increase in 10 year mortality was seen, compared to the Danish background population of the same age and sex. This increase was most pronounced in the microalbuminuria group, and it can be concluded that microalbuminuria predicts early mortality and proteinuria in maturity onset diabetes. Further work obviously needs to be done, and the underlying factors are now being investigated with the perspective of intervention.

STAGES IN DIABETIC NEPHROPATHY

Table 5 and Figure 18 summarize the changes in the kidney in insulin-dependent diabetes. Stage I is the early hyperfunction hypertrophy stage found at diagnosis. Increase in glomerular and kidney size are prominent findings. Microalbuminuria may be present, but is readily reversible by insulin

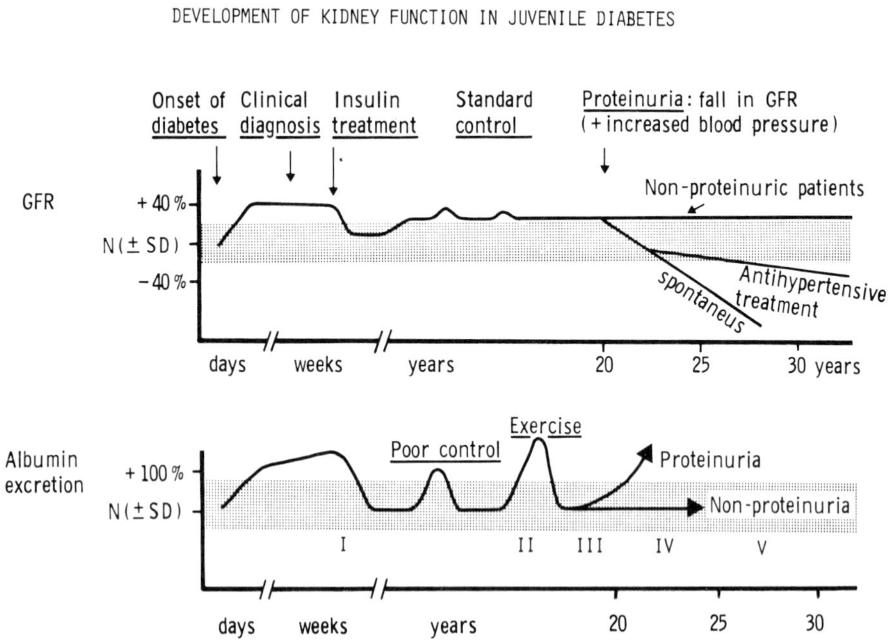

Figure 18 Development of kidney function in juvenile diabetes, indicated by the main parameters: GFR and albumin excretion, measured by radioimmunoassay

treatment. GFR is high in these patients; also this abnormality is reversible. Stage II is the renal-lesion-without-clinical-signs-stage. It is found after 2 years of diabetes, and a number of patients continue in this stage for many, many years. The glomerular basement membrane is thickened and the mesangial regions are expanded in volume. Microalbuminuria is present in poor metabolic control and at exercise. Most often, however, excretion rates are quite normal. GFR is significantly increased in this stage.

Stage III is the stage of incipient diabetic nephropathy, typically found after 10–15 years. Probably more advanced changes with respect to morphology are found, and microalbuminuria steadily increases. However, GFR is still high. Blood pressure starts to increase in this stage and is aggravated by physical exercise.

Stage IV is the well known stage with clinical nephropathy, found in 30–40% of patients after 15–20 years of diabetes. It is characterized by the classical morphological lesions, but the diagnosis is made on clinical findings. Microalbuminuria has developed into clinical proteinuria (>0.5 g/24 h), and GFR is declining. Fall rate in GFR can be reduced by effective antihypertensive treatment.

Stage V is end-stage renal failure, a stage found after many years of diabetes and characterized by glomerular closure and very low GFR. During the present decade diabetic nephropathy has become one of the most common, or even the most common renal disorder, responsible for end-stage renal failure in the Western world.

Effective treatment of this entity is now possible, following the general lines of treatment for end-stage renal failure, irrespective of its original cause, as outlined later in this volume.

References

1. Mogensen, C. E. (1972). Kidney function and glomerular permeability to macro molecules in juvenile diabetes. With special reference to early changes. *Dan. Med. Bull.,* **19,** (Suppl. 3), 1
2. Mogensen, C. E. (1976). Renal function changes in diabetes. *Diabetes,* **25,** 872
3. Mogensen, C. E. (1979). La microangiopathie glomérulaire functionelle. In *Journées Annuelles de Diabétologie de l'Hotel Dieu,* pp. 19–34. (Paris: Flammarion Médicine-Sciences)
4. Mogensen, C. E. (1981). Pathophysiology of diabetic complications. Abnormal physiological processes in kidney. In Brownlee, M. (ed.). *Handbook of Diabetes, Vol. 4: Biochemical Pathology,* pp. 23–85. (New York: London: Garland STPM Press)
5. Mogensen, C. E., Østerby, R. and Gundersen, H. J. G. (1979). Early function and morphological vascular renal consequences of the diabetic state. *Diabetologia,* **17,** 71
6. Viberti, G. C. (1979). Early functional and morphological changes in diabetic nephropathy. *Clin. Nephrol.,* **12,** 47
7. Deckert, T. and Poulsen, J. E. (1981). Diabetic nephropathy. Fault of destiny. *Diabetologia,* **21,** 178
8. McCrary, F. F., Pitts, T. O. and Puschett, J. B. (1981). Diabetic nephropathy. Natural course, survivorship, and therapy. *Am. J. Nephrol.,* **1,** 206
9. Friedman, E. A. (1982). Nephrology forum. Diabetic nephropathy. Strategies in prevention and management. *Kidney Int.,* **21,** 780
10. Mogensen, C. E. (1980). Preazotemic diabetic nephropathy. Inhibited by antihypertensive treatment. In Friedman, E. A. and L'Esperance, F. A. (eds.). *Diabetic Renal/Retinal Syndrome,* pp. 183–196. (New York: Grune and Stratton)
11. Mogensen, C. E. (1982). Long-term antihypertensive treatment inhibiting progression of diabetic nephropathy. *Br. Med. J.,* **285,** 685
12. Mogensen, C. E. (1983). Reduced progression of diabetic nephropathy by controlling hypertension. *Pract. Cardiol.,* **9,** 156
13. Parving, H.-H., Anderson, A. R., Smidt, U. M., Christiansen, J. S., Oxenbøll, B. and Svendsen, P. Aa. (1983). Diabetic nephropathy and arterial hypertension – the effect of antihypertensive treatment. *Diabetes,* **32,** (Suppl. 2), 83–87
14. Parving, H.-H., Andersen, A. R., Smidt, U. M. and Svendsen, P. Aa. (1983). Early and aggressive antihypertensive treatment reduces the rate of decline in kidney function in diabetic nephropathy. *Lancet,* **1,** 1175
15. Koivisto, V. A., Huttunen, N. P. and Vierikko, P. (1981). Continuous subcutaneous insulin infusion corrects exercise-induced albuminuria in juvenile diabetes. *Br. Med. J.,* **282,** 778
16. Lauritsen, T., Frost-Larsen, K., Svendsen, P. Aa., Larsen, H.-W., Deckert, T., Christiansen, J. S., Parving, H.-H., Binder, C., Nerup, J., Deckert, M., Larsen, A., Lorup, B., Bojsen, J. and Beck Jensen, L. (1982). Effect of six months of strict metabolic control on eye and kidney function in insulin-dependent diabetics with background retinopathy. *Lancet,* **i,** 121
17. Viberti, G. C., Pickup, J. C., Bilous, R. W., Keen, H. and MacKintosh, D. (1981). Correction of exercise-induced microalbuminuria in insulin-dependent diabetics after 3 weeks of subcutaneous insulin infusion. *Diabetes,* **30,** 818
18. Mogensen, C. E. (1982). Introduction. Diabetes mellitus and the kidney. *Kidney Int.,* **21,** 673
19. Friedman, E. A. (1982). Is diabetic microangiopathy preventable? A billion dollar question. *Diabetic Nephropathy,* **1,** 1
20. Drury, L. (1983). Diabetes and arterial hypertension. *Diabetologia,* **24,** 1

21. Mogensen, C. E. (1982). Hypertension in diabetics and the stages in diabetic nephropathy. *Diabetic Nephropathy,* **1,** 2
22. Mogensen, C. E., Christensen, C. K., Christensen, N. J., Gundersen, H. J. G., Jacobsen, F. K., Pedersen, E. B. and Vittinghus, E. (1981). Renal protein handling in normal, hypertensive, and diabetic man. *Contr. Nephrol.,* **24,** 139
23. Mogensen, C. E., Christensen, C. K. and Vittinghus, E. (1983). The stages in diabetic renal disease. With emphasis on the stage of incipient nephropathy. *Diabetes,* **32** (Suppl. 2), 64
24. Østerby, R. (1983). Basement membrane morphology in diabetes mellitus. In Ellenberg, M. and Rifkin, H. (eds.). *Diabetes Mellitus. Theory and Practice,* 3rd edn., pp. 323–341. (New York: Medical Examination Publishing Co.)
25. Keen, H. and Chlouverakis, C. (1963). An immunoassay method for urinary albumin at low concentrations. *Lancet,* **ii,** 913
26. Miles, D. W., Mogensen, C. E. and Gundersen, H. J. G. (1970). Radioimmunoassay for urinary albumin using a single antibody. *Scand. J. Clin. Lab. Invest.,* **26,** 5
27. Mogensen, C. E. Sølling, K. and Vittinghus, E. (1981). Studies on mechanisms of proteinuria using amino acid-induced inhibition of tubular reabsorption in normal and diabetic man. *Contr. Nephrol.,* **26,** 50
28. Viberti, G. C., and Vergani, D. (1982). Detection of potentially reversible diabetic albuminuria: a three-drop agglutination test for urinary albumin at low concentration. *Diabetes,* **31,** 973
29. Hermansson, G. and Ludvigsson, J. (1980). Renal function and blood-pressure reaction during exercise in diabetic and non-diabetic children and adolescents. *Acta Paediatr. Scand.,* (Suppl. 283), 86
30. Huttunen, N. P., Kaar, M. L., Puukka, R. and Akerblom, H. K. (1981). Exercise induced proteinuria in children and adolescents with type I (insulin dependent) diabetes. *Diabetologia,* **21,** 495
31. Mogensen, C. E., Christensen, C. K. and Vittinghus, E. (1982). Changes in renal function and blood pressure control in diabetes mellitus. With special reference to exercise-induced changes in albumin excretion and blood pressure. In Friedman, E. A. and L'Esperance, F. A. (eds.). *Second Diabetic Renal/Retinal Syndrome,* pp. 41–58. (New York: Grune and Stratton)
32. Mogensen,. C. E. and Vittinghus, E. (1975). Urinary albumin excretion during exercise in juvenile diabetes. A provocation test for early abnormalities. *Scand. J. Clin. Lab. Invest.,* **35,** 295
33. Poortmans, J., Dorchy, H. and Toussaint, D. (1982). Urinary excretion of total proteins, albumin, and 2-microglobulin during rest and exercise in diabetic adolescents with and without retinopathy. *Diabetes Care,* **5,** 617
34. Viberti, G. C., Jarrett, R. J., McCartney, M. and Keen, H. (1978). Increased glomerular permeability to albumin induced by exercise in diabetic subjects. *Diabetologia,* **14,** 293
35. Vittinghus, E. and Mogensen, C. E. (1981). Albumin excretion and renal haemodynamic response to physical exercise in normal and diabetic man. *Scand. J. Clin. Lab. Invest.,* **41,** 627
36. Vittinghus, E. and Mogensen, C. E. (1982). Graded exercise and protein excretion in diabetic man and the effect of insulin treatment. *Kidney Int.,* **21,** 725
37. Mogensen, C. E. (1968). The glomerular permeability determined by dextran clearance using sephadex gel filtration. *Scand. J. Clin. Lab. Invest.,* **21,** 77
38. Mogensen, C. E. (1968). Chromatographic evidence by sephadex gel filtration of the unrestricted glomerular filtration of inulin. *Scand. J. Clin. Lab. Invest.,* **22,** 203
39. Mogensen, C. E. (1971). Glomerular filtration rate and renal plasma flow in short-term and long-term juvenile diabetes. *Scand. J. Clin. Lab. Invest.,* **28,** 91
40. Mogensen, C. E. (1971). Maximum tubular reabsorption capacity for glucose and renal haemodynamics during rapid hypertonic glucose infusion in normal and diabetic man. *Scand. J. Clin. Lab. Invest.,* **28,** 101
41. Mogensen, C. E. (1976). High blood pressure as a factor in the progression of diabetic nephropathy. *Acta Med. Scand.,* (Suppl. 602), 29
42. Mogensen, C. E. (1976). Progression of nephropathy in long-term diabetics with proteinuria and effect of initial hypertensive treatment. *Scand. J. Clin. Lab. Invest.,* **36,** 383
43. Parving, H.-H., Smidt, U. M., Friisberg, B., Bonnevie-Nielsen, V. and Andersen, A. R. (1981). A prospective study of glomerular filtration rate and arterial blood pressure in

insulin dependent diabetics with diabetic nephropathy. *Diabetologia,* **20,** 457
44. Viberti, G. C., Bilous, R. W., MacKintosh, D. and Keen, H. (1983). Monitoring glomerular function in diabetic nephropathy. A prospective study. *Am. J. Med.,* **74,** 256
45. Jacobsen, F. K., Christensen, C. K., Mogensen, C. E., Andreasen, F. and Heilskov, N. S. C. (1979). Pronounced increase in serum creatinine concentration after eating cooked meat. *Br. Med. J.,* **1,** 1049
46. Viberti, G. C., Keen, H. and MacKintosh, D. (1981). Beta-2-microglobulinaemia: a sensitive index of diminishing renal function in diabetics. *Br. Med. J.,* **282,** 95
47. Andreasen, F., Christensen, C. K., Jacobsen, F. K., Jansen, J., Mogensen, C. E. and Lederballe-Pedersen, O. (1982). The individual variation in pharmacokinetics and pharmacodynamics of furosemide in young normal male subjects. *Eur. J. Clin. Invest.,* **22,** 247
48. Christensen, C. K. (1983). Rapidly reversible albumin and beta-2-microglobulin hyper-excretion in recent severe essential hypertension. *J. Hyperten.,* **1,** 45
49. Christensen, J. J., Gundersen, H. J. G., Mogensen, C. E. and Vittinghus, E. (1980). Intravenous insulin decreases urinary albumin excretion in long-term diabetics with nephropathy. *Diabetologia,* **18,** 285
50. Christiansen, J. S., Frandsen, M. and Parving, H.-H. (1981). The effect of intravenous insulin infusion on kidney function in insulin-dependent diabetes mellitus. *Diabetologia,* **20,** 199
51. Christiansen, J. S., Frandsen, M. and Parving, H.-H. (1981). Effect of intravenous glucose infusion on renal function in normal man and in insulin-dependent diabetics. *Diabetologia,* **21,** 368
52. Christiansen, J. S., Gammelgaard, J., Frandsen, M., Ørskov, H. and Parving, H.-H. (1982). Kidney function and size in insulin-dependent diabetics before and during growth hormone administration for one week. *Diabetologia,* **22,** 333
53. Christiansen, J. S., Gammelgaard, J., Tronier, B., Svendsen, P. Aa. and Parving, H.-H. (1982). Kidney function and size in diabetics, before and during initial insulin treatment. *Kidney Int.,* **21,** 683
54. Ciavarella, A., Flammini, M., Stefoni, S., Borgnino, L. C., Forlani, G., Bacci, L. and Vannini, P. (1982). Kidney function after improved metabolic control in newly diagnosed diabetes and in diabetic patients with nephropathy. *Diabetes Care,* **5,** 624
55. Mogensen, C. E. (1971). Glomerular filtration rate and renal plasma flow during elevation of blood sugar in normal and diabetic man. *Scand. J. Clin. Lab. Invest.,* **28,** 177
56. Mogensen, C. E., Christensen, C. K., Christensen, N. J., Gundersen, H. J. G. and Gjøde, P. (1980). Renal protein handling in man modified by insulin administration, stress situations and hypertension. *Int. J. Biochem.,* **12,** 181
57. Mogensen, C. E., Christensen, J. J. and Gundersen, H. J. G. (1980). The acute effect of insulin in heart rate, plasma noradrenaline and urinary albumin excretion: the role of changes in blood glucose. *Diabetologia,* **18,** 453
58. Mogensen, C. E., Christensen, J. J. and Gundersen, H. J. G. (1978). The acute effect of insulin on renal haemodynamics and protein excretion in diabetics. *Diabetologia,* **15,** 153
59. Mogensen, C. E. and Sølling, K. (1977). Studies on renal tubular protein reabsorption: Partial and near complete inhibition by certain amino acids. *Scand. J. Clin. Lab. Invest.,* **37,** 477
60. Mogensen, C. E., Vittinghus, E. and Sølling, K. (1975). Increased urinary albumin, light chain, and beta-2-microglobulin excretion after intravenous arginine administration in normal man. *Lancet,* **ii,** 581
61. Parving, H.-H., Noer, I., Deckert, T., Evrin, P. E., Nielsen, S. L., Lyngsø, J., Mogensen, C. E., Rørth, M., Svendsen, P. Aa., Trap-Jensen, J. and Lassen, N. A. (1976). The effect of metabolic regulation on microvascular permeability to small and large molecules in short-term diabetes. *Diabetologia,* **12,** 161
62. Parving, H.-H., Noer, I., Kehlet, H., Mogensen, C. E., Svendsen, P. Aa. and Helding, L. (1977). The effect of short-term glucogen infusion on kidney function in normal man. *Diabetologia,* **13,** 323
63. Parving, H.-H., Noer, I., Mogensen, C. E. and Svendsen, P. Aa. (1978). Kidney function in normal man during short-term growth hormone infusion. *Acta Endocrinol. (Copenh.),* **89,** 796
64. Viberti, G. C., Mogensen, C. E., Keen, H., Jacobsen, F. K., Jarrett, R. J. and Christensen,

C. K. (1982). Urinary excretion of albumin in normal man. The effect of water loading. *Scand. J. Clin. Lab. Invest.*, **42**, 147

65. Parving, H.-H., Jensen, H. Æ., Mogensen, C. E. and Evrin, P. E. (1974). Increased urinary albumin excretion rate in benign essential hypertension. *Lancet*, **i**, 1190
66. Pedersen, E. B. and Mogensen, C. E. (1976). Effect of antihypertension treatment on urinary albumin excretion, glomerular filtration rate and renal plasma flow in patients with essential hypertension. *Scand. J. Clin. Lab. Invest.*, **36**, 231
67. Pedersen, E. B., Mogensen, C. E. and Larsen, J. S. (1981). Effects of exercise on urinary excretion of albumin and beta-2-microglobulin in young patients with mild essential hypertension without treatment and during long-term propranolol treatment. *Scand. J. Clin. Lab. Invest.*, **41**, 493
68. Damsgaard, E. M., Nielsen, J. R. and Mogensen, C. E. (1983). Increased glomerular permeability to albumin in Type II diabetics before and after exercise. *Diabetologia* (abstract), (In press)
69. Mogensen, C. E. (1983). Microalbuminuria in maturity onset, primarily type II diabetes, predicts clinical proteinuria and early mortality. *Diabetologia* (abstract) (In press)
70. Mogensen, C. E. (1971). Urinary albumin excretion in early and long-term juvenile diabetes. *Scand. J. Clin. Lab. Invest.*, **28**, 183
71. Viberti, G. C., MacKintosh, D., Bilous, R. W., Pickup, J. C. and Keen, H. (1982). Proteinuria in diabetes mellitus: role of spontaneous and experimental variation of glycaemia. *Kidney Int.*, **21**, 714
72. Viberti, G. C., Pickup, J. C., Jarrett, R. J. and Keen, H. (1979). Effect of control of blood glucose on urinary excretion of albumin and beta-2-microglobulin in insulin-dependent diabetes. *N. Engl. J. Med.*, **300**, 638
73. Mogensen, C. E. (1971). Urinary albumin excretion in diabetes. (Letter to the Editor). *Lancet, ii,* 601
74. Mogensen, C. E. (1973). Urinary albumin excretion and dextran clearance in the development of diabetic glomerulosclerosis. In Peeters, H. (ed.). *Protides of the Biological Fluids, 21st Colloquium,* pp. 463–466. (Oxford, New York: Pergamon Press)
75. Mogensen, C. E. (1971). Kidney function and glomerular permeability in early juvenile diabetes. *Scand. J. Clin. Lab. Invest.*, **28**, 79
76. Mogensen, C. E. (1981). Renal plasma flow in juvenile diabetes. *Acta. Endocrinol. (Copenh.)*, **94** (Suppl. 242), 33
77. Christiansen, J. S., Gammelgaard, J., Frandsen, M. and Parving, H.-H. (1981). Increased kidney size, glomerular filtration rate and renal plasma flow in short-term insulin-dependent diabetics. *Diabetologia*, **20**, 451
78. Mogensen, C. E., Andersen, M. J. F. (1973). Increased kidney size and glomerular filtration rate in early juvenile diabetes. *Diabetes*, **22**, 706
79. Mogensen, C. E. and Andersen, M. J. F. (1975). Increased kidney size and glomerular filtration rate in untreated juvenile diabetics. Normalization by insulin treatment. *Diabetologia*, **11**, 221
80. Brøchner-Mortensen, J., Ditzel, J., Mogensen, C. E. and Rødbro, P. (1979). Microvascular permeability to albumin and glomerular filtration rate in diabetic and normal children. *Diabetologia*, **16**, 307
81. Mogensen, C. E. (1972). Glomerular filtration rate and renal plasma flow in long-term juvenile diabetics without proteinuria. *Br. Med. J.*, **4**, 257
82. Mogensen, C. E. (1973). Elevated glomerular filtration rate in insulin treated short-term diabetes. Non-dependence of the actual blood sugar level. *Acta. Med. Scand.*, **194**, 559
83. Christensen, C. K. (1983). Early or incipient diabetic nephropathy and effect of antihypertensive treatment. *Diabetologia* (abstract), (In press)
84. Parving, H.-H., Oxenbøll, B., Svendsen, P. A., Christiansen, J. S. and Andersen, A. R. (1982). Early detection of patients at risk of developing diabetic nephropathy. A prospective study of urinary albumin excretion. *Acta Endocrinol. (Copenh.)*, **100**, 550
85. Viberti, G. C., Hill, R. D., Jarrett, R. J., Argyropoulos, A., Mahmud, Y. and Keen, H. (1982). Microalbuminuria as a predictor of clinical nephropathy in insulin-dependent diabetes mellitus. *Lancet*, **i**, 1430
86. Parving, H.-H., Andersen, A. R., Smidt, U. M., Friisberg, B. and Svendsen, P. Aa. (1981). Reduced albuminuria during early and aggressive antihypertensive treatment of insulin-dependent diabetic patients with diabetic nephropathy. *Diabetes Care*, **4**, 459

87. Brenner, B. M. (1983). Hemodynamically mediated glomerular injury and the progressive nature of kidney disease. *Kidney Int.,* **23,** 647
88. Mogensen, C. E. (1979). Diabetes and hypertension. (Letter to the Editor). *Lancet,* **,i,** 388
89. Viberti, G. C., Bilous, R. W., MacKintosh, D., Bending, J. J. and Keen, H. (1983). Long term correction of hyperglycaemia and progression of renal failure in insulin dependent diabetes. *Br. Med. J.,* **286,** 598
90. Mogensen, C. E., Vittinghus, E., Gundersen, H. J. G. and Christensen, N. J. (1981). Diabetes and urinary albumin excretion as measured by radioimmunoassay. *Pediat. Adolesc. Endocr.,* **9,** 318
91. Deckert, T., Parving, H.-H., Andersen, A. R., Christiansen, J. S., Oxenbøll, B., Svendsen, P. Aa., Telmer, S., Christy, M., Laurtizen, T., Thomsen, O. F., Kreiner, S., Andersen, J. R., Binder, C. and Nerup, J. (1982). Diabetic nephropathy. A clinical and morphometric study. In Eschwege, E. (ed.). *Advances in Diabetes Epidemiology. INSERM Symposium No. 22,* pp. 235–243. (Amsterdam, Oxford: Excerpta Medica)
92. Mauer, S. M., Steffes, M. W., Sutherland, D. E. R., Brown, D. M. and Goetz, F. C. (1983). Structural–functional relationships in diabetic nephropathy. *J. Clin. Invest.,* (In press)

5
The impact of haemodynamic factors on the development and progression of diabetic nephropathy

H.-H. PARVING

Hyperfiltration and elevated urinary albumin excretion are present in newly diagnosed and short term insulin-dependent diabetics, particularly during poor metabolic control. Strict metabolic control induces near normalization in both variables. Elevated glomerular plasma flow and increased transglomerular hydraulic pressure gradient are suggested as the major determinants of hyperfiltration and microalbuminuria.

Clinical observations and investigations in diabetic man and animals support the haemodynamic concept advocated by several investigators, suggesting that intrarenal hypertension is an important factor in the development and progression of diabetic nephropathy. The beneficial effect of antihypertensive treatment on the progression of kidney function in diabetic nephropathy supports this concept. Glomerular filtration rate (GFR) is abnormally high in newly diagnosed and short term insulin-dependent diabetics (IDDM), particularly during poor metabolic control[1-3]. Improved metabolic control induces a reduction, but not a normalization of GFR[1-3]. Recent investigations have suggested that hyperglycaemia[4], hyperglucagonaemia[5] and growth hormone elevation[6] contribute to the rapid reversible part of the GFR elevation in IDDM. The enlargement of the kidney and of the glomerular filtration surface area[7-10] have been suggested as major factors of the slowly reversible part of the GFR elevation in IDDM.

Glomerular filtration rate is determined by four factors: renal plasma flow (RPF) transglomerular pressure gradient ($\overline{\Delta P}$), oncotic pressure and the ultrafiltration coefficient (*Kj*)[11]. A reversible increase in RPF and filtration fraction (by inference $\overline{\Delta P}$) has been demonstrated in IDDM[1,3]. Plasma albumin concentration (oncotic pressure) is normal in short-term IDDM[12].

Recent studies of glomerular haemodynamics in insulin treated streptozotocin diabetic rats strongly supports the view that the enhanced GFR of IDDM patients is due to elevated RPF and $\bar{\Delta}P$[13,14]. The contribution from *Kj* remains uncertain.

Increased transglomerular passage of plasma proteins and dextrans is demonstrable at the time of diagnosis of IDDM, before measurable thickening of the glomerular basement membrane has occurred[1,15]. Near-normalization of blood glucose for a few days induces a reduction in both resting and exercise-provoked urinary albumin excretion[1,2,16]. Alterations in the size or charge-selective properties of the glomerular membrane cannot account for increased transglomerular passage of macromolecules[1,2]. The demonstrated increase in transglomerular pressure appears to be the most likely explanation.

Intrarenal hypertension markedly accelerates the development of diabetic glomerulopathy in man and animals[17-19]. Elevated arterial blood pressure is frequently present in young IDDM patients with diabetic nephropathy and normal serum creatinine[20]. Early aggressive antihypertensive treatment reduces albuminuria and the rate of decline in glomerular filtration rate in young patients with diabetic nephropathy[21-23]. The simplest explanation of these findings may, therefore, be the correct one: a reduction of glomerular capillary pressure induced by the antihypertensive treatment. Arterial blood pressure may thus stand in complex relationship with diabetic nephropathy, both being raised by it and also accelerating its course.

The above mentioned findings suggest intrarenal hypertension as a possible link between early and late diabetic nephropathy.

ACKNOWLEDGEMENTS

This study was supported by grants from the Danish Medical Research Council and the Danish Diabetes Association.

References

1. Mogensen, C. E. (1972). Kidney function and glomerular permeability to macromolecules in juvenile diabetes. *Dan. Med. Bull.,* **19** (Suppl. 3), 1
2. Parving, H.-H. (1976). Increased microvascular permeability to plasma proteins in short- and long-term juvenile diabetics. *Diabetes,* **25** (Suppl. 2), 884
3. Christiansen, J. S., Gammelgaard, J., Tronier, B., Svendsen, P. Aa. and Parving, H.-H. (1982). Kidney function and size in diabetics, before and during initial insulin treatment. *Kidney Int.,* **21**, 683
4. Christiansen, J. S., Frandsen, M. and Parving, H.-H. (1981). Effect of intravenous glucose infusion on renal function in normal man and in insulin-dependent diabetics. *Diabetologia,* **21**, 368
5. Parving, H.-H., Christiansen, J. S., Noer, I., Tronier, B. and Mogensen, C. E. (1980). The effect of glucagon infusion on kidney function in short-term insulin-dependent juvenile diabetics. *Diabetologia,* **19**, 350
6. Christiansen, J. S., Gammelgaard, J., Frandsen, M., Ørskov, H. and Parving, H.-H. (1982). Kidney function and size in Type I (insulin-dependent) diabetic patients before and during growth hormone administration for one week. *Diabetologia,* **22**, 333

7. Mogensen, C. E. and Andersen, M. J. E. (1973). Increased kidney size and glomerular filtration rate in early juvenile diabetes. *Diabetes,* **22,** 706
8. Christiansen, J. S., Gammelgaard, J., Frandsen, M. and Parving, H.-H. (1981). Increased kidney size, glomerular filtration rate and renal plasma flow in short-term insulin-dependent diabetics. *Diabetologia,* **20,** 451
9. Kroustrup, J. P., Gundersen, H. J. G. and Østerby, R. (1977). Glomerular size and structure in diabetes mellitus. III. Early enlargement of the capillary surface. *Diabetologia,* **13,** 207
10. Hirose, K., Tsuchida, H., Østerby, R. and Gundersen, H. J. G. (1980). A strong correlation between glomerular filtration rate and filtration surface in diabetic kidney hyperfunction. *J. Lab. Invest.,* **43,** 434
11. Brenner, B. M. and Humes, H. O. (1977). Mechanisms of glomerular ultrafiltration. *N. Engl. J. Med.,* **297,** 148
12. Parving, H.-H. and Rasmussen, S. M. (1973). Transcapillary escape rate of albumin and plasma volume in short- and long-term juvenile diabetics. *Scand. J. Clin. Lab. Invest.,* **32,** 81
13. Hostetter, T. H., Troy, J. L. and Brenner, B. M. (1981). Glomerular hemodynamics in experimental diabetes. *Kidney Int.,* **19,** 410
14. Jensen, P. K., Christiansen, J. S., Steven, K. and Parving, H.-H. (1981). Renal function in diabetic rats. *Diabetologia,* **21,** 409
15. Parving, H.-H., Rutili, F., Granath, K., Noer, J., Deckert, T., Lyngsøe, J. and Lassen, N. A. (1979). Effect of metabolic regulation on renal leakiness to dextran molecules in short-term insulin-dependent diabetics. *Diabetologia,* **17,** 157
16. Viberti, G. C., Pickup, J. C., Bilous, R. W. and Keen, H. (1981). Correction of exercise-induced microalbuminuria in insulin-dependent diabetics after 3 weeks of subcutaneous insulin infusion. *Diabetes,* **30,** 818
17. Berkman, J. and Rifkin, H. (1973). Unilateral diabetic glomerulosclerosis (Kimmelstiel–Wilson). Report of a case. *Metab. Clin. Exp.,* **22,** 715
18. Steffes, M. W., Brown, D. M., Mauer, S. M. (1978). Diabetic glomerulopathy following unilateral nephrectomy in the rat. *Diabetes,* **27,** 35
19. Mauer, S. M., Steffes, M. W., Azar, S., Sandberg, S. K. and Brown, D. M. (1978). The effect of Goldblatt hypertension on development of the glomerular lesions of diabetes mellitus in the rat. *Diabetes,* **27,** 738
20. Parving, H.-H., Andersen, A. R., Smidt, U. M., Oxenbøll, B., Edsberg, B. and Christiansen, J. S. (1983). Diabetic nephropathy and arterial hypertension. *Diabetologia,* **24,** 10
21. Mogensen, C. E. (1982). Long-term antihypertensive treatment inhibiting progression of diabetic nephropathy. *Br. Med. J.,* **285,** 685
22. Parving, H.-H., Andersen, A. R., Smidt, U. M., Christiansen, J. S., Oxenbøll, B. and Svendsen, P. Aa. (1983). Diabetic nephropathy and arterial hypertension – the effect of anti-hypertensive treatment. *Diabetes,* **32** (Suppl. 2), 83
23. Parving, H.-H., Andersen, A. R., Smidt, U. M. and Svendsen, P. Aa. (1983). Early aggressive antihypertensive treatment reduces the rate of decline in kidney function in diabetic nephropathy. *Lancet,* **i,** 1175

Discussant

J. JERVELL

Dr Jervell (Norway): Being a clinician, and not having done research myself in this clinically very important field I should like to raise three questions.

First, it is often said that only about 30%, or perhaps in New York 50%, type I diabetics get proteinuria and terminal renal failure. If this is so, it is very important to discover what these protective factors are. I should like to suggest that the statement is untrue, and I shall present some old clinical material.

First, a study from Sweden. Dr Jonsson compared people who got diabetes during the first years after the discovery of insulin, when only multiple daily dose soluble insulin was available and dietary treatment was still considered important with those treated with the long-acting insulin preparations and free diet which came along later. He looked at these patients in the late 1950s and found that those who got diabetes in the early phase, just after the discovery of insulin, fared much better in terms of retinopathy and proteinuria than those who got it in the period of free diet and long-acting insulins once daily.

Fourni in Switzerland followed a small group of children whom he put on a peculiar protein-poor diet. After 16 years all these children had proteinuria and after 22 years all were dead, although perhaps not from nephropathy.

There is another question that I should like to raise. When does the renal process of diabetes become irreversible? When is the point of no return? It is somewhere between the phase of micro- and of macroproteinuria. Clinicians need measures that can tell us when we are approaching this point of no return, so that we can intensify our care of these patients. When they pass the point of no return, then perhaps antihypertensive treatment is what is most important, preparing for the phase of terminal failure, and maintaining optimum fitness for dialysis or transplantation.

The third question, the $64 000 question at the moment, is, What degree of glycaemic or metabolic control is necessary to prevent microangiopathy and clinical diabetic nephropathy? Is it complete normalization, perhaps to be achieved possibly in only a very few, or the near normalization with insulin pumps or multiple injections? My suggestion is that for the majority of diabetics the optimal conventional treatment using haemoglobin A1 and home glucose monitoring as aids in getting good metabolic control is necessary.

I have spoken to more than a hundred diabetic transplant patients, and as a group they had been given very poor health care. Most of them had no regular diabetic clinic; indeed, no regular doctor. They have had no dietary instruction, and practically all of them, for long periods of their lives, have been on one injection of long-acting insulin.

Professor Ritz: Dr Jervell has posed questions which tear people out of their intellectual complacency and, like Socrates needling the Athenians, he has put questions to the audience which probably at this point in time no one can answer.

6
Determinants of renal failure in the diabetic patient

G. C. VIBERTI

INTRODUCTION

Great improvement has been achieved over the last few years in the rate of success of renal transplantation and of both haemo- and peritoneal dialysis treatment for the uraemic diabetic[1], however these therapies are costly, still often fail and in a proportion of cases are unable to provide an enjoyable quality of life for the patient. These considerations have prompted a number of studies, particularly in insulin-dependent diabetics, directed at examining whether end-stage renal failure in the diabetic can be delayed, arrested or even prevented.

STUDIES IN OVERT CLINICAL DIABETIC NEPHROPATHY

Classically, the clinical diagnosis of diabetic nephropathy is made when a persistently positive Albustix (i.e. total urinary protein excretion >0.5 g/24 h) develops in an insulin-dependent diabetic with retinopathy, more than 10 years duration of diabetes, absence of cardiac failure, severe hypertension, urinary tract infection and of a history of non-diabetic renal disease[2]. The importance of such definition is highlighted by the epidemiological studies of Deckert *et al*[3], who showed that the percent survival of insulin-dependent diabetics with persistent proteinuria is markedly reduced compared with that of a control population of both non-diabetics or diabetics without proteinuria. The glomerular filtration rate (GFR), that can be normal or even high at diagnosis of Albustix positive proteinuria, begins its relentless decline[4–6]. The rate of decline varies from patient to patient with a mean of about 1 ml min^{-1} $month^{-1}$ but is strikingly linear in each individual. The proteinuria becomes heavier as the

GFR falls, and there is a highly significant inverse correlation between the clearance of both albumin and IgG and the GFR[7]. Interestingly, the clearance of IgG increases proportionally more than that of albumin for GFRs below 20 ml/min/1.73 m^2. There is, therefore, a change from a high selectivity proteinuria, where predominantly albumin is filtered, at GFRs above 80 ml/min/1.73 m^2, to a low selectivity proteinuria at markedly reduced GFRs, the selectivity index (clearance of IgG/clearance of albumin) rising from 0.133 to 0.620[8]. This change in the restrictive properties of the glomerular membrane has been investigated by Myers *et al*[9,10] using fractional clearance of neutral dextran with a wide range of Einstein–Stokes radii. These authors showed that the clearance of dextran with Stokes radii ranging from 5 to 6.4 nm is facilitated in advanced nephropathy, whereas no differences were seen between normals and patients with 'minimal nephropathy' (i.e. intermittent or persistent light proteinuria). They interpreted these findings as evidence for the existence of a discrete second population of large pores. This bimodal distribution of pores could readily explain the loss of selectivity with relatively more IgG, a virtually neutral molecule of Stokes radius of 5.5 nm, being filtered. The clearance of neutral dextran only explores the size selective properties (pore size/number) of the glomerular membrane and interestingly, the clearance of dextran with Stokes radius of 3.6 nm, the same as albumin, is not different in diabetics with significant albuminuria and in non-diabetic, non-proteinuric controls. As the filtration of albumin, a polyanion, is regulated not only by pore size/number but also by the electrical properties of the glomerular filter[11], these findings clearly suggest that the albuminuria of diabetic nephropathy is likely to be due to a loss of the charge selective properties of the glomerular membrane. Thus, the proteinuria of established diabetic nephropathy could be explained, at least in part, by a loss of the restrictive properties (charge and size) of the glomerular barrier to filtration of plasma proteins. Haemodynamic factors are also likely to play an important role as glomerular hyperfusion, hyperfiltration, and intraglomerular hypertension are likely to develop in the surviving glomeruli in an attempt to compensate for the loss of sclerosed nephrons[12]. The fractional clearances (clearance protein/GFR) of albumin and IgG increase as the GFR declines[6] indicating a massive glomerular filtration of these proteins per functioning nephron. That the proteinuria of established nephropathy is glomerular in origin is derived, firstly, from the fact that the tubular reabsorptive capacity is likely to be completely saturated under conditions of heavy proteinuria[13] and therefore urinary excretion of a protein is a reflection of its glomerular filtration, and, secondly, from the finding that the excretion rate of low molecular weight proteins, charactistically increased in tubular dysfunction, is normal until the GFR falls below 40 ml/min/1.73 m^2[7,14]. The increased urinary excretion rates of β_2-microglobulin and lysozyme with marked reduction of GFR may however be interpreted in different ways. The plasma concentration of these proteins increases as the GFR falls[6], and it is possible that an increased urinary excretion rate be the result, not of tubular damage, but of protein overload per surviving nephron with saturation of tubular reabsorptive capacity and overspill of the protein into the urine. As the GFR starts its decline the blood pressure (BP) begins to rise[5]. This seems to occur early in the course of nephropathy and not be simply the result of end-stage renal failure.

The effect of correction of hyperglycaemia and raised blood pressure

The search for a relation between metabolic control on the one hand and GFR, rate of GFR decline and excretion rates or clearances of plasma proteins on the other has produced negative results[6,7]. Moreover, correction of hyperglycaemia for up to 2 years in six insulin-dependent diabetics with nephropathy has not been able to either arrest the decline of the GFR (Figure 1) or to change significantly the rate of increase of plasma protein filtration[15]. The

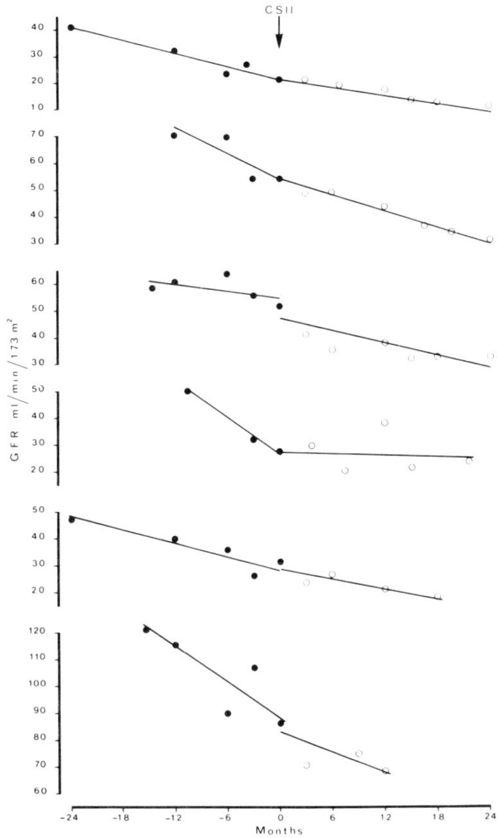

Figure 1 Individual glomerular filtration rates before (●) and after (○) continuous subcutaneous insulin infusion (CSII) induced near-normoglycaemia in six insulin-dependent diabetics with clinical diabetic nephropathy. (Reproduced with permission from Viberti, G.C. *et al.* (1983). *Br. Med. J.*, **286**, 598)

interrelationship between blood pressure and deterioration of renal function seems closer at this stage. A correlation between diastolic blood pressure and rate of decline of GFR has been described by Mogensen[4], even though this has not been confirmed by others[5,6]. Vigorous treatment of raised blood pressure seems capable of checking the progressive increase in the clearance of albumin and of slowing the rate of decline of GFR in some patients[16]. However, no arrest in the progression of nephropathy has ever been demonstrated. It would thus appear that in established diabetic nephropathy the process leading to end-stage renal failure is independent of the metabolic disturbance of diabetes, but that its rate of progression is, to a certain extent, affected by the BP. This would support the view that haemodynamic factors have become predominant in late nephropathy as determinants of progression of damage[12]. There is evidence that the adaptive response to loss of nephrons with the development of glomerular hyperperfusion, hyperfiltration and intraglomerular hypertension becomes a self-destructive process eventually leading to the occlusion of more glomeruli with further reduction of the GFR and kidney size[12]. This downward spiral, once begun, cannot be arrested, let alone reversed, and only the strict control of BP holds out hopes of delaying the time to achievement of end-stage renal failure.

This therapeutic impotence in established diabetic nephropathy calls for earlier intervention, and indeed the natural history of renal involvement in diabetes seems to start well before the appearance of Albustix positive proteinuria.

STUDIES OF RENAL FUNCTION IN INSULIN-DEPENDENT DIABETICS WITHOUT CLINICAL NEPHROPATHY

Renal abnormalities are in fact evident at diagnosis of diabetes. Glomerular filtration rate and renal plasma flow (RPF) may be elevated, the increase of GFR outweighing that of RPF and almost invariably resulting in elevation of the filtration fraction[17]. The kidney size may also be increased in diabetes[17]. These changes in the untreated diabetic are promptly reduced and in many cases normalized by the initial insulin treatment[17]. However, approximately 20–30% of insulin-dependent diabetics maintain a GFR above the normal range and large kidneys for several years during ordinary insulin injection treatment[18].

A disturbance in the urinary excretion of large molecular weight plasma proteins has also been found early in diabetes. The use of sensitive radioimmunoassays for albumin in urine has demonstrated elevated levels (though still well below the detection limits of the Albustix test) for urinary albumin excretion in newly diagnosed diabetics[17]. The institution of insulin treatment promptly reverses this microalbuminuria of untreated diabetes. However, during conventional insulin injection treatment a proportion of 30–45% of

Albustix negative insulin-dependent diabetics maintain an excretion rate of albumin and IgG above the normal range[7,19]. In these same patients the urinary excretion rate of β_2-microglobulin, a sensitive indicator of tubular reabsorptive capacity, is normal. This and other experimental and theoretical considerations[20] suggest that the microalbuminuria and IgGuria are glomerular in origin and reflect an increased transglomerular flux of these proteins. Under conditions of average glycaemic control patients with normal resting albumin excretion rate also show an excessive albuminuric response to physical exercise in comparison with matched non-diabetic controls[21]. This excessive exercise-induced albuminuria is also likely to be of glomerular origin because of concomitantly normal β_2-microglobulin excretion rates, and it is probably mediated by an abnormally high intraglomerular pressure in response to exercise. The absolute values in filtration fraction obtained during exercise appear to be considerably higher in diabetics than in normals[22]. The significance of these physiological changes in responses to moderately strenuous physical activity is at present unknown. The microalbuminuria and IgGuria under resting conditions are also likely to be mediated, at least in part, by increases in transglomerular pressure gradient. A cross-sectional study of insulin-dependent diabetics with different degrees of microalbuminuria has recently shown that the selectivity index (SI = clearance of IgG/clearance of albumin) of patients with albumin excretion up to 30 μg/min is unchanged compared with that of non-diabetic controls with albumin excretion rates between 1 and 12 μg/min[8]. This indicates that the charge and size selectivity properties of the glomerular barrier that restrict the filtration of albumin, a polyanion of 3.6 nm, and IgG, a neutral molecule of 5.5 nm, are intact and that the raised transglomerular flux can only be due to an elevated transglomerular pressure gradient driving these two proteins in unchanged proportions through the glomerular filter. Micropuncture studies in the moderately hyperglycaemic diabetic rat have confirmed significant elevation in the transglomerular pressure gradient[23]. As the microalbuminuria increases toward levels of detectability by Albustix, the SI falls. This is due to a preferential increase in the filtration of albumin, while the filtration of IgG remains virtually unmodified[8]. This strongly suggests a change in the charge selectivity properties of the glomerular membrane with loss of the fixed negative charge that normally restricts the filtration of albumin. Loss of membrane polyanions would have little effect on the filtration of IgG that is controlled by the size selectivity properties of the membrane (i.e. pore size/number) and by the intraglomerular pressure.

We have reached here the transitional phase to Albustix positive proteinuria with the institution of a high selectivity proteinuria.

The effect of correction of hyperglycaemia

Many studies have succeeded in relating these early phenomena to the metabolic control. A good relationship has been shown between urinary excretion of albumin and IgG on the one hand and glycosylated haemoglobin on the other, and the elevation of both these proteins during the average control of conventional insulin treatment is promptly corrected, at least in the short term, by radical metabolic improvement[7,19]. The raised GFR of the established, averagely controlled insulin-treated diabetic, is also near-normalized by several months of optimal glycaemic control with continuous subcutaneous insulin infusion.

The significance of these early changes is that of a metabolically dependent set of abnormalities which appears, within certain limits, to be reversible.

Thus, we are confronted here with two sets of observations: one, the late changes, beyond reasonable recovery and the other, the early changes, well responsive to metabolic correction. The heart of the problem is to establish whether we are dealing with two different entities or with two phases of the same process.

STUDIES ON THE TRANSITION BETWEEN EARLY AND LATE RENAL CHANGES IN DIABETES

For many years doubts have been raised as to whether a connection between early and late phenomena exists at all.

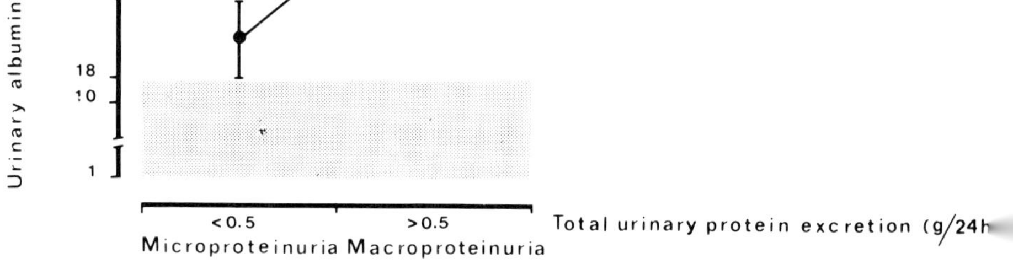

Figure 2 Diagrammatic representation of the relationship between microproteinuria and persistent Albustix positive proteinuria (macroproteinuria). Approximately 80% of Albustix test negative diabetics with urinary albumin excretion rate (AER) from 50 to 200 mg/24 h but only 4% with AER from 18 to 50 mg/24 h or less will become Albustix positive within 6–14 years. Stippled area represents the range (mean ± 2 SD) of AER in non-diabetics. AERs in the range predictive of persistent macroproteinuria are potentially reversible by strict glycaemic control. (Adapted from Viberti, G. C. *et al.* (1982). *Lancet*, **i**, 1430 and Parving, H.-H. *et al.* (1982). *Acta Endocrinol.*, **100**, 550)

Recent longterm prospective studies[24,25] have been able to connect these two phases and have demonstrated that diabetic patients with urinary albumin excretion from 50 to 200 mg/24 h have approximately a 20-fold higher risk of developing Albustix positive proteinuria (Figure 2). Thus certain degrees of microalbuminuria (Albustix test negative) appear strongly predictive of later persistent Albustix positive proteinuria, a reliable precursor of renal failure. The available evidence does not fully illuminate the factors responsible for the microalbuminuria nor the time course of the passage from one stage to the other. Preliminary data, however, indicate that the time taken to develop Albustix positive proteinuria differs from patient to patient and blood glucose and blood pressure levels may combine to influence the rate of this passage. Patients in the upper microproteinuric range show higher BP values and poorer glycaemic control[26]. The findings of these longitudinal studies strongly suggest that the early and the late proteinuric changes are not distinct entities, but are two phases of the same process culminating in end-stage renal failure. One could also speculate that the diabetics with high GFR and large kidneys suffer from what has been termed a hyperperfusion and hyperfiltration syndrome[12]. The high filtration fraction found in these patients could reflect intraglomerular hypertension. These haemodynamic changes combined with increased glomerular filtration of plasma proteins could produce mesangial expansion and glomerulosclerosis and lead, over several years, to the establishment of clinical diabetic nephropathy.

Detection of markers such as microalbuminuria of a certain degree (i.e. in excess of 50 mg/24 h) would identify a group of patients at high risk of renal failure. As these early predictive indicators may be corrected by careful control of glycaemia and arterial pressure, the stage appears to be set for an attempt at the prevention of diabetic nephropathy.

ACKNOWLEDGEMENTS

I wish to thank all those who made these studies possible, and in particular Professor H. Keen for his help and encouragement.

References

1. Goetz, F.C. and Kjellstrand, C.M. (1979). The treatment of diabetic kidney disease. *Diabetologia,* **17,** 267
2. Ireland, J.T., Viberti, G.C. and Watkins, P.J. (1982). The kidney and the urinary tract. In Keen, H. and Jarrett, J. (eds.). *Complications of Diabetes.* pp. 137–178. (London: Edward Arnold)
3. Deckert, T., Poulsen, J.F. and Larsen, M. (1978). Prognosis of diabetics with diabetes onset before the age of thirty-one. *Diabetologia,* **14,** 363
4. Mogensen, C.E. (1976). Progression of nephropathy in long-term diabetics with proteinuria and effect of initial anti-hypertensive treatment. *Scan. J. Clin. Lab. Invest.,* **36,** 383
5. Parving, H.-H., Smidt, U.M., Friisberg, B., Bonnevie-Nielsen, V. and Anderson, A.R.

(1981). A prospective study of glomerular filtration rate and arterial blood pressure in insulin-dependent diabetics with diabetic nephropathy. *Diabetologia,* **20,** 457
6. Viberti, G. C., Bilous, R. W., Mackintosh, D. and Keen, H. (1983). Monitoring glomerular function in diabetic nephropathy. A prospective study. *Am. J. Med.,* **74,** 256
7. Viberti, G. C., Mackintosh, D., Bilous, R. W., Pickup, J. C. and Keen, H. (1982). Proteinuria in diabetes mellitus: Role of spontaneous and experimental variation of glycaemia. *Kidney Int.,* **21,** 714
8. Viberti, G. C., Mackintosh, D. and Keen, H. (1983). Determinants of the penetration of proteins through the glomerular barrier in insulin-dependent diabetes mellitus. *Diabetes* (In press)
9. Carrie, B. J. and Myers, B. D. (1980). Proteinuria and functional characteristics of the glomerular barrier in diabetic nephropathy. *Kidney Int.,* **17,** 669
10. Myers, B. D., Winetz, J. A., Chui, F. and Michaels, A. S. (1982). Mechanisms of proteinuria in diabetic nephropathy: A study of glomerular barrier function. *Kidney Int.,* **21,** 633
11. Brenner, B. M., Hostetter, T. H. and Humes, H. D. (1978). Molecular basis of proteinuria of glomerular origin. *N. Engl. J. Med.,* **298,** 826
12. Hostetter, T. H., Rennke, H. G. and Brenner, B. M. (1982). The case for intrarenal hypertension in the initiation and progression of diabetic and other glomerulopathies. *Am. J. Med.,* **72,** 375
13. Landwehr, D. M., Garvalho, J. S. and Oken, D. E. (1977). Micropuncture studies of the filtration and absorption of albumin by nephrotic rats. *Kidney Int.,* **11,** 9
14. Farr, M., Wardle, E. N. and Wilkinson, K. (1976). Lysozymuria in diabetes. *Br. Med. J.,* **1,** 624
15. Viberti, G. C., Bilous, R. W., Mackintosh, D., Bending, J. J. and Keen, H. (1983). Long-term correction of hyperglycaemia and progression of renal failure in insulin-dependent diabetes. *Br. Med. J.,* **286,** 598
16. Mogensen, C. E. (1982). Long-term antihypertensive treatment inhibiting progression of diabetic nephropathy. *Br. Med. J.,* **285,** 685
17. Mogensen, C. E. (1976). Renal function changes in diabetes. *Diabetes,* **25,** 872
18. Mogensen, C. E., Østerby, R. and Gundersen, H. J. G. (1981). Early functional and morphologic vascular renal consequences of the diabetic state. *Diabetologia,* **17,** 71
19. Viberti, G. C., Pickup, J. C., Jarrett, R. J. and Keen, H. (1979). Effect of control of blood glucose on urinary excretion of albumin in β_2-microglobulin in insulin-dependent diabetes. *N. Engl. J. Med.,*, **300,** 638
20. Deen, W. M. and Satvat, B. (1981). Determinants of glomerular filtration of proteins. *Am. J. Physiol.,* **241,** F162
21. Viberti, G. C., Jarrett, R. J., McCartney, M. and Keen, H. (1978). Increased glomerular permeability to albumin induced by exercise in diabetic subjects. *Diabetologia,* **14,** 293
22. Vittinghus, E. and Mogensen, C. E. (1981). Albumin excretion and renal haemodynamic response to physical exercise in normal and diabetic man. *Scand. J. Clin. Lab. Invest.,* **41,** 627
23. Hostetter, T. H., Troy, J. L. and Brenner, B. M. (1981). Glomerular haemodynamics in experimental diabetes mellitus. *Kidney Int.,* **19,** 410
24. Viberti, G. C., Hill, R. D., Jarrett, R. J., Argyropoulos, A., Mahmud, U. and Keen, H. (1982). Microalbuminuria as a predictor of clinical nephropathy in insulin-dependent diabetes mellitus. *Lancet,* **i,** 1430
25. Parving, H.-H., Oxenbøll, B., Svendsen, F. Aa., Christiansen, J. S. and Anderson, A. R. (1982). Early detection of patients at risk of developing diabetic nephropathy. A longitudinal study of urinary albumin excretion. *Acta Endocrinol.,* **100,** 550
26. Viberti, G. C., Wiseman, M. J., Mackintosh, D., Jarrett, R. J. and Keen, H. (1983). The correlates of microalbuminuria in insulin-dependent diabetes mellitus. *17th Annual Meeting European Society for Clinical Investigation.* Travemünde. April 1983.

Open discussion

Professor Ritz: Dr Viberti mentioned that in this age of scientific tourism he and Dr Mogensen meet each other quite frequently. I am still content that some differences in emphasis and some facts have not been papered over, so that we can hope for a lively discussion in which some blood will flow, at least verbally.

Professor G D'Amico (Italy): Working in Italy, it is my experience that in our population of diabetic patients – in my opinion at least, and I believe in that of many of my colleagues from Italy – the incidence of renal failure is less than in other countries, specifically the Scandinavian countries. I am wondering if there is some genetically determined difference which might favour or retard the appearance of renal failure in an average diabetic population.

Genetics is one possibility. Diet is another. Could different dietary habits act as determinants of at least the speed of progression to renal failure once microalbuminuria appears?

Dr Viberti: I do not know what the incidence is of clinical diabetic nephropathy in Italy, which makes my answer more difficult. Could Professor D'Amico tell me?

Professor D'Amico: There are no statistical data. It is a personal impression.

Dr Viberti: Then the first question is unanswerable. We should start to collect proper data.

On the second question, it is possible that there are genetic differences. People have looked at it in England and in the Scandinavian countries. People have looked at the genetic markers that we now use – there may be other genetic markers that we do not know about – and they could find no clear relation between HLA-type and diabetic nephropathy or renal failure.

As to the second question on dietary habits, it is a very important question. A lot of people are looking to see whether low-protein diets slow the progression to end-stage renal failure once proteinuria has appeared. I do not know whether the English eat a diet that is particularly high in protein. I would doubt it. Or whether there is a difference in protein intake between an English diet and an Italian diet. That is very difficult to tell.

Professor Keen will correct me, I am sure.

Professor H Keen (UK): It is an extraordinarily important question which covers the genetic and the environmental determinants and we know very little about either.

There has been a comparison of the frequency of clinical proteinuria using a standardized test method in comparable groups of diabetics from fourteen countries. In the WHO-sponsored multinational study, the frequency of proteinuria, defined as light and heavy was compared in carefully-selected matched groups of diabetics. From that came one extraordinary difference in the comparison between the Hong Kong and the Tokyo diabetic populations. The frequency of heavy proteinuria was about five times as high in the Japanese sample as it was in Hong Kong and this was seen in all duration groups.

There is always the question of observer variation even with the use of a standard methodology, but the conclusion was reinforced by the fact that the frequency of severe retinopathy, essentially retinitis proliferans, was also several times higher in the Japanese than in the Hong Kong population.

Ethnically they are fairly comparable Chinese stock. Dietetically I suspect they are similar. So there is this, a fivefold difference in the frequency of a major microvascular complication of diabetes which is unexplained.

Dr Jervell: I believe that until recently the Japanese were not allowed to give themselves insulin. They had to go to the outpatient clinic every morning. That makes for poor diabetic control.

The incidence of diabetes is certainly lower in Southern Europe than in Scandinavia. I believe we have about the highest in the world. Clinically I work in two settings. One is a large outpatient Type I diabetic clinic, and working there I would believe that diabetic nephropathy is a very rare disease. If one looks after one's diabetics, in a large population this will be a rare occurrence.

But, working in the hospital setting at the transplant centre, I think all diabetics have nephropathy.

Professor P Lefebvre (Belgium): I should be covering heredity in my own lecture (Chapter 10). There have been several studies about the possible role of heredity. Two studies have claimed that there is an association with severe nephropathy and some HLA groups, and Dr Jervell's study has been negative. I shall be presenting the details.

In the experience of Dr Mogensen and Dr Viberti, how reproducible is the exercise-induced increase in albuminuria in patients having a similar degree of control, being in a similar stage of their disease? In our experience the exercise-induced rise seems to vary from day to day.

Dr Mogensen: We recently re-examined patients studied five years ago and they appear to have approximately the same pattern. There may be a variation from day to day, and that may be partly explained by a variation in the degree of control, because degrees of control are very important in that respect.

The day-to-day variation was measured over one month. We measured only the microalbuminuric patients, and there was very good reproducibility.

Professor Lefebvre: A single patient cannot switch from one group to another because two weeks have elapsed?

Dr Mogensen: It is possible to have a normal test on Day 1 and then an abnormal test on Day 40. That is certainly possible. But as a whole there is no increase in exercise-induced albuminuria.

Dr Viberti: One must be very careful here about standardization of procedures. Training, glycaemic control, perhaps diet or other factors can influence the response to an exercise test, or difference in blood pressure for that matter. It is easier to get good reproducibility of data in a normal person, and in normals it is quite good. It is much more difficult in diabetics because so many can change at the same time.

The problem with exercise-induced microalbuminuria is that we still do not know what it means; whether it has any predictive value as does the resting or overnight microalbuminuria, which comes out from three different centres as having a very strong predictive value. I do not know what exercise-induced microalbuminuria means in the very early stages.

Professor M Legrain (France): The speakers have not discussed the so-called hyperviscosity syndrome, the hypothesis raised by Simpson. What do they think about that?

Dr Parving: Hyperviscosity is only slightly elevated in diabetes. We have to remember that - about 5–10%.

The hypothesis according to Simpson is that this viscous blood actually blocks the capillaries, which would imply that the blood flow, with everything else being equal, should go down. In a tube with viscous blood at the same blood pressure the flow will decrease. Everybody knows that.

But the condition in diabetes is not so. Blood flow is always elevated in muscle tissue, subcutaneous tissue, skin, kidney, eye, brain - whatever. In every tissue where it is possible to measure blood flow it is increased. So, personally I cannot see how this viscous blood can be so harmful.

Furthermore, even if we accept this hypothesis from Simpson, he is actually saying the same thing as we are saying today, that viscous blood works by raising the pressure within the small capillaries. I do not think that that is how it happens but I think we are right about the pressure.

Professor N Lameire (Belgium): Treating hypertension in diabetic nephropathy with the slowing of the deterioration of renal function – is that not also a common observation in other renal diseases? Have either Dr Mogensen or Dr Parving compared other glomerular diseases in non-diabetics and the effect of treating hypertension on proteinuria and on the deterioration of renal function? What is so specific about this intervention?

Dr Mogensen: I would agree that it is a generalized concept and everybody believes that it is so, but to my knowledge it has not been previously documented in other kinds of nephropathies.

Professor Lameire: It is quite well known that treating hypertension in any other kidney disease will slow the deterioration of GFR and decrease proteinuria. I do not think it is a very specific finding.

What is the mechanism of speculation on the mechanism of the increase in GFR in early diabetes? It is obvious that it is haemodynamic, and that if glucose can be controlled the haemodynamics will change. What is the cause and is there any speculation on that? Is it an osmotic effect of the glucose, or a volume expansion, or something else?

Dr Parving: On the first question, there is a huge difference between clinical impressions and good scientific experiment. Most trained doctors know that if they keep blood pressure at a good level, then the kidney will probably have a better run and the proteinuria will be less. But I have never seen a published study in non-diabetic nephropathy demonstrating this and if someone has a reference I would be very happy.

If any hypertensive patient is reasonably treated for his hypertension, the blood pressure will go down. That is for sure. We know that. But I do not think we know if treating other types of glomerulopathies will modify the rate of renal decline. Personally I think it does but it should be demonstrated, so somebody should go and do it.

On the other question, with initial hyperfiltration we have to realize that there are two phases. There is the rapid reversible part which I showed today. With this part there is no change in kidney size. We know that several hormones may participate. An increase in blood glucose itself elevates GFR. That has been demonstrated in man and animals. Elevation in glucagon, which is present in the diabetic state, also raises GFR and so does elevated growth hormone, which is also present in poorly-controlled diabetics. Insulin decreases GFR if blood sugar is allowed to go down but if blood sugar is kept constant and a lot of insulin is given, then nothing happens. So the insulin effect is glucose-dependent.

There are other candidates. Prostaglandins have been suggested. I know of studies at Guy's, and elsewhere. However, we have not been able to demonstrate any effect of blocking prostaglandin synthesis in newly-diagnosed diabetics.

The GFR can be reduced by treatment of diabetes but it cannot be normalized. It is still raised even if blood sugar is kept completely normal for a week or more. This part of the elevation may well be due to the enlarged kidney, so that we have a fast and a slow reversible part of hyperfiltration.

Dr G A Cinotti (Italy): My first question was exactly the same as the question just posed; namely, do we think that the evolution of renal disease may be different when hypertension is controlled in diabetic patients with nephropathy and in the other nephropathies?

My second question is perhaps the reciprocal of that. If the hypertension plays a major role in the hyperfunction of the kidney and in the hyperfiltration process, why in an essential hypertensive patient is the evolution of renal damage so different?

Dr Parving: Dr Cinotti is right in questioning the effect of pressure *per se*. The studies so well carried out in Minneapolis using unilaterally nephrectomized non-diabetic animals showed that this type of animal has only a minor acceleration of structural lesions in the remaining kidney. If the litter mates are made diabetic, unilateral nephrectomy is seen to cause a very pronounced acceleration.

I quite agree that hypertension *per se* is not capable of producing diabetic glomerulosclerosis, but on the other hand, we have to remember that the main theory of the morphogenesis or the pathogenesis of hypertensive vascular lesions, i.e. arteriolonecrosis and hyalinosis is that the increased pressure as an initial event causes an increased exudation of plasma proteins into the vessel walls, the concept that Lendrum called plasmatic vasculosis. At present it is the main concept on the evolution of hypertensive vascular disease.

Professor M Berger (Germany): We are running round in circles somewhat because we are confused about how much the involvement of hypertension plays any role here. When I saw the figures, almost none of the patients getting so-called antihypertensive treatment was hypertensive. Mostly they were normotensive. Our friends from Denmark should not really talk about antihypertensive treatment. Rather they should talk about supernormalization of blood pressure or something. Someone who is not hypertensive cannot be given antihypertensive treatment. Thus, some of the earlier arguments on hypertensive patients do not really apply.

I have a question to the two speakers from Denmark. Are they suggesting to us, based on their six patients in Aarhus and nine out of ten patients in Copenhagen, that we should treat all those patients with incipient diabetic nephropathy with drugs that lower blood pressure, even though the patients are not hypertensive? Is the evidence there to do it? From the practical point of view this is the important question to be answered.

Dr Mogensen: All our patients with overt diabetic nephropathy had significantly increased blood pressure, and they were at about the levels accepted by the WHO. More important, blood pressure levels were much higher than the values seen in normal young people.

One point on the generally accepted values used for treatment of hypertension. It is of great importance to note that if pressure values are compared with quite normal young people, there is an increase of 20–30% in overt diabetic nephropathy. The ranges used in ordinary antihypertension treatment may not apply in diabetic nephropathy. Still it makes sense to use a blood pressure level of 140/90 for the start of treatment, and that is in agreement with most studies. It is not a minute elevation of blood pressure. It is a rather dramatic increase in blood pressure in young people.

One must also add that these patients already have severe morphological lesions in the kidney, and then an additional damaging effect, namely increase in blood pressure, is added.

Professor Ritz: Of course if we talk first about cardiovascular events, there is a grave risk. An increment of 10 mm mercury, as was recently pointed out by McGregor in the *Lancet*, will have a huge impact on the total incidence of vascular accidents.

More important with respect to diabetes, at least for retinopathy. Knowles, in his study on Pima Indians could show that it did make a difference whether a patient was in the upper normal or in the lower normal range, as patients within blood pressure between 125 and 140, well within the accepted range of the WHO norms, had a higher *de novo* incidence of retinal haemorrhages and exudates than did those below. So the concept is sound but we still lack the data.

Professor C Jacobs (France): Dr Viberti showed beautiful data about the strongly predictive effect of microalbuminuria at rest in early diabetics. Given that, to what extent would he advise our colleagues – I mean the clinicians – to look for this parameter systematically in young diabetics, considering, too, the economics discussed in Session 1.

Dr Viberti: I am a bit more cautious than my Danish friends and I am always reluctant to lay down recommendations. Having shown that there is a relationship between microalbuminuria and the Albustix-positive proteinuria, and that one is a predictive marker of the other, it does not mean that if we correct one we shall prevent the second.

I am prepared to go as far as to say that people should investigate this problem very carefully and very thoroughly in a prospective manner. If a randomized prospective study were to come up in three or five years' time, that showed that people with microalbuminuria left on conventional treatment would develop Albustix-positive proteinuria, and people with microalbuminuria brought under very strict control would not, then a case would have been made out for applying that test on a larger scale. But it has to be proved. We only demonstrated an association between the two factors; a very important one, I think, but not definitive proof that by correcting the first we would stop the second.

Professor Ritz: Pythagoras once said one should stop one's life when it is at its best. I would extrapolate and say one should stop the discussion when it is at its height. We should end it here.

Session Three

CLINICAL MANAGEMENT AND PREVENTION OF COMPLICATIONS

Chairmen:
J. MIROUZE and N. LAMEIRE

7
The case for control

H. KEEN

INTRODUCTION

There can be no doubt of the advantages to the diabetic patient of a life free of wild metabolic fluctuations, between the malaise and torpor of ketotic hyperglycaemia on the one hand and the embarrassments and the sudden perils of symptomatic hypoglycaemia on the other. Even coarse control of this sort is not achieved by all insulin-treated diabetics and failure to obtain it may arise from many causes[1]. Regrettably and avoidably, inadequate or inaccurate understanding by the patient often lies at the root; failure of motivation on the part of both the patient and the attendants may be major contributors. In a very few patients, sometimes called brittle diabetics, control may be lost through poorly understood disturbances of endogenous glucoregulatory mechanisms or abnormalities of insulin absorption or action. Wilful, deliberate and ingenious malefaction must always be considered when seeking explanations.

It is the fine tuning of the diabetes that has now become much more a matter of concern to clinicians – the attempt to return the 'glycaemic profile' of the diabetic to one much more closely resembling that of the non-diabetic. It is this goal, with its attendant difficulties and dangers, for which a case must be made. Its costs are clearly apparent – a greatly increased concern of patient and doctor with the minutiae of management, the need for relatively expensive equipment and consumables, the risk of hypoglycaemia. Its benefits are, at present, largely unproven but of tremendous potential importance. They aspire to the preservation of vision, of renal function, of tissue integrity, even of life itself.

DEFINITIONS

Control, a seemingly innocent, straightforward word, acquires complex connotations when applied to the care of the human diabetic. In everyday clinical usage, it is usually restricted to the effort to return circulating glucose concentrations to the 'normal' range but of course the term 'control' also applies to correction of the whole complex of disturbances of substrates, hormones and enzymes which characterizes the diabetic state[2]. Glycaemia in the non-diabetic is very tightly regulated and held within remarkably narrow limits. Rapidly acting regulatory mechanisms promptly resist perturbations of concentration, positive and negative. Measures of control (or, better, uncontrol) must therefore at least denote both the success with which the 'setting level' of glycaemia is maintained and the degree, duration, direction and frequency of fluctuations from the expected level. While there is a strong conviction that it is departure from normoglycaemia which is responsible for the specific delayed complications of diabetes, there is little evidence as to whether it is the chronic elevation of the setting level, the size and frequency of hyperglycaemic excursions or both of these abnormalities which is most pathogenic. As discussed later, it cannot, in any case, be hyperglycaemia alone which determines the advent or evolution of diabetic complications. Other presently ill-discerned factors, genetic perhaps, also determine the liability of the individual diabetic to complications. Hyperglycaemia is always necessary but not always sufficient for development of the complications of diabetes.

ASSESSMENT OF CONTROL

No intelligent assessment of control can be made without a full understanding of the regime of insulin injections, food intake, vigorous physical activity and perhaps emotional life of the patient. Time, type and site of insulin administration, time and composition of meals are minimum data for the understanding (and regulation) of control[3,4]. In the insulin-dependent diabetic (IDD) patient, fine assessment of control without strategically and accurately placed blood glucose measurement is hopeless. Urine tests may be adequate for coarse control[5]; blood glucose measurement is vital for fine tuning. Several indices have been recommended to express the level of glycaemic control in numerical terms. They differ to a greater or lesser degree in what they convey[6,7]. No single figure or index can signify the complexity of the departures from normoglycaemia so no one index is 'best', though some are more informative than others.

Indices of uncontrol

The mean daily blood glucose (MBG) itself will give some information though it will not, of course, indicate the degree of fluctuation around it and interpretation will be influenced by the timing and frequency of blood samples:

$$\mathrm{MBG} = \frac{\Sigma(\mathrm{BG})}{n}$$

There are several indices which summarize the variability of blood glucose.

Schlichtkrull *et al*[8] devised an '*M*' value which is essentially a mean of the weighted deviations of blood glucose from a preselected desired value (e.g. 90 mg/dl, 5 mmol/l). Thus it embodies both deviations below (hypoglycaemic) and above (hyperglycaemic) the chosen value, the weighting giving numerical advantage to the former:

$$\text{`}M\text{'} = \frac{\sum\left(10\log_{10}\frac{\mathrm{BG}}{x}\right)^3}{n}$$

where x is the chosen 'setting' value (e.g. 90 mg/dl or 5 mmol/l), BG the actual blood glucose, n the number of measurements and Σ means 'sum of'.

The simplest is the range, the difference between the highest and lowest values recorded in a nominated time period. This, like all other measures of variability, will depend for its accuracy and representativeness for the individual upon the number of samples and the times at which they are taken. A good index is the standard deviation of the mean (SD) which, when expressed as a proportion of the mean value, is known as the coefficient of variation (CV).

$$\mathrm{SD} = \left[\frac{\Sigma(\mathrm{BG}^2) - \frac{(\Sigma\mathrm{BG})^2}{n}}{n-1}\right]^{\frac{1}{2}}; \ \mathrm{CV}\% = \frac{\mathrm{SD}}{\mathrm{MBG}} \times 100$$

Many pocket calculators have 'wired-in' programmes to calculate these statistics very simply. (Statisticians may object to the use of the SD for a variate like BG which departs notably from the normal distribution; however, its empirical misuse in this way is actually valuable in practice). Somewhat more demanding and sophisticated is Service's mean amplitude of glycaemic excursions[9] (MAGE), which sums in concentration units all the unidirectional swings in glucose concentration which exceed 1SD of the mean during the 24 hours and divides this sum by the number of such swings:

$$\mathrm{MAGE} = \frac{\text{Unidirectional swings (peak to trough)} > 1\mathrm{SD}}{\text{No. of unidirectional swings}}$$

Day-to-day variation can be estimated by comparison of daily MBGs or by the mean of daily differences (MODD)[10] which averages the differences between concentrations taken at the same time point on different days:

$$\text{MODD} = \frac{\Sigma\{(\text{BG}(a_1) - \text{BG}(a_2)) + (\text{BG}(b_1) - \text{BG}(b_2)) + \ldots + (\text{BG}(n_1) - \text{BG}(n_2))\}}{n}$$

where a_1 and a_2 are the same time point on day 1 and 2, b_1 and b_2 another time point on the two days, etc., and n the number of time points. Similar, more time-focussed measures can be obtained from a series (e.g. 10) of samples all taken at the same time of day, calculating mean, SD and CV[11]. Several other indices such as the area of excess glycaemia (the area of the day curve of glycaemia exceeding some selected value or profile) and the indices of meal excursions (extent and timing of blood glucose rise and recovery with meals[12]) have also been described. Like the other indices, they may be useful for systematic studies of different treatment regimes or comparisons between patients but are little used in day-to-day clinical practice. For the latter, there is little to better the practice of systematic analytical scrutiny of the carefully timed and graphed record of test results in the context of injections and meals, preferably in consultation with the patient, arriving at joint decisions on the nature of changes required in insulin dose, type or timing and the quantity and form of mealtime carbohydrate.

Other measures of control should be included here for completeness. Glycosylated haemoglobin (GHb, 'HbA_{lc}')[13] and perhaps other circulating glycosylated proteins (e.g. albumin)[14] are increasingly used as an integrated measure of long-term control. GHb is a useful measure but is a supplement to and certainly not a substitute for the much more informative blood glucose profile. The proportion of BG results exceeding or falling short of selected control threshold values also gives valuable information of effectiveness of therapy over long periods of time. The urine test for glucose has some value and testing for ketones is still of great importance if major loss of control is suspected from greatly raised blood glucose, heavy glycosuria or symptoms of thirst, polyuria and torpor. Hypoglycaemia can best be categorized by grade into biochemical (low BG value, e.g. below 2 mmol/l without symptoms), symptomatic (low values with symptoms but not requiring assistance) and severe (low values requiring assistance with or without disturbance of consciousness). Finally, frequency of hospital admissions per unit time (e.g. year) will distinguish the truly hyperlabile, brittle patient.

Longterm assessment

Even more difficult to evaluate for the purpose of analytical studies is the level of control over long periods of time, for instance the 20 or 30 years of diabetes that may precede the appearance of severe organ or tissue damage in the diabetic. As with short-term variability, there are problems in aggregating and expressing control in patients who suffer intermittent periods of severe uncontrol superimposed on a more stable background and distinguishing them from those who are continuously moderately bad. So-called brittle or metabolically hyperlabile diabetics have variously been alleged to be more, or less, susceptible to microangiopathy. A further assertion has been that diabetics who were well controlled in the first few years of their diabetes are less susceptible than the others to long-term complications despite poor control later on in their course. This might point to some protective influence of the retention of a degree of endogenous insulin secretory capacity which is an important contribution to 'good control'; it may even be a statistical artefact caused by the selective early removal from a starter cohort of patients who do badly from the beginning, leaving as survivors only those with a shorter history of bad control.

MEANS FOR MONITORING CONTROL

Technical advances in blood glucose self-measurement[15,16] have made the greatest contribution to the achievement of glycaemic control and have created conditions which make far higher standards of near normalization feasible. This rapidly developing field is well reviewed[3,4,17,18] and familiar to most diabetologists and their patients. Descriptions of glucose-sensitive strips and meters would be out of place (and probably out of date) here. What must be said, however, is that the provision of such impedimenta has limited value unless it is part of a comprehensive scheme of patient education. Realistic goals of treatment, recognition of failures, measures to deal with them and a fair working knowledge of how insulin preparations act are a necessity for the patient if the potential of these techniques is to be fully realized. Only by efficient organization of such facilities, staffed by informed and selected communicators working full-time with diabetics, with adequate accommodation, time and commitment, can these important goals be achieved. Their provision must be given the highest priority in diabetes health care expenditure in societies that can afford them. Self-measurement of blood glucose is central to control strategies but there is also some place for an independent laboratory check on the glycaemic profile from time to time. The use of the Sarstedt capillary tubes for self-collection (though not self-testing) of finger prick blood samples by the patient is a valuable 'quality control' on self-measurement[19]. Samples so collected can be brought in by the patient or mailed to the laboratory and have an important place in improving and maintaining control. A useful first application of a continuous implantable glucose sensor will be as a ready source of quantitative BG information to the patient, supplemented by audible alarms to indicate when glucose concentration is dangerously low or high.

CONTROL AND COMPLICATIONS

The evidence

The notion that better diabetic control will lower the risk of the retinal, renal, neural and perhaps arterial complications of diabetes has grown steadily, encouraged by results of animal experiments and carefully collected observations on clinical groups of patients. Only recently has experimental study in man become possible and proper. The evidence in human diabetes falls short – far short one might say – of conclusive. There are clear ethical limits to the possibilities of applying scientifically valid experimental designs to man to compare the long-term effects of good versus bad diabetic control. Only limited access to tissues and secretions for detailed study of mechanisms and interventions is possible. Many animal models have been developed in which a diabetic state, induced with B-cell toxins, is associated with vascular changes resembling those of the long-term human counterpart. These changes can be largely reversed by correction of the diabetic state. Particularly noteworthy are the elegant studies of glomerular pathology and its reversal in the diabetic rat[20] and the retinal microvascular responses to different levels of diabetic control in experimentally diabetic dogs[21]. However encouraging these findings may be, one must critically question the authenticity of the animal models for the diabetic complications of man. No example of experimental diabetic renal failure or retinopathic blindness, the major consequences in man, has yet been produced in the animal. Early, partial or analogous changes in animals may not represent the organ-damaging processes which are the target of concern in the diabetic patient.

Clinical studies in man

Until recently almost all of the evidence in man came from studies of groups of diabetic patients, usually hospital-based, in whom the presence or severity of more or less well defined 'complications' were related to some more or less well defined index of 'control'. Such studies have proved a happy hunting ground for generations of enthusiastic protagonists but also for sophisticated critics who have pointed out the major possibilities of erroneous conclusions. These arise from errors in design, operation of major selection, ascertainment and interpretative biases, imprecision of definitions and criteria and inappropriate strategies in data analysis and statistical testing of 'effects'. Knowles[22] summarized and reviewed these studies up to the early 1960s and Tchobroutsky[23] further updated them in a broad assessment. A critical review of clinical studies of this sort accompanied the impressive study of 4400 diabetic patients, observed personally over twenty-five years, published by Pirart[24], a monumental work which is among the best of the unrandomized clinical observation studies. There were many inescapable weaknesses even of this study (e.g. patients not randomized to different levels of control but settling there spontaneously perhaps because of different degrees or mechanisms of diabetes, observers aware of control when assessing complications, massive losses to follow-up ascertainment, use of technically untested measures of control variables and pathological endpoints, a varying composition of the study cohort during the observation period with many 'drop-ins' as well as 'drop-outs'). It is, however, difficult totally to reject the conclusion that there was some broad direct relationship between the general level of glycaemia as assessed and the risk of serious damage to retinal, renal and neurological structure and function. Even if one accepts this important conclusion, it does not answer the key question as to whether the *imposition* of improved control will reduce the complication risk. Inspection of the Pirart data reveals many important messages. Among the most telling is that, even in the best 'control' group (i.e. that with the lowest glycaemia), some diabetics developed complications after only a few years while, in the worst 'control' group, a substantial proportion (of the survivors) was recorded as free of them after 25 years of 'poorly controlled' diabetes. Even granted that the level of glycaemia (or some metabolic process closely associated with it) is a major determinant of angiopathic risk, these anomalous patients demonstrate that hyperglycaemia is clearly not the only factor. Some independent characteristic of the patient, ('susceptibility/resistance factor') is also very likely to be involved as well. At present, we have little or no information as to how the inherent resistance or susceptibility of the diabetic individual to the pathogenic consequences of sustained hyperglycaemia is constituted[25]. The most direct clinical statement to that effect was made by Deckert and Poulsen[26] in an important paper entitled 'Diabetic nephropathy: fault or destiny', a case–control study in which they matched 21 IDD patients in renal failure with 21 diabetics who had survived 32 years or more of the disease without clinical evidence of renal involvement. They concluded after comparing their clinical courses that, although they did not 'believe that diabetic control is irrelevant to the development of nephropathy, . . . destiny rather than faults in the treatment seem to be of importance in the development of nephropathy in insulin dependent diabetics'. This is no snap judgement but the carefully considered opinion of workers long and deeply concerned with the problem of diabetic complications. Their study is not beyond criticism; only 21 out of 461 nephropathic patients fulfilled their rigorous out-patient attendance criteria for admission to the trial and only 21 out of the 991 non-nephropathic matched controls. One may question how representative of all nephropaths these assiduous nephropathic clinic attenders were in their diabetic control. The careful matching for clinic attendances may have been the 'over-matching' pitfall which besets all case–control (so-called) studies; if the relevant explanatory variable is inadvertently matched between 'cases' and 'controls', no difference can be found. Though diabetic control was not matched for directly in this study, assiduous clinic attendance may be well enough correlated with it to have partly obscured a metabolic control difference between the groups. In a retrospective study of a cohort of the whole of the 336 patients with juvenile diabetes mellitus registered in a specialist centre in Bucharest, Mincu *et al*[27] came to the conclusion that both metabolic control and individual susceptibility or resistance were important determinants of nephropathy.

Experimental studies in man

These can be only briefly reviewed here and are dealt with at greater length in this volume and elsewhere. The development of improved methods of insulin administration to IDDM patients (multiple mixed dose regimes[3]; continuous subcutaneous insulin infusion[28]) and of blood glucose monitoring[15–18] have created conditions for scientifically more rigorous trials which do not ask the 'forbidden question' (in man) 'is bad control more damaging than good control' but can ask 'is improved control protective compared with ordinarily prevailing levels'. This enables patients to be ethically randomized to levels of *imposed* control and, with suitable safeguards, to make estimates of glycaemic response and microvascular outcome. To date, studies of this sort have largely concentrated upon retinovascular response to treatment since this is much the most available outcome variable for such studies. The publications of Job *et al*[29] and Eschwege *et al*[30] and of the Kroc[31] and Steno[32] study groups have laid the ground for the much larger long-term study along these lines recently inaugurated by the US National Institutes of Health, the Diabetes Control and Complications Trial (DCCT)[33].

A disconcerting feature of the Steno and the Kroc studies has been the suggestion that the imposition of tight control in diabetics with mild background retinopathy may actually provoke deterioration in the photographic appearance of the retina. This change may be the local response of capillary-diseased areas of retina to the fall in tissue hyperperfusion and of substrate concentration which promptly follows metabolic normalization. The crop of new lesions appears to be soon completed without initiating deleterious long-term sequels. In fact, early indications suggest[34] that, after two years of tight control, the retinopathic process has slowed by comparison with the conventionally treated group.

Most of the studies in diabetic renal disease have been relatively short-term, 'in-depth' investigations of the renal response to periods of metabolic normalization achieved with CSII or intensified conventional treatment. The reversal of diabetic microalbuminuria (i.e. urinary albumin excretion above the normal, non-diabetic range but short of levels giving positive clinical Albustix tests) after comparatively short periods of glycaemic correction[35,36] has been confirmed and recently extended by the strong suggestion that microalbuminuria is reduced for up to 8 months in the CSII-treated, compared with the conventional therapy group of the Kroc Collaborative Study[31,37]. The use of CSII in the late renal failure phase of diabetic nephropathy, however, failed to demonstrate a significant slowing of the decline in glomerular filtration rate, the rise in plasma creatinine or the fractional urinary clearance of albumin[38]. Numbers in this study were small and the results cannot (and should not) be taken to *exclude* slowing the erosion of renal function to a clinical useful degree. Further concerted attack on this late phase of diabetic renal disease is of major clinical and potential economic importance.

True primary prevention trials of the effect of control on the *genesis* as distinct from the *evolution* of either nephropathy or retinopathy in IDDM have not as yet been undertaken. They are of major proportion in terms of financial cost, observation time and patient numbers but appear to represent the only convincing approach to establishing the truth. The DCCT has bitten on the bullet and will address this crucial question.

Behind these detailed patient studies and clinical trials lies the poorly defined but highly important question of individual susceptibility (or resistance) to retinopathy and nephropathy; metabolic control factors being equal, not all diabetics appear to run the same risk of developing blindness or renal failure. In the present state of knowledge, it is difficult to know whether the subjects of our studies are those destined to escape or to fall prey to the organ damage of long-term diabetes. At the least, this means that in studies of control and complications its effects on the susceptibles will be 'diluted out', perhaps even obscured, by the resistant majority whom we are presently unable to distinguish. This would seem to place further search for the markers (and perhaps, therefore, the mechanisms) of susceptibility/resistance high on the priority list for scientific investigation.

CONCLUSION

The case for control is easy to make but the reality of tight control much more difficult to achieve[39]. It seems likely that, to bring the susceptible diabetic out of the danger zone for renal and retinal complications, physiological normality of blood glucose concentration must be approached and maintained for long periods[40]. There is as yet no convincing evidence in man that, even if this is achieved, it will succeed in obviating or reducing microangiopathic risk. Circumstantial and indirect studies point in that direction as do animal experiments. We can now achieve more with patient treatment than we thought possible even a decade ago but not all diabetics receive this high level of care. It makes demands upon patient, doctor and social resources. Not until we have better evidence of its long-term efficacy will we be able to press unreservedly for the universal application of these approaches and the resources required for their implementation. Until this evidence is to hand in man, the case for control, though strong, cannot be considered complete.

References

1. Tattersall, R. (1977). Brittle diabetes. In Tattersall (ed.). *Clinics in Endocrinology and Metabolism*. Vol. 6, No. 2, pp. 403–419. (London: W. B. Saunders)
2. Alberti, K. G. M. M. and Press C. M. (1982). The biochemistry of the complications of diabetes mellitus. In Keen, H. and Jarrett, J. (eds.). *Complications of Diabetes*, 2nd Edn. pp. 231–270. (London: Edward Arnold)
3. Tattersall, R. and Gale, E. (1981). Patient self-monitoring of blood glucose and refinements of conventional insulin treatment. *Am. J. Med.*, **70**, 177–182
4. Skyler, J. S., Skyler, D. L., Seigler, D. E. and O'Sullivan, M. J. (1981). Algorithms for adjustments of insulin dosage by patients who monitor blood glucose. *Diabetes Care*, **4**, 311–318

5. James, R.C. and Chase, G.R. (1974). Evaluation of some commonly used semi-quantitative methods for urinary glucose and ketone determinations. *Diabetes*, **23**, 474–479
6. Molnar, G.D., Marien, G.J., Hunter, A.N. and Harley, C.H. (1979). Methods of assessing diabetic control. *Diabetologia*, **17**, 5–10
7. Service, F.J. and Nelson, R.L. (1980). Characteristics of glycemic stability. *Diabetes Care*, **3**, 58
8. Schlichtkrull, J., Munck, O. and Jersild M. (1965). The M-value, an index of blood sugar control in diabetes. *Acta Med. Scand.*, **177**, 95
9. Service, F.J., Molnar, G.D., Rosevear, J.W., Ackerman, E., Gatewood, L.C. and Taylor, W.F. (1970). Mean amplitude of glycaemic excursions, a measure of diabetic instability. *Diabetes*, **18**, 644–655
10. Molnar, G.D., Taylor, W.F. and Ho, M.M. (1972). Day-to-day variation of continuously monitored glycaemia: a further measure of diabetic instability. *Diabetologia*, **6**, 342–348
11. Molnar, G.D., Taylor, W.F. and Langworthy, A. (1980). On measuring the adequacy of diabetic regulation: comparison of continuously monitored blood glucose patterns with values at selected time points. *Diabetologia*, **10**, 139–143
12. Service, F.J. (1981). Parameters for the assessment of glycemic control. In Irsigler, K., Kuntz, K.N., Owens, D.R. and Regal, H. (eds.). *New Approaches to Insulin Therapy*. pp. 237–244. (Lancaster: MTP Press)
13. Gonen, B. and Rubenstein, A.H. (1978). Haemoglobin A1 and diabetes mellitus. *Diabetologia*, **15**, 1–8
14. Bunn, H.F. (1981). Nonenzymatic glycosylation of protein: Relevance to diabetes. *Am. J. Med.*, **70**, 325–330
15. Sonksen, P.H., Judd, S.L. and Lowy, C. (1978). Home monitoring of blood glucose. *Lancet*, **1**, 729–732
16. Walford, S., Gale, E.A.M., Allison, S.P. and Tattersall, R.B. (1978). Self-monitoring of blood glucose. *Lancet*, **1**, 732–735
17. Symposium on home glucose monitoring (1980). *Diabetes Care*, **3**, 57
18. Peacock, I. and Tattersall, R. (1982). Methods of self-monitoring of diabetic control. In Johnston, D.G. and Alberti, K.G.M.M. (eds.). *New Aspects of Diabetes; Clinics in Endocrinology and Metabolism*. pp. 485–502. (London: W.B. Saunders)
19. Clark, A.J.L., Bilous, R.W., Keen, W.L. and Keen, H. (1982). Capillary tubes for blood glucose sampling. *Diabetologia*, **23**, 539–540
20. Mauer, S., Steffes, M.W., and Brown, D.M. (1981). The kidney in diabetes. *Am. J. Med.*, **70**, 603–612
21. Engerman, R., Bloodworth, T.M.B. and Nelson, S. (1977). Relationship of microvascular disease in diabetes to metabolic control. *Diabetes*, **26**, 760–769
22. Knowles, H.C. Jr., Guest, G.M., Lampe, J., Kessler, H. and Skillman, T.G. (1965). The course of juvenile diabetes treated with unmeasured diet. *Diabetes*, **14**, 239
23. Tchobroutsky, G. (1978). Relation of diabetic control to development of microvascular complications. *Diabetologia*, **15**, 143–152
24. Pirart, J. (1977). Diabète et complications dégénératives. Présentation d'une étude prospective portant sur 4400 cas observés entre 1947 et 1973. *Diab. Metab.*, **3**, 97. Translated as Pirart, J. (1978). Diabetes mellitus and its degenerative complications. A prospective study of 4400 patients observed between 1947 and 1973. *Diabetes Care*, **1**, 168–188; 252–263
25. Cudworth, A.G. and Bodansky, H.J. (1982). Genetic and immunological factors in diabetic complications. In Keen, H. and Jarrett, J. (eds.). *Complications of Diabetes*, 2nd Edn. pp. 1–12. (London: Edward Arnold)
26. Deckert, T. and Poulsen, J.E. (1981). Diabetic nephropathy: fault or destiny? *Diabetologia*, **21**, 178–183
27. Mincu, I., Ionescu-Tirgoviste, C., Santu, E., Cheta, D. and Lacatis, D. (1982). The renal complications of juvenile diabetes mellitus. Study of 336 cases. *Dt. Gesundh-Wesen*, **37**, 1290–1292
28. Pickup, J.C. and Keen, H. (1980). Continuous subcutaneous insulin infusion: a developing tool in diabetes research. *Diabetologia*, **18**, 1–6
29. Job, D., Eschwege, E., Guyot-Argenton, C., Aubry, J.P. and Tchobroutsky, G. (1976). Effect of multiple daily insulin injections on the course of diabetic retinopathy. *Diabetes*, **25**, 463–469

30. Eschwege, E., Job, D., Guyot-Argenton, C., Aubry, J. P. and Tchobroutsky, G. (1979). Delayed progression of diabetic retinopathy by divided insulin administration: a further follow-up. *Diabetologia*, **16**, 13–15
31. Kroc Collaborative Study Group (1983). Near normal glycaemic control does not slow progression of mild diabetic retinopathy. *Diabetes*, **32** (Suppl. 1), 10A (Abstr.)
32. Steno Study Group (1982). Effect of 6 months of strict metabolic control on eye and kidney function in insulin-dependent diabetics with background retinopathy. *Lancet*, **1**, 121–124
33. National Institute of Arthritis, Metabolism and Digestive Diseases (1981). Request for research cooperative agreement applications: clinical centers for a collaborative clinical trial on the relationship between blood glucose control and vascular complications of insulin-dependent diabetes mellitus. R. F. A. NIAMDD 81–01.
34. Lauritzen, T., Frost-Larsen, K., Larsen, H.-W., Deckert, T., Keiding, N. and Nelson, G. (1983). Continuous subcutaneous insulin. *Lancet*, **2**, 1445–1446
35. Viberti, G. C., Pickup, J. C., Jarrett, R. J. and Keen, H. (1979). Effect of control of blood glucose on urinary excretion of albumin and β_2 microglobulin in insulin dependent diabetes. *N. Engl. J. Med.*, **300**, 638
36. Viberti, G. C., Pickup, J. C., Bilous, R. W., Mackintosh, D. and Keen, H. (1981). Correction of exercise induced microalbuminuria in insulin dependent diabetics after 3 weeks of subcutaneous insulin infusion. *Diabetes*, **30**, 818–823
37. Kroc Collaborative Study (1983). A randomised controlled study of the effects of CSII in retinal and renal complications of diabetes (In preparation)
38. Viberti, G. C., Bilous, R. W., Mackintosh, D., Bending, J J. and Keen, H. (1983). Long term correction of hyperglycaemia and progression of renal failure in insulin dependent diabetes. *Br. Med. J.*, **286**, 598–602
39. Cahill, G. F. Jr., Etzwiler, D. D. and Frenkel, N. (1976). 'Control' and diabetes. *N. Engl. J. Med.*, **294**, 1004–1005
40. Viberti, G. C., Haycock, G. B., Pickup, J. C., Jarrett, R. J. and Keen, H. (1980). Early functional and morphologic vascular renal consequences of the diabetic state. *Diabetologia*, **18**, 173–175

Discussant

M. BERGER

Professor Berger (Germany): Whilst I was pleased, indeed grateful, to be asked to come to this excellent meeting and to visit this equally magnificent city, I find myself right now in a somewhat unusual position; to try to act as an official discussant.

First I thought I had been hired as somebody whom the Americans would call a cheer leader. Following Professor Keen's talk it is obvious to me, and to everybody else, that that is really unnecessary. Having heard Professor Keen's magnificent lecture, there is no need to motivate his audience to cheer or to applaud.

Secondly, I thought I should motivate delegates to enter into a critical discussion on what has been discussed so far, but I see from the programme there is no room for discussion at this point in the proceedings. So, the only thing I can do right now is to take the standpoint of a clinical diabetologist, very much like Dr Jervell in an earlier session, and raise two or three points, bringing them again to the attention of participants.

One point has already been made, and it is a very important question for a clinical diabetologist faced with patients with incipient or manifest nephropathy; do we have to lower their blood pressure even though their blood pressure readings may not exceed the limits of borderline hypertension? If the blood pressure is below 140/90, equal to a mean arterial pressure of 115 - if I have calculated correctly - do we still have to lower that, say from 110 to 95, as was done in some of the patients from Copenhagen? It is an important question because it has a number of consequences, as any drug treatment has.

The second, and maybe even more important point for the clinical diabetologist is what do we do as far as glycaemic control is concerned with the patient who has already developed manifest diabetic nephropathy? Dr Viberti and Dr Keen have told us that it is very important to strive for normoglycaemia to prevent nephropathy, or to treat microalbuminuria, but it might not be necessary, or it might even be harmful if we think of retinopathy, to strictly normalize the glycaemia when the patient has already developed manifest nephropathy.

On the other hand, there are a lot of patients, and we see them every week, almost every day these days, who have developed nephropathy and who realize that they have been neglected, due to their fault, due to the fault of their doctors, due to the fact that they have not been really informed or educated about their disease in the decades before. They feel that they have not really paid enough attention to glycaemic control but they want to do it now. What do we tell them? That it is too late? That they should forget about it? That it may even be harmful for them to strive for normoglycaemia? Or should they be encouraged in these goals? For a clinical diabetologist these are pertinent and important questions, and I hope we shall have a chance to address them later on.

8.1
Optimized conventional treatment

I. H. DE LEEUW

Previous chapters in this book have drawn attention to two facts:

(1) Chronic complications of diabetes arise early in the natural history of the disease when classical management is applied.

(2) Improved control can often stabilize and possibly reverse the malignant evolution of some complications.

The natural conclusion from these statements is that prevention of complications has to start from the onset of the disease, and has to be maintained throughout the life of the diabetic.

For this reason little can be expected from special control efforts applied in Type II diabetics where the real duration of the disease is mostly unknown, and the diagnosis often is concomitant with the discovery of already present complications. Therefore all energy to obtain optimized control has to be concentrated on Type I juvenile-type true insulin-dependent diabetics where the life expectancy and the quality of life can possibly be influenced by a dynamic treatment programme. During the past few years most diabetologists[1] have agreed on the level of blood glucose which has to be maintained to limit the diabetic risk:

	Ideal	*Acceptable*
Fasting	60–90 mg/dl	60–130 mg/dl
Before meals	60–150 mg/dl	60–130 mg/dl
1 h after meals	max 140 mg/dl	max 180 mg/dl
2 h after meals	max 120 mg/dl	max 150 mg/dl

To reach this goal patient self-monitoring of blood glucose (SMBG) is a must. It provides the ability to document the blood sugar levels throughout the day and permits the patient to adjust the treatment on a continuous basis depending on the variability of practical life. The importance of this procedure is well documented in a work of Schiffrin *et al*[2] where the stopping of monitoring and self control procedures was followed by a worsening of the diabetic control in the short period of 3 months. Re-establishing SMBG restored the degree of previous control. On the contrary, urine testing for glucose has been proved to be an unreliable and unsensitive marker of the control level. A recent paper by Daneman *et al*[3] shows that an intense effort to obtain a significant larger number of negative urine tests in diabetic children was insufficient to lower the levels of HbA_1. The basis for optimized conventional treatment (OCT) will therefore be an *algorithm* system able to adjust insulin treatment to actual glycaemia. This system has to be adapted to the specific insulin regimen prescribed for the patient on a physiological basis[1].

Clinical research with open- and closed-loop devices had indeed fixed the rules of modern insulin treatment:

(1) Approximately half of the daily insulin has to be given as 'basal insulin' in order to maintain a continuous level of insulinaemia.

(2) The remaining half is given as meal-related shots, knowing that more insulin is needed for breakfast than for lunch and supper.

(3) In some patients a 'dawn phenomenon' exists, requiring higher basal insulin before the consumption of breakfast.

All these rules can be perfectly programmed in mechanical devices to deliver insulin but *can the same degree of control be obtained by intensified conventional therapy*? Basal insulin can be given as one dose of very long acting Ultralente or two injections of intermediate acting (NPH, Monotard, Lente) insulin while a meal-related bolus can be added several times a day as quick acting regular insulin.

Several authors have compared the degree of control obtained by such a regimen with continuous subcutaneous insulin infusion (CSII) in matched patients (Champion[4], Barbosa[5], Reeves[6], Schiffrin[7], Calabrese[8], Home[9] and Buysschaert[10]. Most studies involving inpatient short-term comparisons have demonstrated equivalent glycaemic control with both methods, but in outpatient studies often better control was obtained with the CSII.

The rate of success in OCT is indeed determined by a *progressive individualized teaching* of the patient and a *strict control by the physician.* Treatment has to be scheduled on the following basic rules:

(1) An activity profile fixes the energy expenditure during work, week-end, sports etc.

(2) Meal-planning and caloric distribution is discussed with the patient and his family.

(3) An adapted insulin regimen is chosen as a function of the most convenient solution for the patient.

(4) Intensive teaching and training is started for:
   (a) perfect insulin injection technique,
   (b) SMBG and urine testing for acetonuria,
   (c) carbohydrate exchange and meal-planning.
(5) Teaching in adjustment of insulin dosage as a function of hyper- and hypoglycaemia.

(6) Regular contact with teaching-nurse, dietitian and diabetologist to correct the first scheme in order to maintain a HbA_1 value below 9%.

The physician has to be aware of a few caveats:

(1) Nocturnal hypoglycaemia especially in pregnant women and patients with a deficiency in counterregulatory responsiveness,
(2) absorption problems in the presence of local reactions to insulin or with the use of slow-acting insulins,

(3) timing and composition of the meals in patients with delayed absorption due to sympathic neuropathy, the use of starch-blockers or a high fibre diet, and

(4) the presence of a remaining endogenous insulin secretion giving more flexibility to the insulin regimen in the early period of the disease.

In 1980 with the help of a well-trained staff we started an OCT programme in 130 Type I diabetics (mean age 27 years, mean duration of diabetes less than 10 years) without clinically detectable complications. After 3 years (end 1982) only 20 patients were found to be able to continuously maintain the 'acceptable' blood sugar levels and a total HbA_1 value of lower than 9%. Since good to excellent control has to be maintained during the whole life to offer a protection against complications we think that OCT is feasible, but highly time, personal and money consuming, and is limited to a selected number of patients able to understand and apply the self-control techniques, to follow a strict way of life and to have the economical possibility to pay for it. However, we remain convinced that the method is valid and useful, but at present the facilities to apply the method are not always available for the patients.

References

1. Skyler, J.S., Skyler, D.L., Seigler, D.E. and O'Sullivan, M.J. (1981). Algorithms for adjustment of Insulin dosage by patients who monitor blood glucose. *Diabetes Care,* **4**, 311
2. Schiffrin, A. and Belmonte, M. (1982). Multiple daily self-glucose monitoring: its essential role in long-term glucose control in insulin-dependent diabetic patients treated with pump and multiple subcutaneous injections. *Diabetes Care,* **5**, 749
3. Daneman, D., Epstein, L.H., Siminerio, L., Beck, S., Farkas, G., Figueroa, J., Becker, D.J. and Drash, A.L. (1982). Effects of enhanced conventional therapy on metabolic control in children with insulin-dependent diabetes mellitus. *Diabetes Care,* **5**, 472
4. Champion, M.C., Shepherd, G., Rodger, N.W. and Dupre, J. (1980). Continuous subcutaneous infusion of insulin in the management of diabetes mellitus. *Diabetes,* **29**, 206
5. Barbosa, J., Menth, L., Eaton, J., Sutherland, D., Freier, E. and Najarian, J. (1981). Long-term ambulatory, subcutaneous insulin infusion versus multiple daily injections in brittle diabetic patients. *Diabetes Care,* **4**, 269

6. Reeves, M.L., Seigler, D.E., Ryan, E.A. and Skyler, J.S. (1982). Glycemic control in insulin-dependent diabetes mellitus: comparison of outpatient intensified conventional therapy with continuous s.c. insulin infusion. *Am. J. Med.,* **72,** 673
7. Schiffrin, A. and Belmonte, M.M. (1982). Comparison between continuous subcutaneous insulin infusion and multiple injections of insulin. A one year prospective study. *Diabetes,* **31,** 255
8. Calabrese, G., Bueti, A., Santeusanio, F., Giombolini, A., Zega, G., Angeletti, G., Cartechini, M. and Brunetti, P. (1982). Continuous subcutaneous insulin infusion treatment in insulin-dependent diabetic patients: a comparison with conventional optimised treatment in a long-term study. *Diabetes Care,* **5,** 457
9. Home, P.D., Capaldo, B., Burrin, J.M., Worth, R. and Alberti, K.G.M.M. (1982). A cross-over comparison of continuous subcutaneous insulin infusion (CSII) against multiple insulin injections in insulin-dependent diabetic subjects: improved control with CSII. *Diabetes Care,* **5,** 466
10. Buysschaert, M., Marchand, E., Ketelslegers, J.M. and Lambert, A. (1983). Comparison of Plasma Glucose and Plasma free insulin during CSII and Intensified Conventional Insulin Therapy. *Diabetes Care,* **6,** 1

Discussant

A. TEUSCHER

Professor Teuscher (Switzerland): I shall make two comments, one on long-term control of diabetes and one on short-term.

We heard from Professor Keen that apparently once complications of diabetes arise, intensive treatment does not change the outcome of nephropathy. So, I have tried to summarize the views we hold on treatment. In the early phase we tried to administer insulin so that patients would be asymptomatic, but later, when we had wide fluctuations we decided in the second phase to intensify treatment. However, we have not seen any arrest in the rate of decline of the glomerular filtration rate.

It seems to me that in the future, intensive treatment will have to start at the very beginning of diabetes, and that we shall have to optimize control to keep glomerular filtration at a normal level. These points have been made by Professor Keen and Professor De Leeuw, in order to emphasize the importance of early treatment.

Professor Keen has also mentioned a very important point; whether glycaemic control is the central factor, or whether we should look for other problems. Perhaps multiplicity of insulin injections might be as important as glycaemic control. In our Swiss Group in the multinational study of vascular disease in diabetics we have 534 patients whom we are separating into two groups; one with multiple daily injections and one with a single injection. These are age, sex and duration matched groups of diabetics. As yet there are no results from the follow-up study undertaken eight years after the primary examination.

I shall finish with a third comment on the short-term and early phases of treatment in two diabetics I have been following for several years. With the first, treated with an early regimen, the patient is still alive, without any complications, some 42 years after her diabetes started at the age of 4. The regimen was given to her in 1947, and it requires regular calculation of the daily intake of fats, proteins, and carbohydrates.

This patient came under my observation in 1954 when I did an appendicectomy on her as a resident in surgery, and she has been under my care ever since. This patient has injected insulin four times a day throughout her life. I have followed another such uncomplicated longterm patient who has tested her urine and injected her insulin four times a day since her diabetes began; she would never go on a longer-acting insulin.

What can we learn from these two patients? Perhaps we need a four-point programme:

- early instruction;
- possibly old-fashioned diabetes diet instruction;
- insulin four times a day;
- a quantum of good luck.

8.2
Continuous subcutaneous insulin infusion: a means to obtain near-normal glycaemic control

W. V. TAMBORLANE, Jr., J. E. PUKLIN, M. C. PRESS, E. L. ETKIND and R. S. SHERWIN

ADVANCES IN INSULIN DELIVERY USING MECHANICAL DEVICES

The failure of conventional treatment to normalize blood glucose levels in diabetes provided the impetus for development of a true mechanical endocrine pancreas. With such a system, blood glucose levels are maintained within a target range by the infusion of insulin at a variable rate adjusted by online monitoring of blood glucose levels[1]. Use of monitored systems, however, has been limited due to technical problems in developing an implantable glucose sensor. Since none of the miniaturized glucose sensors designed for implantation work effectively *in vivo*, presently available systems utilize extracorporeal sensors which are bulky and require attachment of the patient to an intravenous line with continuous blood withdrawal.

Due to the difficulties encountered in the development of a glucose sensor, attention turned to the use of insulin delivery systems that mimic normal insulin secretory patterns, but do not depend on minute-to-minute monitoring of blood glucose levels. Initial attempts to simulate diurnal plasma insulin profiles with battery powered infusion pumps used the intravenous route of insulin delivery[2,3]. It was felt that mealtime boluses of insulin would be absorbed too slowly if given subcutaneously. While glucose control could be markedly improved with continuous intravenous infusion, use of these systems is limited by problems with infection, thrombosis, occlusion and breakage of the intravenous catheter.

Conventional treatment of Type I diabetes with one or two daily injections of insulin rarely, if ever, lowers plasma glucose values to normal levels. This failure is partially accounted for by the non-physiologic nature of standard insulin replacement. In non-diabetics, insulin release can be roughly divided into two phases: continuous basal insulin secretion between meals and during the night, and bursts of insulin secretion with each meal. Basal insulin secretion is important in restraining hepatic production of glucose in the fasting state, and may also play a role in the normal suppression of endogenous glucose production which accompanies meal ingestion. Prandial bursts of insulin stimulate disposal of ingested carbohydrate by the liver and peripheral tissues.

The failure of conventional insulin treatment to normalize blood glucose levels in diabetes can be attributed, at least in part, to difficulties in maintaining adequate basal insulin levels. Insufficient basal insulinization leads to hepatic overproduction of glucose and fasting hyperglycaemia. Subsequent meal ingestion leads to a marked postprandial glycaemic excursion which can only be overcome by an excessive amount of rapid acting insulin. The latter often overshoots the mark and leads to hypoglycaemia prior to the next meal.

In comparison to the intravenous route, continuous subcutaneous insulin infusion (CSII) offers a number of practical advantages. In addition, maintainance of adequate basal insulin levels can be readily accomplished using this route of insulin delivery. Pickup and colleagues were the first to employ a preprogrammed insulin pump delivery system which used the subcutaneous route of administration[4]. These and other investigators demonstrated in short-term, inpatient studies that normal or near-normal glucose control could be achieved by CSII in diabetic subjects who had previously been difficult to control outside the hospital[4,5]. While such results were encouraging, it remained to be determined whether CSII would be effective in the management of Type I diabetic subjects in their usual home, work or school environment where factors such as diet, activity and emotional stress are more variable.

LONGTERM OUTPATIENT SUBCUTANEOUS INSULIN INFUSION: YALE EXPERIENCE

To determine whether CSII would be effective in the outpatient setting, we have studied 27 patients with Type I diabetes for more than 3 years. The patients ranged in age from 13 to 46 years, and in known duration of diabetes from 2 to 29 years at the start of study. Seven patients had no evidence of microvascular disease, while 20 had diabetic retinopathy of varying severity.

All patients were admitted to the hospital at the start of the study. During the first 2 days, baseline assessments were performed while the patients were maintained on their usual insulin regimen. Treatment with the insulin infusion pump (Figure 1) (model AS6C, Auto-Syringe, Inc., Hooksett, New

Hampshire) was then initiated. Basal infusion rate and premeal bolus doses were adjusted over the next 5–7 days in order to achieve the following target blood glucose values:

Fasting and preprandial:	70–120 mg/dl
Peak postprandial:	< 180 mg/dl
0300 h:	> 65 mg/dl

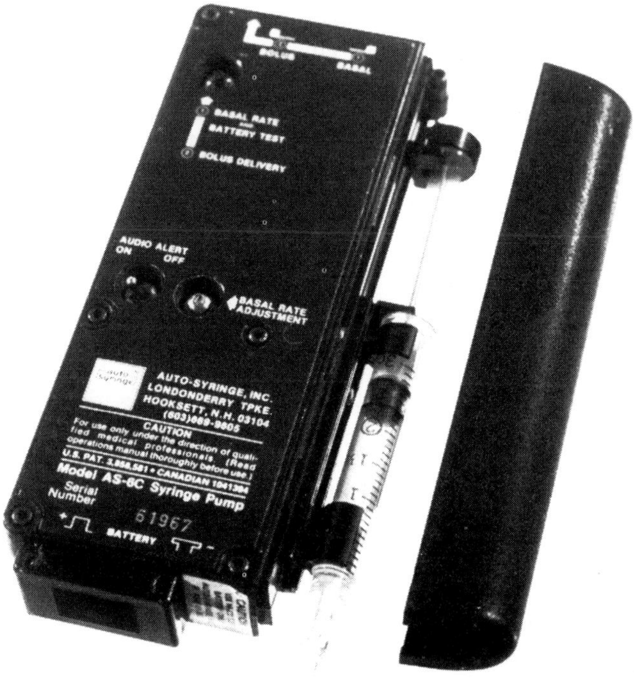

Figure 1 Infusion pump used for continuous subcutaneous infusion

Patients were instructed on how to manage the pump system and to measure blood glucose levels accurately using both visual and reflectance meter methods. In addition to developing technical skills, patients were taught how to make alterations in the treatment regimen based on changes in premeal blood glucose levels, meal size and anticipated exercise.

During outpatient CSII treatment, frequent contact was maintained via the telephone. Patients were seen weekly in the outpatient clinic until stable, then once a month. Self-blood glucose monitoring data was collected during outpatient visits, and blood obtained for measurement of glycosylated haemoglobin. Before and at regular intervals after starting CSII, all patients had complete ophthalmologic evaluations, including non-simultaneous stereoscopic fundus photography. The stereoscopic fundus photographs were read and graded in a masked fashion at the end of the study by a modification of the Early Treatment Diabetic Retinopathy Study System[6]. This modification added a group labelled as 'no classifiable retinopathy (NCR)' to account for mild background changes insufficient to meet the lowest grade of the ETDRS system.

The effect of CSII on blood glucose levels is shown in Figure 2a. Mean plasma glucose levels during conventional treatment (prepump) is compared to the average blood glucose value determined by the patients at home before and after meals during CSII. Blood glucose levels fell sharply during the first year of CSII. More importantly, blood glucose levels remained reduced even after 3 years of outpatient treatment. The improvement in glucose control was also reflected in a marked reduction in glycosylated haemoglobin (HbA_1) levels (Figure 2b). HbA_1 levels exceeded the upper limits of normal in all subjects during conventional treatment. During the first year of CSII, mean values fell to levels within the normal range and remained reduced throughout the study.

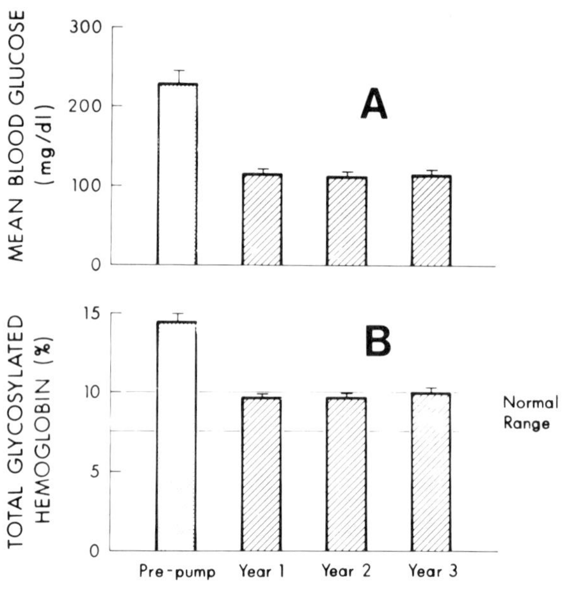

Figure 2 This shows the effect of CSII on glucose regulation. 2a shows the effect on blood glucose, 2b shows the effect on total glycosylated haemoglobin

In addition to lowering blood glucose levels, CSII has been shown to correct a variety of other metabolic, functional and structural abnormalities which characterize poorly controlled diabetes. Such treatment has been shown to reverse hyperamino-acidaemia[7], elevations of circulating lipids[7], excessive urinary losses of calcium and phosphate[8] and increases in plasma catecholamines[9], growth hormone[9] and glucagon[10]. High density lipoproteins[11] and somatomedin-C levels[12] have been shown to increase with improved glycaemic control. Even in the absence of clinical complications, CSII has been shown to increase nerve conduction velocity[13] and reduce vitreous fluorescein leakage[14], microalbuminurea[15] and capillary basement membrane thickness[16].

CSII fails to halt progression of diabetic retinopathy

While changes in capillary permeability and basement thickening which accompany strict metabolic control are noteworthy, these alterations have not been definitely linked with the retinal and renal complications of diabetes. One must still rely on well established, quantifiable clinical endpoints to evaluate diabetic microangiopathy. Our experience with the 27 patients recruited for longterm outpatient CSII therapy indicates that CSII does not halt progression of diabetic retinopathy. As shown in Figure 3, 16 of 54 eyes (29.6%) showed progression of diabetic retinopathy after 2–3 years of CSII. One of 14 eyes without retinopathy developed minimal background retinopathy, 11 of 25 eyes (44%) with background retinopathy worsened including 2 eyes that developed proliferative changes; 4 of 15 eyes (27%) with proliferative changes

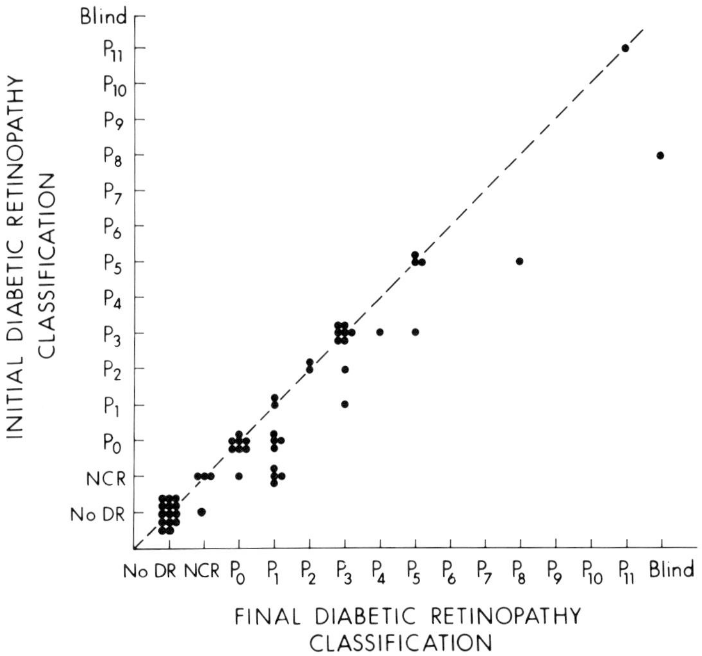

Figure 3 The initial modified ETDRS classification of each eye (Y-axis) is plotted against the final modified ETDRS classification (X-axis). Dots falling on the 45 ° line represent no change; those below the line represent a progression of retinopathy

progressed. However, there was no substantial visual loss noted over the course of follow-up. These observations are similar to those made by other investigators who have reported a progression of both diabetic retinopathy[17] and nephropathy[18] during CSII. Thus, longterm, controlled, randomized clinical trials are urgently needed to determine whether CSII can provide the requisite degree of metabolic improvement to prevent the development or delay the progression of diabetic retinopathy and nephropathy.

Who should wear a pump? (risks *vs* benefits)

Attempts to achieve blood glucose values which approximate non-diabetic levels are not without risk. The major risk of intensive insulin treatment with either CSII or multiple injections is hypoglycaemia. Self blood glucose monitoring techniques help to minimize, but do not eliminate, this problem. Nocturnal hypoglycaemia may be particularly difficult to avoid due to fluctuations in basal insulin requirements. In many patients, basal insulin requirements reach a nadir at 0300 h and rise steadily between 0500 h and 0800 h, this has been termed the 'Dawn Phenomenon'[19]. Factors which predispose to hypoglycaemia must be considered in the estimation of risk of CSII. Diabetics appear to be particularly vulnerable to hypoglycaemia since they characteristically fail to show an appropriate rise in plasma glucagon during hypoglycaemia. While this defect is generally not sufficient to impair glucose counterregulation by itself, it becomes important when other factors coexist. Specifically, diminished release of growth hormone, cortisol or catecholamines; autonomic neuropathy; or treatment with β-adrenergic blocking agents increase the risk of hypoglycaemia. In addition, patients receiving CSII may be at increased risk for development of diabetic ketoacidosis if the infusion of rapid acting insulin is interrupted due to catheter leakage or pump malfunction.

Because the major issue concerning control and complications is not yet proven, it is difficult to make generalized pronouncements concerning which patients should wear a pump. The known and potential benefits must be weighed against the risks for the individual patients. In patients who are found suitable, however, the results are often quite gratifying. Improvement in metabolic control is accompanied by an increased sense of well-being in the majority of patients. The investment in time and effort by patients and medical staff would pay even greater dividends if such treatment is found to reduce the risk of developing the degenerative complications of diabetes.

ACKNOWLEDGEMENTS

The authors thank the nurses and staff of the Clinical Research Centers, Susan Bates, RN, and Jo Ann Ahern, RN, for the excellent care given to our patients. We are grateful to Helen Black for her expert assistance in completing the manuscript.

This research was supported by grants PR 125 and EY 00785 from the National Institutes of Health and grants from the Juvenile Diabetes Foundation and Connecticut Lions Research Foundation.

References

1. Albisser, A. M., Leibel, B. S., Ewart, T. G. *et al.* (1974). Clinical control of diabetes by the artificial pancreas. *Diabetes,* **23,** 397
2. Slama, G., Hautecouverture, M., Assan, R. and Tchobroutsky, G. (1974). One to five days of continuous intravenous insulin infusion on seven diabetic patients. *Diabetes,* **23,** 732
3. Irsigler, K. and Kritz, H. (1979). Long-term continuous intravenous insulin therapy with a portable insulin dosage-regulating apparatus. *Diabetes,* **28,** 196
4. Pickup, J. C., Keen, H., Parsons, J. A. *et al.* (1978). Continuous subcutaneous insulin infusion: an approach to achieving normoglycaemia. *Br. Med. J.,* **1,** 204
5. Tamborlane, W. V., Sherwin, R. S., Genel, M. and Felig, P. (1979). Reduction to normal of plasma glucose in juvenile diabetics by subcutaneous administration of insulin with a portable infusion pump. *N. Engl. J. Med.,* **300,** 573
6. *Early Treatment Diabetic Retinopathy Study: Manual of Operations* (1980). Bethesda, MD., Public Health Service, Department of Health, Education & Welfare, National Institutes of Health
7. Tamborlane, W. V., Sherwin, R. S., Genel, M. and Felig, P. (1979). Restoration of normal lipid and amino-acid metabolism in diabetic patients treated with a portable insulin-infusion pump. *Lancet,* **i,** 1258
8. Gertner, J. M., Tamborlane, W. V., Horst, R. L., Sherwin, R. S., Felig, P. and Genel, M. (1980). Mineral metabolism in diabetes mellitus: changes accompanying treatment with a portable subcutaneous insulin infusion system. *J. Clin. Endocrinol. Metab.,* **50,** 862
9. Tamborlane, W. V., Sherwin, R. S., Koivisto, V., Hendler, R., Genel, M. and Felig, P. (1979). Normalization of the growth hormone and catecholamine response to exercise in juvenile onset diabetics treated with a portable insulin infusion pump. *Diabetes,* **28,** 785
10. Raskin, P., Pietri, A. and Unger, R. (1979). Changes in glucagon levels after four to five weeks of glucoregulation by portable insulin infusion pumps. *Diabetes,* **29,** 1033
11. Dunn, F. L., Pietri, A. and Raskin, P. (1981). Plasma lipid and lipoprotein levels with continuous subcutaneous insulin infusion in Type I diabetes mellitus. *Ann. Intern. Med.,* **95,** 426
12. Tamborlane, W. V., Hintz, R. L., Bergman, M., Genel, M., Felig, P. and Sherwin, R. S. (1981). Insulin infusion pump treatment of diabetes: influence of improved metabolic control on plasma somatomedin levels. *N. Engl. J. Med.,* **305,** 303
13. Pietri, A., Ehle, A. L. and Raskin, P. (1980). Changes in nerve conduction velocity after six weeks of glucoregulation with portable insulin infusion pumps. *Diabetes,* **29,** 668
14. White, N. H., Waltman, S. R., Krupin, T. and Santiago, J. (1982). Reversal of abnormalities in ocular fluorophotometry in insulin-dependent diabetes after five to nine months of improved metabolic control. *Diabetes,* **31,** 80
15. Viberti, G. C., Pickup, J. C., Jarrett, R. J. and Keen, H. (1979). Effect of control of blood glucose on urinary excretion of albumin and β_1-microglobulin in insulin-dependent diabetics. *N. Engl. J. Med.,* **300,** 638
16. Raskin, P., Pietri, A. O., Unger, R. H. and Shannon, W. A. (1982). The effect of meticulous diabetes control on quadriceps capillary basement membrane thickness in Type I diabetes mellitus. *Clin. Res.,* **30,** 878A
17. Lauritzen, T. and the Stino Study Group (1983). Effect of 1 year of near-normal blood glucose levels on retinopathy in insulin-dependent diabetics. *Lancet,* **i,** 200
18. Viberti, G. C., Bilous, R. W., Keen, H. and MacKintosh, D. (1982). Failure of long-term correction of hyperglycaemia to affect the progression of clinical diabetic nephropathy. *Diabetes,* **31** (Suppl.), 11A
19. Schmidt, M. I., Hadji-Georgopoulos, A., Rendell, M., Margolis, S. and Kowarski, A. (1981). The Dawn Phenomenon, an early morning glucose rise: implications for diabetic intraday blood glucose variation. *Diabetes Care,* **4,** 579

8.3
Alternatives to continuous subcutaneous insulin infusion: the other routes of insulin administration

G. SLAMA

The most widely used route of insulin administration by pump is undoubtedly the subcutaneous one. One of the main reasons for this success, which are summarized in Table 1, is the good results obtained with this route in terms of blood glucose control and patient acceptability. This is particularly due to the fact that insulin-treated patients are used to injecting themselves, insertion of a butterfly needle being not so different from a syringe needle. However the s.c. route of insulin administration is far from being totally satisfactory due to various drawbacks.

The main drawback is that there are many indications in the literature[1,2] that the kinetics (and hence the efficacy) of insulin injected as a bolus by a pump before a meal do not differ from those observed after a conventional injection with a syringe. In addition, in a recent survey[3], cutaneous complications (which can lead to a local abscess and, in one case, a fatal endocarditis) affected approximately 10% of the patients treated by s.c. pump in one year.

This explains both the prevalence of the s.c. route when using a pump and the need to continue the research on other routes of continuous insulin administration by devices.

Table 1 S.c. infusions

Advantages	*Drawbacks*
Efficient	Kinetics of resorption comparable to that of s.c. injections
Easy to handle by the patient him/herself	Cutaneous risks Insulin degradation
Permits transient disconnection	Bolus injections done before meals

The other possibilities are the intravenous (i.v.), the intramuscular (i.m.), the intraportal (i.po.) and the intraperitoneal (i.p.) routes of insulin administration.

THE INTRAVENOUS ROUTE

This route is the first one to have been utilized in continuous insulin infusion[4] because only intravascular administration can mimic the physiological pattern and the minute-to-minute variations of insulin secretion.

Table 2 gives the main advantages and disadvantages of this route of insulin administration.

Table 2 I.v. infusions

Advantages	*Drawbacks*
Highly efficient	Surgical procedure
Instant flexibility	Infection risks
Prandial dose taken after the meal	Disconnection not permitted (clotting)
Diet liberalization	Limited duration
Bioavailability of the insulin	

Its great efficacy apart, we should note its flexibility: for instance the prandial dose of insulin is administered *after* the meal (10 to 20 min), when blood glucose starts to rise; this permits a good correlation between the total amount of carbohydrate in a meal and the amount of insulin administered[5]; this also allows the patient to interrupt a meal or to eat much more or much less than he initially planned. The disadvantages of such a continuous i.v. infusion are obvious, the main ones being the risks of infectious phlebitis and the inability for the patient to disconnect the pump without a risk of catheter obturation. Moreover, the catheter can only be inserted (for long term treatment) under surgical procedure with a 20 to 40 cm s.c. tunnelization of the catheter before penetration and catheterization of a central vein.

The i.v. route of insulin administration is thus very seldom used nowadays for external pumps. One of its best indications could be the state of insulin resistance due to massive s.c. insulin degradation.

THE INTRAMUSCULAR ROUTE

For many reasons this route of insulin administration, first described by Pickup *et al*[6], is also seldom used. The main advantage of the s.c. route is a better insulin absorption with less degradation; the disadvantages are that there is a muscle fibrosis around the catheter and that the cannula is cumbersome to insert.

THE INTRAPORTAL ROUTE

This route has only been used in experimental studies on animals[7,8]. The serious risks of a pylephlebitis in a human being carrying an external pump make it unethical to use such a route (Table 3).

Table 3 I.po. infusions (only experimental animals)

Advantages	*Drawbacks*
Physiological (maintains the portal–suprahepatic gradient of insulin avoiding peripheral hyperinsulinism)	Portal thrombosis
	Pylephlebitis
Net balance: Future?	

However there is no doubt that this route is the only one which permits a perfect mimicking of physiological events, with the conservation of the portal–suprahepatic gradient of insulin. This lack of peripheral hyperinsulinism might have a very important impact on the incidence of macrovascular complications in diabetes[9].

This explains why this route has never been used in humans up to now, but in the future and for *implantable* devices such an approach will certainly be carefully investigated.

THE INTRAPERITONEAL ROUTE

This route has been the most recent one utilized and the Montpellier team has certainly the widest experience in this field[10]. The (more or less theoretical) advantages and possible drawbacks of the method are summarized in Table 4. The main superiority of this route, apart from the fact it approaches the physio-

Table 4 I.p. infusions

Advantages	*Drawbacks*
Partly absorbed through the portal system	Peritonitis? (fibrosis or infectious)
Kinetics intermediate between i.v. and s.c.	Ethics (for external pumps)
Large cavity with easy access	Limited duration
No clotting problems	

logical state as an (unknown) proportion of the insulin is absorbed through the portal system, is its effectiveness in brittle diabetics, when conventional intensive, s.c. and i.v. routes of insulin administration have failed.[10].

The very rapid insulin resorption[11], much faster than with the s.c. route, makes this approach very flexible and efficient. The need for a permanent catheter in the peritoneal cavity makes this route for connecting an external pump only valid for very severely affected patients when other methods have failed.

No doubt in the future the i.p. route will be the best choice for implantable devices, as it has already been done in 53 diabetic patients in the world[12].

The two main questions which should be answered at this point are to determine which route is best among the s.c., i.v., i.m., i.po. and i.p. routes of insulin administration and, secondly, to evaluate the results obtained with pump therapy as compared to conventional treatment.

INDICATIONS FOR THE DIFFERENT ROUTES IN INSULIN ADMINISTRATION

Taking into account what has been previously said, it is evident that no one method is totally satisfactory. The choice must be made after balancing the risks encountered by the patients and the advantages of the treatment they can expect. If we accept that the i.m. route is quite cumbersome and the i.po. route unethical to use for the moment in patients wearing an external pump, the choice has to be made between the s.c., the i.v. and the i.p. routes.

– At the present time, due to its ease of use, the s.c. route is certainly the first choice.

– The i.v. route is usually reserved for limited indications in some centres.

– The i.p. route should only be used when other approaches have failed and an improvement is mandatory. For the future the i.p. route appears the most promising one.

RESPECTIVE INDICATIONS OF CONVENTIONAL AND PUMP THERAPY

The questions are:

– Does a pump give better metabolic results than conventional therapy?

– Does a pump have any other advantages over conventional therapy?

Answering these points is not easy, looking at the literature.

The difficulties lie in large differences between centres when defining the type of diabetic treated (stable or brittle), the tool utilized (in particular the quality of the information (education) given to a patient is difficult to assess), the therapeutic goals chosen, the type of population treated (American, European, etc) and the results usually reached in each centre. For example the mean fasting blood glucose values in a non-selected diabetic population can be between 250 and 300 mg/100 ml in one centre[13], between 200 and 250 in another[3], and between 150 and 200 in another. The mean fasting blood glucose value in a study done in our centre on an unselected diabetic population was 1.48 mg/100 ml[14].

Obviously, comparing conventional therapy and pump treatment, the quality of metabolic control can show dramatic differences in a study and small or no differences in another[15].

However it could be said that, even when conventional therapy permits good or very good results, pump treatment can in *some patients* not only (slightly) improve metabolic control but can also greatly improve the quality of life[15].

The main improvement is the smaller risk of severe hypoglycaemic attacks and the greater flexibility in meal time, size and content.

References

1. Murat, A. and Slama, G. (1981). Plasma free insulin levels during continuous subcutaneous insulin infusion (CSII) by pump. *Diabetologia,* **21,** 307
2. Kobayashi, T., Sawano, S., Itoh, T., Kosaka, K., Hirayama, H. and Kasuya, Y. (1983). The pharmacokinetics of insulin after continuous subcutaneous infusion or bolus subcutaneous injection in diabetic patients. *Diabetes,* **32,** 331–336
3. Mecklenburg, R. S., Benson, J. W., Jr., Becker, N. M., Brazel, P. L., Fredlund, P. N., Metz, R. J., Nielsen, R. L., Sannar, C. A. and Steenrod, W. J., Jr. (1982). Clinical use of the insulin infusion pump in 100 patients with Type I diabetes. *N. Engl. J. Med.,* **307,** 513–518
4. Slama, G., Hautecouverture, M., Assan, R., Tchobroutsky, G. (1974). One to five days of continuous intravenous insulin infusion on seven diabetic patients. *Diabetes,* **23,** 732–738
5. Slama, G., Klein, J. C., Delage, A., Ardila, E., Lemaignen, H., Papoz, L. and Tchobroutsky, G. (1981). Correlation between the nature and amount of carbohydrate in meal intake and insulin delivery by the artificial pancreas in 24 insulin-dependent diabetics. *Diabetes,* **30,** 101–105
6. Pickup, J. C., Home, P. D., Bilous, R. W. *et al* (1981). Management of severely brittle diabetics by continuous subcutaneous and intramuscular insulin infusions: evidence for a defect in subcutaneous insulin absorption. *Br. Med. J.,* **282,** 347–349
7. Poulsen, J. S. D., Smith, M., Deckert, M. and Deckert, T. (1980). Comparison of intraperitoneal, intraportal and intravenous insulin infusion. *Acta Endocrinol.,* **95,** 500–504
8. Stevenson, R. W., Parsons, J. A. and Alberti, G. M. M. (1981). Comparison of the metabolic responses to portal and peripheral infusions of insulin in diabetic dogs. *Metabolism,* **30,** 745–752
9. Stout, R. W. (1979). Diabetes and atherosclerosis – the role of insulin. *Diabetologia,* **16,** 141–150
10. Selam, J. L., Slingeneyer, A., Hedon, B., Mares, P., Beraud, J. J. and Mirouze, J. (1983). Long-term ambulatory peritoneal insulin infusion of brittle diabetes with portable pumps: comparison with intravenous and subcutaneous routes. *Diabetes Care,* **6,** 105–111
11. Balducci, A., Slama, G., Rottembourg, J., Baumelou, A. and Delage, A. (1981). Intraperitoneal insulin in uraemic diabetics undergoing continuous ambulatory peritoneal dialysis. *Br. Med. J.,* **283,** 1021–1023

12. Irsigler, K., Kritz, H., Najemnik, C., Hagmuller, G. and Lovett, R. (1983). Pompes implantables à débit continu invariable dans le diabète de type I (Diabète insulino-dépendant). In *Journées Diabetol. Hotel-Dieu,* pp. 65–78. Vol. 1 (Paris: Flammarion Med. Sci. Ed.)
13. Tamborlane, W. V., Sherwin, R. S., Genel, M. *et al* (1979). Normalization of plasma glucose in juvenile diabetics by subcutaneous administration of insulin with a portable infusion pump. *N. Engl. J. Med.,* **300,** 573–576
14. Basdevant, A., Costagliola, D., Lanoe, J. L., Goldgewicht, C., Triomphe, A., Metz, F., Denys, H., Eschwege, E., Fardeau, M. and Tchobroutsky, G. (1982). The risk of diabetic control: a comparison of hospital versus general practice supervision. *Diabetologia,* **22,** 309–314
15. Grimm, J. J., Haardt, M. J., Thibult, N., Levy, A., Goicolea, I., Elgrably, F. and Slama, G. (1983). Metabolic control and psychosocial implications of CSII in non-highly selected Type I diabetics. *EASD Meeting,* Oslo, Sept. 1983 (submitted for publication)

Discussant

U. KELLER

Professor Keller (Switzerland): I should like to make some short comments on Professor Tamborlane's and Professor Slama's papers and to put them in perspective of what we think in Basel is the current role of the insulin pump in the clinical management of diabetics.

Dr Tamborlane's paper demonstrated that long-term improvement of diabetic control by subcutaneous insulin infusions is feasible. In addition he showed that optimized therapy by pumps improved almost all the metabolic and endocrine abnormalities of diabetes. The question we should now discuss is when to use insulin pumps clinically. Should we use them in all insulin-dependent diabetics, or in none?

There are diabetologists who deny any clinical benefit of pump therapy and they usually bring up two arguments against the pump on which I shall comment in more detail. The first argument against the pump relates to the fact that several controlled trials have failed to demonstrate beneficial effects of the pumps. These studies demonstrated that insulin pumps and intensified conventional insulin injection therapy were equally effective in improving glycaemic control in non-selected diabetics who were not well-controlled. However, this kind of trial does not rule out the possibility that selected patients, particularly diabetics with insufficient glycaemic control, in spite of multiple injections and their best effort, will benefit from pump therapy.

Conventional insulin injections have, as we have heard, inherent limitations regarding optimal insulinization throughout the whole day, and we shall never be able to fine-tune insulin availability as required in all situations.

A further factor which has not been discussed which may limit the ability of conventional therapy to normalize glycaemic control is the poor reproducibility of absorption of long-acting insulin. Insulin delivery devices may therefore be a tool to improve bioavailability of insulin because insulin delivery is better controlled. The issue is therefore the selection of patients who do not do well on multiple injections and who do better during controlled delivery of insulin using pumps.

The second point is the fact that the pump may involve certain risks. Cases of sudden death possibly related to hypoglycaemia have been reported. Candidates for pump therapy have therefore to be selected to avoid this problem, and only diabetics who are able to manage their pump and who are compliant in monitoring should be given a pump. In addition, physicians should instruct the patients in its proper use, and physicians should provide continued assistance if necessary.

Taken together, the two injections to pump therapy tell us that not all insulin-treated patients should receive a pump, and that we should make appropriate selection of patients.

One further point has been brought up. Although widely used, subcutaneous infusions have their limitations because of the absorption barrier of the subcutaneous tissue. As Dr Slama pointed out, direct access to the vascular system or to the peritoneum will improve control of insulin delivery. But, from the outside, all these approaches imply a considerable risk, both of infections and of thromboembolic complications. These risks are the reasons why these alternative routes have not found widespread use, but it may be that in certain patients, for instance those who degrade insulin in subcutaneous tissue, these routes may be beneficial.

Taken together, it appears to us that pump therapy is a valuable alternative in patients who do not do well on conventional therapy, in spite of their best efforts. In addition, it may help us to answer some of the questions on the relationship between metabolic control and diabetic complications.

9

Glycohaemoglobin – a measure of glycaemic cruising altitude

K. H. GABBAY

INTRODUCTION

In the past decade, investigations of the structure and biosynthesis of glycosylated haemoglobins have provided a means for objective assessment of the average level of glycaemia in the diabetic patient. The difficulty in accurately assessing the level of long-term glycaemia had in part contributed to the lack of a consensus on a convincing long-term relationship of the glycaemia of diabetes to the development of diabetic complications. Although methodological problems and difficulties in interpretation of results still exist, the use of glycosylated haemoglobin levels as an integrated index of long-term blood glucose levels represents a significant weapon in our research and therapeutic armamentarium. Furthermore, the non-enzymatic reaction between glucose and haemoglobin has served as a model for the non-enzymatic interaction of many other small molecules with haemoglobin and other proteins (e.g. carbamylated haemoglobin in uraemia). This chapter will review the conceptual and practical frameworks that are basic to the understanding and use of this tool.

STRUCTURE AND FORMATION OF GLYCOHAEMOGLOBIN

Cation exchange chromatography of haemolysates of red blood cells resolves four minor haemoglobin components from the main Hb A fraction. These minor components (Hb A_{1a1}, Hb A_{1a2}, Hb A_{1b}, and Hb A_{1c}), collectively referred to as the Hb A_1 fraction, result from post-translational non-enzymatic modification of Hb A by a variety of small molecular weight substances (e.g. glucose, cyanate, phosphorylated sugars, aspirin, etc.), and comprise about 7% of the total haemoglobin in normal subjects. Each of these chromatographically determined components is thus not homogeneous, and may be composed of many different entities. For instance, the Hb A_{1c} peak is composed of haemoglobin modified by various reactants. The major component of the Hb A_{1c} peak (about 70% in normal subjects) is glycosylated haemoglobin. Glycosylated haemoglobin, or glycohaemoglobin, is formed when a glucose molecule attaches to the N-terminal amino group of the β chains to form a Schiff base, which subsequently undergoes an Amadori rearrangement to a stable ketoamine linkage form[1]. It is present in increased amounts in patients with diabetes mellitus as a consequence of the increased blood glucose levels. The post-translational glycosylation of Hb A occurs continuously within the red blood cell throughout its 120-day life span in the circulation.

The attachment of glucose to haemoglobin occurs non-enzymatically via a two-step mechanism (Figure 1). In the initial rapid and reversible condensation, the Schiff base (aldimine) is formed and slowly undergoes the Amadori rearrangement to the more stable ketoamine form. The Schiff base formation is rapid, dependent on the concentration of glucose, and is readily reversible upon dialysis of the reaction mixture, or lowering of the glucose concentration. The ready reversibility of the Schiff base accounts for the reversible 'fast glycosylation' phenomenon described by many authors, since the Schiff base form of Hb A_{1c} elutes from a cation exchange resin with the same mobility as the more stable ketoamine form.

Although the ketoamine form is the more stable configuration, an equilibrium exists between the two forms which strongly favours the ketoamine. One indication of the Amadori rearrangement is found upon mild acid hydrolysis of HbA_{1c}[2], which liberates 5-hydroxymethylfurfural (5-HMF). The formation of 5-HMF (Figure 2), identified by the characteristic spectrum of the adduct formed with thiobarbituric acid, is specific for

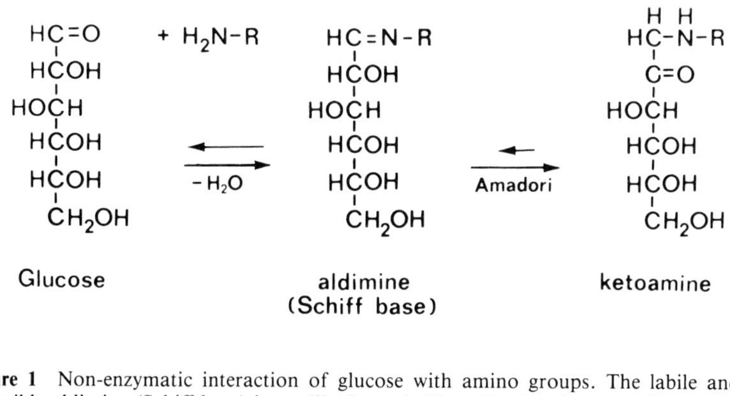

Figure 1 Non-enzymatic interaction of glucose with amino groups. The labile and easily reversible aldimine (Schiff base) is readily formed. The aldimine slowly enolizes to form the more stable ketoamine configuration via an Amadori rearrangement

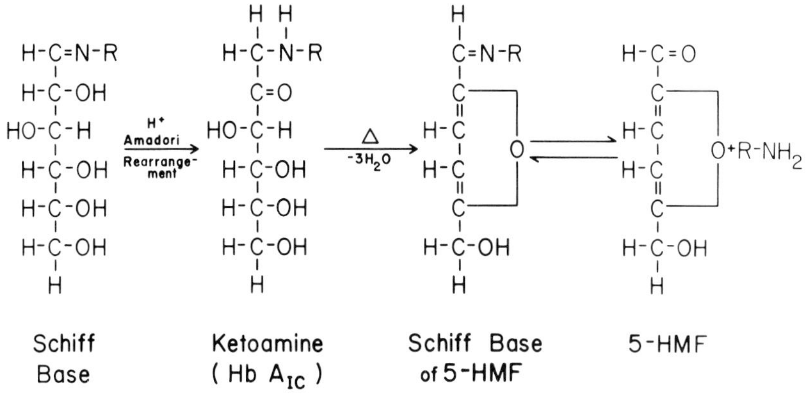

5-HMF + 2-Thiobarbituric Acid ⟶ Adduct
(Abs_{max} 443 nm)

Figure 2 Chemistry of the TBA colorimetric test for detection of glycosylation. Only the ketoamine rearranged form reacts to yield 5-hydroxymethylfurfural (5-HMF). The latter is detected by forming an adduct with thiobarbituric acid

ketoamine-linked hexoses and forms the basis for a specific chemical method to detect total ketoamine glycosylation of proteins (see below).

Hb A_{1a1} and Hb A_{1a2} are predominantly the β chain N-terminal adducts of fructose-1, 6-diphosphate, and glucose-6-phosphate respectively, while Hb A_{1b} is thought to be possibly related to Hb A_{1c}. In addition, glycosylation also occurs at the α chain N-terminal amino group as well as the ϵ-amino groups of lysine residues in both α and β chains. The extent of glycosylation at the various sites increases proportionately, indicating that haemoglobin glycosylation is a general and non-specific process, with its extent determined primarily by the prevailing glucose concentration and the relative reactivities of the various amino groups[2].

RELATION OF GLYCOHAEMOGLOBIN LEVELS TO DIABETIC HYPERGLYCAEMIA

From the structural and biosynthetic information available, it is clear that glycohaemoglobin is formed slowly and almost irreversibly by the condensation of two abundant reactants within the red blood cell, namely glucose and haemoglobin. With continuous accumulation of glycohaemoglobin, it is evident that the amount of this component should be a reflection of the average glucose concentration seen by the red blood cells during their life span.

Direct evidence for this relationship derives from at least three lines of investigations, which include: (1) a reduction in glycohaemoglobin levels after diabetic patients are brought under optimal blood glucose control; (2) a plethora of studies which demonstrate a relationship between glycohaemoglobin levels and a variety of diabetic glycaemia indices, and (3) excellent correlations between clinical evaluation of the patient's level of control and glycohaemoglobin levels (for detailed reviews, see references 3 and 4).

MEASUREMENT OF GLYCOHAEMOGLOBIN LEVELS

Haemoglobin glycosylation is currently estimated by two basic methods which operate on different principles and yield independent results that are nonetheless related. The chromatographic methods depend on a net change in the charge of the haemoglobin molecule when the N-terminal position of the β chain is modified. Thus, the components Hb A_{1a-c} are eluted readily from a cation exchange resin and can be quantitated and expressed as a percentage of total haemoglobin. Haemoglobin molecules glycosylated at sites other than the β N-termini do not have sufficiently altered net charge to enhance their mobilities and are hence not measured by these techniques. These chromatographic separations are exquisitely sensitive to minor changes in buffer pH and temperature which can significantly affect the values obtained.

Separation based on a charge difference is the basis for the standard Biorex-70 column chromatography, iso-electric focusing, high performance liquid chromatography, and the popular commercial minicolumn kits. The latter columns measure the sum of Hb A_{1a-c} (referred to by the trivial name 'fast haemoglobins'), and are unfortunately particularly sensitive to temperature and pH changes. In general, the methods that depend on charge change are not readily amenable to standardization and long-term quality control procedures.

The other general type of method involves direct chemical measurement of total glycosylation. In the TBA method[2,5], furfural compounds are generated from the ketoamine-linked carbohydrated moieties upon heating under acidic conditions and are quantitated colorimetrically with 2-thiobarbituric acid (see Figure 2). This test has advantages in that it is easily performed, provides a reliable assessment of total glycosylation, is specific for the stable ketoamine form, and is particularly suited to quality control procedures and laboratory standardization[2,4–6].

A variety of new methods which may have future promise has recently become available. We described a very sensitive method for the determination of total glycosylation in very small amounts of protein, e.g. 0.5 mg haemoglobin. The method[7] depends on the fluorometric detection of formaldehyde released upon periodate oxidation of the protein.

A promising new chromatographic method was recently described by

Garlick *et al*[8], which is distinctly different from previous chromatographic procedures. The method uses large pore beads (GlycoGel B) with immobilized phenylboronic acid. The boronic acid side chains form reversible complexes with vicinal hydroxyl groups of carbohydrate moeities (either aldimine or ketoamine-linked hexose) present on proteins with resultant selective retention of glycosylated proteins. The glycosylated proteins can then be eluted from the beads with a sugar such as glucose or sorbitol. Results obtained with this method suggest that glycosylation accounts for only about 70% of the Hb A_{1c} peak isolated by cation exchange chromatography of a haemolysate. This would be consistent with the finding of a variety of non-glucose substances that can modify the N-terminal amino acid of the β chain (e.g. carbamylation, see below). The phenylboronic affinity chromatography method has the potential drawbacks of reactivity with both the aldimine and ketoamine forms of glycohaemoglobin, as well as a narrow range of buffer pH, and sensitivity to the geometric design and flow characteristics of the columns.

GLYCOHAEMOGLOBIN AND HAEMOGLOBIN CARBAMYLATION IN URAEMIA

Both Hb A_{1c} and Hb A_1 fractions, chromatographically determined, have been reported to be elevated in uraemic subjects[9]. This increase is now known[10] to result from haemoglobin carbamylation occuring via the condensation of urea-derived cyanate with the N-terminal amino groups of the haemoglobin chains (Figure 3). This form of non-glycosylated haemoglobin is detected by column chromatography, but not by the TBA method which is specific for the detection of glycosylation (Figure 4). The increased HbA_1 level in uraemia correlates with the BUN level. We have identified valine hydantoin which is released from the carbamylated N-termini of the haemoglobin chains upon acid hydrolysis, and showed that the valine hydantoin levels correlate with the time-averaged BUN of the previous 2–3 months in haemodialysed and stable

$$NH_2-\overset{O}{\overset{\|}{C}}-NH_2 \rightleftharpoons NH_4^+ + {}^-NCO \qquad (I)$$

$$R-NH_2 + HN=C=O \longrightarrow R-\overset{H}{\overset{|}{N}}-\overset{O}{\overset{\|}{C}}-NH_2 \qquad (II)$$

Figure 3 Formation of cyanate from urea and its reaction with an amino group (reprinted from Fluckiger *et al* (1981), by kind permission of *N. Engl. J. Med.*, **304,** 823–827

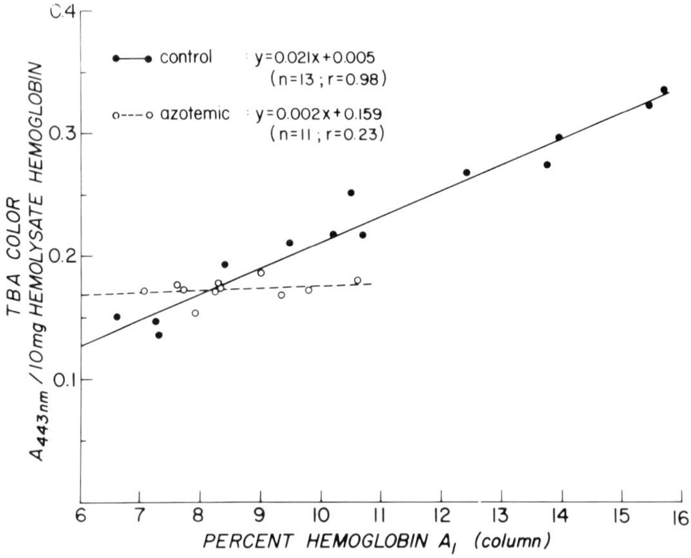

Figure 4 Relation of chemical estimates (TBA color) to column chromatographic estimates (Hb A_1 values) of haemoglobin glycosylation in 11 patients with uraemia ('uraemic') and 13 patients without uraemia ('control'). The TBA values did not increase in uraemia despite elevations in Hb A_1 levels (reprinted from Fluckiger *et al* (1981), by kind permission of *N. Engl. J. Med.*, **304,** 823–827

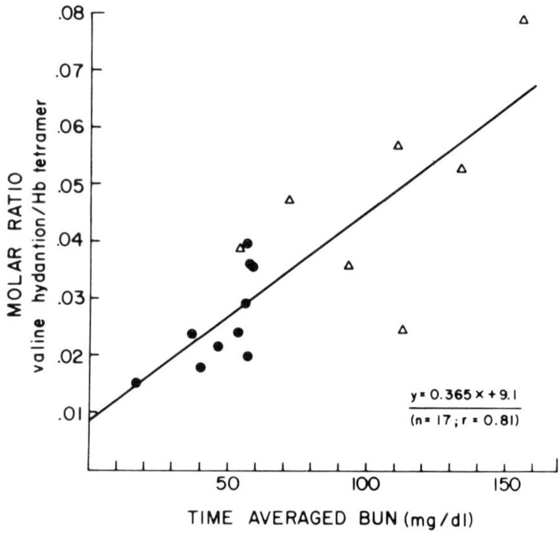

Figure 5 Relation of haemoglobin-derived valine hydantoin to time-averaged BUN in 17 patients with uraemia. Ten patients received long-term haemodialysis (circles) and seven did not (triangles). Haemoglobin carbamylation correlated significantly ($r = 0.81$, $p < 0.001$) with the time-averaged BUN of the previous two months (reprinted from Fluckiger *et al* (1981), by kind permission of *N. Engl. J. Med.*, **304,** 823–827

non-dialysed uraemic patients (Figure 5). The carbamylated haemoglobin level thus appears to integrate the BUN levels over a long period of time – a situation analogous to that seen for glycohaemoglobin levels in diabetic patients. Therefore, the assessment of true glycohaemoglobin levels in *diabetic* uraemic patients must be performed by the specific chemical TBA method.

LIMITATIONS OF THE ASSAY

Table 1 lists a number of situations in which chromatographic-type procedures lead to falsely abnormal values. Conditions such as uraemia, aspirin intake, antibiotic therapy and alcohol intake can all lead to falsely elevated glycosylated haemoglobin levels by the chromatographic techniques. These effects are caused by changes in charge of the haemoglobin molecule brought about by post-translational modifications occurring via mechanisms other than glycosylation. As mentioned above, carbamylated haemoglobin species lead to falsely elevated values for Hb A_1 in uraemia by the chromatographic techniques, but are not measured by the TBA colorimetric procedure. Similar considerations apply to aspirin, antibiotic and alcohol intakes. The presence of fetal haemoglobin (Hb F), and certain other unusual negatively charged haemoglobin variants such as Hb H and Hb I, also leads to marked elevation of Hb A_1 values because of the altered molecular charges. In contrast, patients with variant haemoglobins such as Hb S, C or D have falsely low values because these more positively charged haemoglobins bind more tightly to the cation exchange resin[11]. It should be kept in mind that glycohaemoglobin levels (by any method) will be significantly reduced in patients with decreased red cell

Table 1

I – Conditions leading to false elevation of Hb A_1

A. *Chromatographic abnormalities:*
1. Hyperlipidaemia – due to lactescence
2. Elevated temperature and/or buffer pH
3. Negatively charged Hb variants – e.g. Hb F
4. Acute hyperglycaemia – 'fast glycosylation'

B. *Other post-translational Hb modifications:*
1. Aspirin – acetylation
2. Antibiotics – penicilloylation
3. Alcohol – 5-deoxy-xylulose-1-phosphate
4. Uraemia – carbamylation

II – Conditions leading to falsely low Hb A_1 values

A. *Chromatographic abnormalities:*
1. Low temperature and/or buffer pH
2. Positively charged Hb variants – e.g. Hb S, C

B. *Altered red blood cell dynamics:*
1. Increased destruction – e.g. haemolytic anaemia
2. Active erythropoeisis – e.g. pregnancy
3. Recent transfusions

life span (e.g. anaemia, uraemia) or patients with active erythropoiesis (e.g. pregnancy).

It is now common practice directly to chromatograph whole blood haemolysates which may give rise to artefacts in two circumstances. In hyperlipaemic blood samples, an increased 'fast' haemoglobin fraction may result from interference by lactescence. In addition, when rapid column methods are used to measure Hb A_1, variable amounts of the labile aldimine species of Hb A_{1c} will be measured along with the stable ketoamine Hb A_{1c}. This problem does not arise if the haemolysates are adequately dialysed prior to chromatography. Specific determination of total haemoglobin glycosylation by chemical means (e.g. TBA method) circumvents all the above complications with the exception of the effect resulting from the decreased red blood cell life span.

INDICATIONS FOR USE OF GLYCOHAEMOGLOBIN

Clearly, estimation of glycohaemoglobin levels provides an important tool for clinical research in diabetes, particularly in the insulin-dependent diabetic patients where blood glucose levels may be subject to wide fluctuation. Such fluctuation in blood glucose seldom occurs in non-insulin-dependent diabetic individuals under dietary and/or oral hypoglycaemic agent therapy. The overall degree of glucose intolerance in such patients can be readily and more economically estimated by fasting blood glucose measurements. Of course, glycohaemoglobin levels can always be measured with the patient in the fed, non-fasting state and, hence, may be more convenient in the management of diabetic patients in general, and in office practice in particular.

Glycohaemoglobin levels have an important role to play in the routine management of insulin-dependent diabetic patients. For the first time, the physician can independently and objectively assess average diabetic glycaemia with minimal patient cooperation. Similarly, objective results may have a positive motivating influence on the patient by providing a target number for average blood glucose control. Comparisons of different treatment regimens or patient groups are now facilitated. As a diagnostic tool, estimations of glycohaemoglobin levels are not as discriminating in detecting subclinical, borderline diabetes as the standard oral glucose tolerance test or even the fasting blood glucose level. Nevertheless, its convenience and lack of acute dependence on such variables as patient cooperation, time of day, stress, exercise, food intake, and renal threshold makes it an attractive screening test for unequivocal diabetes in population studies.

ACKNOWLEDGEMENT
Supported by grants AM-15019 and HL-20539 from the National Institutes of Health.

References

1. Bunn, H.F., Haney, D.N., Gabbay, K.H. and Gallop, P.M. (1975). *Biochem. Biophys. Res. Commun.,* **67,** 103
2. Gabbay, K.H., Sosenko, J.M., Banuchi, G.A., Mininsohn, M.J. and Fluckiger, R. (1979). *Diabetes,* **28,** 337–340
3. Bunn, H.F., Gabbay, K.H. and Gallop, P.M. (1978). *Science,* **200,** 21–27
4. Bunn, H.F. (1980). In Gordon, A. S., Silber, R. and LoBue, J. (eds.). *Contemporary Hematology.* (New York: Plenum Press)
5. Fluckiger, R. and Winterhalter, K. (1978). *FEBS Lett.,* **71,** 356–360
6. Pecoraro, R.E., Graf, R.J., Halter, J.B., Beiler, H. and Porte, D. (1979). *Diabetes,* **28,** 1120–1125
7. Gallop, P.M., Fluckiger, R., Hanneken, A., Mininsohn, M.M. and Gabbay, K.H. (1981). *Anal. Biochem.,* **117,** 427–432
8. Garlick, R.L., Mazer, J.S., Higgins, P.J. and Bunn, H.F. (1983). *J. Clin. Invest.,* **71,** 1062–1072
9. Saibene, J.V., Brembilla, L., Bertoletti, A., Bolognani, L. and Pozza, G. (1979). *Clin. Chem. Acta,* **93,** 199–205
10. Fluckiger, R., Harmon, W., Meier, W., Loo, S.W. and Gabbay, K.H. (1981). *N. Engl. J. Med.,* **304,** 823–827
11. Sosenko, J.M., Fluckiger, R., Platt, O.S. and Gabbay, K.H. (1980). *Diabetes Care,* **3,** 590–593

10
Non-glycaemic determinants of diabetic complications

P. J. LEFÈBVRE

INTRODUCTION

After decades of hesitations in the literature, few, if any, diabetologists now question the predominant role that chronically excessive blood glucose levels play in the pathogenesis of the diabetic complications. As already reviewed in detail in this Symposium, the natural history of diabetic complications in experimental models and in man, as well as the beneficial effects of tight control, both support such a concept.

However, there is some evidence that factors other than blood glucose may, to a certain extent, have an influence on the incidence and/or severity of diabetic complications. These factors include heredity, insulin antibodies, circulating immune complexes and hormones. Their role has been reviewed recently and masterly by the late Andrew Cudworth together with H. J. Bodansky. Most of the relevant literature can be found in their paper[1].

DOES HEREDITY HAVE AN INFLUENCE ON THE DEVELOPMENT OF THE BASEMENT MEMBRANE DISEASE OF DIABETES?

The paper published in 1968 by Siperstein *et al*[2] has been the starting point of a long controversy about the role that heredity may play in the basement membrane disease of diabetes. In that paper it was reported that the thickness of capillary basement membrane of quadriceps femoris muscle was markedly increased not only in a group of 51 diabetic patients but also in 53% of a group of 30 subjects considered as 'prediabetics' (these subjects had normal glucose tolerance tests but both of their parents were diabetic). It is now generally accepted[3] that the conclusion of Siperstein *et al*[2] that 'thickening of the muscle capillary basement membranes is a characteristic of genetic diabetes mellitus, and further, that the hyperglycemia of diabetes is probably not the factor responsible for the microangiopathy characteristic of diabetes' was not substantiated since (1) basal membrane thickness had been underestimated in the normal, younger control group, and (2) duration of diabetes had not been known precisely in several of the patients included in the diabetic series.

Since it is now accepted that type I, insulin-dependent, and type II, non insulin-dependent, diabetes are indeed different diseases, one has to envisage separately the possible role of heredity on the complications of diabetes.

The role of heredity on the development of diabetic complications in type I diabetes

It is beyond the scope of the present short paper to review the abundant evidence that type I diabetes is strongly associated with certain antigens of the HLA system. As summarized by Cudworth and Bodansky[1], in type I diabetes there appear to be at least two susceptibility genes, or groups of closely related genes associated with the following, not exclusive, HLA specificities:

S1 axis: DW3 - DR3 - B8 - CW7 - A1
S2 axis: DW4 - DR4 - BW62 (major part of B15) - CW3 - A2

It is generally considered that the relative risk for type I diabetes, with a value of 1 in the general population, is 3–4 for the individuals having either DW3 (-DR3) or DW4 (-DR4), while it can raise up to 40 for those having both DW3 (-DR3) *and* DW4 (-DR4). Many studies, reviewed in ref. 1, have attempted to correlate HLA-linked genes to the pathogenesis of the microvascular disease of diabetes, but none has led to unequivocal and universally accepted conclusions, although, in the field of diabetic *nephropathy*, two studies[4,5] have indicated a significant increase in HLA-B8, a finding not confirmed by Jervell and Solheim[6]. Other studies have suggested a possible association of *severe proliferative retinopathy* with HLA-B15 (or DR-4 which is in linkage desequilibrium with B-15).

The role of heredity on the development of diabetic complications in type II diabetes

Although the role of heredity is predominant in type II diabetes, there is no evidence of preferential association with HLA phenotypes. As in type I diabetes, duration and severity of hyperglycaemia undoubtedly play the predominant role in the development of diabetic complications. Over the last few years, Pyke's group at King's College Hospital in London has reported that certain type II diabetic patients exhibit a severe facial 'flush' when ingesting alcohol after having taken chlorpropamide. This chlorpropamide–alcohol flush phenomenon seems to be inherited as a Mendelian dominant trait[7]. Leslie *et al*[8] have reported that diabetic retinopathy and persistent proteinuria were less frequent in the chlorpropamide–alcohol flush positive than in the chlorpropamide–alcohol flush negative patients, and therefore suggested that the patients with a positive test might be, to a certain extent, generically 'protected' against complications of diabetes. This seems to be particularly the case of the patients with maturity-onset diabetes of the youth (MODY) who are often positive in the chloropropamide–alcohol flush tests and who are frequently relatively free of the complications of diabetes. However, further studies are needed to establish that, for a similar degree of hyperglycaemia of similar duration, chlorpropamide–alcohol 'flushers' are indeed less exposed to diabetic microangeiopathy than the 'non-flushers'.

IS THERE A LINK BETWEEN INSULIN ANTIBODY PRODUCTION AND DIABETIC COMPLICATIONS?

That anti-insulin antibodies may be involved in the pathogenesis of diabetic complications has been raised by the early observations of Andersen[9], that patients with retinopathy often exhibit higher insulin binding capacity of their plasma. Two studies[10,11] have reported a possible association of high insulin antibody levels with HLA-B15, which, as already mentioned, has been claimed to be associated with severe proliferative retinopathy. However, in a series of 434 type I diabetic patients, 126 of them having proliferative retinopathy, Bodansky *et al*[12] did not find association between HLA-B15 and high levels of circulating antibodies. Similarly, no correlation has been found between increased antibody titres, capillary basement membrane thickening and proliferative retinopathy by Deckert *et al*[13]. A strong argument against a major role of anti-insulin antibodies in the pathogenesis of diabetic microangiopathy lies in the fact that the latter occurs in patients who have never received insulin injections.

IS THERE A LINK BETWEEN CIRCULATING IMMUNE COMPLEXES AND DIABETIC COMPLICATIONS?

This topic has been recently reviewed by Di Mario *et al*[14]. Increased production and/or decreased removal of immune complexes may be involved to explain the raised levels of immunocomplexes found in some diabetic patients[15]. In a randomly selected population, Di Mario *et al*[16] reported circulating immune complexes to be increased in a small but significant proportion of insulin-treated diabetic patients, particularly in those with at least 11–20 years duration of the disease. Both Irvine *et al*[17] and Ventriglia *et al*[18] reported increased prevalence of immune complexes in patients with microangiopathy. As shown by Andreani *et al*[19], the presence of immune complexes seems to be more closely related to the presence of microangiopathic changes rather than to the duration of the illness or the type of antidiabetic treatment. The extent to which circulating immune-complexes play a role in the initiation or aggravation of microvascular disease or, merely represent a consequence of decreased removal remains to be established[1,14,20].

IS THERE A ROLE FOR HORMONES IN THE PATHOGENESIS OF DIABETIC MICROANGIOPATHY?

Numerous data indicate that *insulin lack* is primarily involved in the pathogenesis of diabetic microangiopathy. As discussed by others in this Symposium, the deleterious effect of insulin lack mainly results from prolonged hyperglycaemia, although other biochemical mechanisms resulting from insulin deficiency have been envisaged. Most forms of chronic aggressive insulin therapy, either conventional or using insulin delivery devices, induce *high peripheral insulin levels*. There is no evidence that this may induce or aggravate microangiopathy, but there is some indication that it may favour macroangiopathy[21]. All forms of known diabetes are accompanied by absolute or relative increased *glucagon* circulating levels (reviewed in reference 22). There is no evidence that glucagon is directly involved in the pathogenesis of microangiopathy, to which it undoubtedly contributes indirectly through its effect on blood glucose. *Growth hormone* is classically considered as deleterious on the diabetic microvascular disease; such a concept has emerged from the beneficial effects that spontaneous pituitary necrosis or pituitary therapeutic ablation have on the course of diabetic retinopathy (reviewed in reference 23) and also from the observation of Merimee[24] that sexual ateliotic dwarfs exhibit marked diminution of glucose tolerance over the years without evidence of microangiopathy. Finally, it is generally accepted that type I diabetes has a slightly higher prevalence in males than in females. Even taking this into account, various statistics indicate that *male* diabetics tend to be more susceptible than *female* patients to develop diabetic microangiopathy. The reason for this situation is unclear, it does not seem to be associated with the HLA - DR3 - A1 haplotype more frequently seen in males[1], and clearly further studies are needed to clarify whether this is an inherited trait or whether it is related to a different hormonal milieu.

ACKNOWLEDGEMENTS

We acknowledge the expert secretarial help of E. Vaessen–Petit.

References

1. Cudworth, A.G. and Bodansky, H.J. (1982). Genetic and immunological factors in diabetic complications. In Keen, H. and Jarrett, J. (eds.). *Complications of Diabetes,* pp. 1–12. (London: Edward Arnold)
2. Siperstein, M.D., Unger, R.H. and Madison, L.L. (1968). Studies of muscle capillary basement membranes in normal subjects, diabetic and prediabetic patients. *J. Clin. Invest.,* **47**, 1973
3. Ross, H., Bernstein, G. and Rifkin, H. (1983). Relationships of metabolic control of diabetes mellitus to long-term complications. In Ellenberg, M. and Rifkin, H. (eds.). *Diabetes Mellitus, Theory and Practice* (3rd edn.). pp. 907–926. (New York: Medical Examination Publishing Co.)

4. Barbosa, J., Noreen, H., Emme, L., Goetz, S., Simmons, R., deLeiva, A., Najarian, J. and Yunis, E. J. (1976). Histocompatibility (HLA) antigens and diabetic microangiopathy. *Tissue Antigens,* **7,** 233
5. Jones, R. H. (1982). cited by Cudworth, A. G. and Bodansky, H. J. (1982). In Keen, H. and Jarrett, J. (eds.). *Complications of Diabetes,* p. 4. (London: Edward Arnold)
6. Jervell, J. and Solheim, B. (1979). HLA-Antigens in long-standing insulin-dependent diabetics with terminal nephropathy and retinopathy with or without loss of vision. *Diabetologia,* **17,** 391
7. Leslie, R. D. G. and Pyke, D. A. (1978). Chlorpropamide–alcohol flushing: a dominantly inherited trait associated with diabetes. *Br. Med. J.,* **2,** 1519
8. Leslie, R. D. G., Barnett, A. H. and Pyke, D. A. (1979). Diabetic retinopathy and chlorpropamide–alcohol flushing. *Lancet,* **i,** 997
9. Andersen, O. O. (1976). Anti-insulin antibodies and later diabetic complications. *Acta Endocrinol.,* **83,** 329
10. Bertrams, J., Jansen, F. K., Grüneklee, D., Reis, H. E., Drost, H., Beyer, J., Gries, F. A. and Kuwert, E. (1976). HLA Antigens and immunoresponsiveness to insulin-dependent diabetes mellitus. *Tissue Antigens,* **8,** 13
11. Schernthaner, G., Ludwig, H., Mayr, W. R. and Frisch, H. (1977). Evidence for genetic control of anti-insulin antibodies in juvenile-onset diabetes mellitus. *Diab. Metab.,* **3,** 117
12. Bodansky, H. J., Wolf, E., Cudworth, A. G., Dean, B. M., Nineham, L. J., Bottazzo, G. F., Matthews, J. A., Kurtz, A. B. and Kohner, E. M. (1982). Genetic and immunologic factors in microvascular disease in type I insulin-dependent diabetes. *Diabetes,* **31,** 70
13. Deckert, T., Egeberg, J., Frimodt-Møller, C., Sander, E. and Svejgaard, A. (1979). Basement membrane thickness, insulin antibodies and HLA-antigens in long standing insulin-dependent diabetics with and without severe retinopathy. *Diabetologia,* **17,** 9
14. Di Mario, U., Iavicoli, M., Pozzilli, P. and Andreani, D. (1982). Immunological aspects of diabetic microangiopathy: the possible role of immune complexes. In Cudworth, A. G., Andreani, D., Bodansky, H. J. and Squadrito, G. (eds.). *Diabetes and its Late Complications,* pp. 27–31. (London: John Libbey)
15. Irvine, W. J., Al-Kateeb, S. F., Di Mario, U., Feek, C. M., Gray, R. S., Edmond, B. and Duncan, L. J. P. (1977). Soluble immune complexes in the sera of newly diagnosed insulin dependent diabetics and in treated diabetics. *Clin. Exp. Immunol.,* **30,** 16
16. Di Mario, U., Iavicoli, M. and Andreani, D. (1980). Circulating immune complexes in diabetes. *Diabetologia,* **19,** 89
17. Irvine, W. J., Di Mario, U., Guy, K., Iavicoli, M., Pozzilli, P., Lumbroso, B. and Andreani, D. (1978). Immune complexes and diabetic microangiopathy. *J. Clin. Lab. Immunol.,* **1,** 187
18. Ventriglia, L., Di Mario, U., Pietravalle, P., Galfo, C. and Iavicoli, M. (1983). Circulating immune complexes in the evolution of late diabetic complications. *Diabetologia.* (In press)
19. Andreani, D., Di Mario, U., Galfo, C., Ventriglia, L. and Iavicoli, M. (1982). Circulating immune complexes in diabetics with severe microangiopathy: evaluation by two different methods. *Acta Endocrinol.,* **99,** 239
20. Di Mario, U., Iavicoli, M. and Andreani, D. (1980). Circulating immune complexes in diabetes. *Diabetologia,* **19,** 89
21. Stout, R. W. (1979). Diabetes and Atherosclerosis - The role of insulin. *Diabetologia,* **16,** 141
22. Lefèbvre, P. J. and Luyckx, A. S. (1979). Glucagon and diabetes: a reappraisal. *Diabetologia,* **16,** 347
23. Joachim, M., Stevenaert, A., Luyckx, A. and Stals, J. (1980). La place de l'hypophysectomie dans le traitement de la rétinopathie diabétique. *Bull. Soc. Belge Ophthalmol.,* **188–189,** 193
24. Merimee, T. J. (1978). A follow-up study of vascular disease in growth-hormone-deficient dwarfs with diabetes. *N. Engl. J. Med.,* **298,** 1217

Open discussion

Professor Lameire: I should like to ask Dr Gabbay a simple, practical question concerning the use of glycosylated haemoglobin in uraemics. He said that there is an artificial elevation due to the chemical reaction with cyanate, and on the other hand there can also be an artificial lowering of the fast haemoglobin due to the shortened red cell survival. How do these two factors cancel out?

Related to that, when a diabetic uraemic patient is treated with a method such as peritoneal dialysis where the uraemia *per se* remains quite stable, can one then say, if there is a change seen in fast haemoglobin, that this is really related to changes in glucose control.

Professor Gabbay: If the thiobarbituric acid method is used, one can get a direct estimate of the glycosylation, regardless of the metabolic state (normal, diabetic or uraemic). Increased haemolysis with a decrease in the haemoglobin will lower the proportion glycosylated.

Professor H. Keen (UK): Can Professor Gabbay give a brief opinion about glycosylation of proteins other than haemoglobin as indicators of diabetic status?

Professor Gabbay: Any protein in the body can get glycoslyated. Albumin has been attracting the most attention. As a way of measuring glycosylation it is valid, but we do not know the half life of albumin in the circulation, and we have no way of looking at states where the albumin level is decreased, for instance, if the turnover is altered. In diabetes, especially if there is any kind of a renal problem, there is an accelerated loss of albumin, so whereas it can be used, we really do not think it can be used in as valid a way as, say, haemoglobin, where we can estimate if there is increased synthesis or destruction of red blood cells.

Some studies have reported that lipoproteins can be glycosylated and it has been suggested that the turnover of these proteins is altered by glycosylation. I tend to think that that is not so, but we are not yet sure. The basement membrane itself can be glycosylated by the kind of chemical reaction that I described. I suspect this plays some part in the basement membrane thickening we see in diabetes.

Dr V Parsons (UK): Professor Gabbay did not have time to mention the effects of his control on platelet function. In most ongoing nephritic diseases there are alterations in the coagulation factors and platelet reactions in the plasma and they may have a part to play in vascular disease.

Professor Gabbay: In our studies of a young juvenile diabetic population that presumably does not have much arteriosclerosis there were, surprisingly, no platelet abnormalities whatsoever. Platelet abnormalities in older diabetics may be due to what I call the rusty pipe syndrome. If the pipes are rusty the platelets will become damaged and their function abnormal.

Dr S B Beardsworth (UK): I suggest a possible reason for the male preponderance of diabetic complications. In non-diabetic renal disease, there appears to be a preponderance in females of the immune disorders, whereas in males there is a preponderance of glomerulonephritis. This may be due to greater exposure of men to hydrocarbons in the environment at work. This may also be the case in male diabetics. Hydrocarbon may be the common link between the two.

Dr E Kohner (London): Platelet abnormalities are not found in early diabetes. They are the result of the abnormalities of the small vessels. They are a reparative process. Dr Massimo Porta from Italy has shown that platelet abnormalities only occur in severe diabetic microvascular disease. They are therefore not a cause. They are an effect.

Professor Lefebvre: Dr Kohner has reviewed, and I believe has participated in those studies showing higher prevalence of some HLA groups in severe proliferative retinopathy. Has she any comment on that?

Dr Kohner: Dr Bodansky's studies were done in our clinic. There were more males than females with both retinopathy and nephropathy but there was no difference in the HLA groups.

Dr Reach (Paris): On the sex distribution of complications, what about the B-cell residual function in males as compared to females?

Professor Lefebvre: I am not aware of any systematic study performed with age-matched groups and duration of diabetes and so on. This clearly merits study.

Professor Gabbay: I wanted to comment on the genetic factors. We are studying a population that has been completely HLA and complement typed so that we are now able to recognize extended haplotypes that involve the entire MHC. As a result we can divide the DR3 individuals into two different subtypes.

We find no relationship whatsoever between any of the things we are measuring, be it the muscle CBMT, the cholesterol levels, or what have you, with the HLA types but the HLA region is only a very small part of the total genome.

Professor Lameire: It must be very disturbing if one looks at the relationship between HLA types and a very common disease like diabetes to take into account the phenomenon of linkage disequilibrium. That means that several loci may be located on one haplotype more frequently than one would expect from statistical analysis. Moreover, this linkage disequilibrium phenomenon is different in different areas of the world, and we must be very cautious in interpreting the data.

Professor Lefebvre: That is true. The point is that it has been long claimed that the association was with HLA-B8 and B15, and now there has been a move, and this is more solid, showing that the association is closer with DR3 or DR4 which are in linkage disequilibrium with the B locus alleles.

DR3 and DR4 exist in the islet cells themselves, so at least there is a potentiality there.

Dr Barsi (Italy): I should like to ask Professor Lefebvre about the sexual distribution of microangiopathy. Is there any difference in the prevalence of chlorpropamide alcohol flush as between males and females?

Professor Lefebvre: Frankly I cannot answer that question. Professor Keen says that there is no difference.

Dr R Bouillon (Belgium): May patients with diabetic nephropathy also have neuropathy, and as a consequence fail to respond with epinephrine and glucagon release after hypoglycaemia? Would Professor Tamborlane consider that a contra-indication for using insulin pump treatment?

Professor Tamborlane: The question is whether there are predictors for patients who may be at greater risk of hypoglycaemia. This is an area of active investigation. Some groups have suggested that certain responses during a hypoglycaemia test may help to predict who may have more trouble with hypoglycaemia than others. Some groups say the tests are good and others say that they are not, so it is still open to question.

Intensive treatment, whether with pumps or multiple injections, may reduce the regulatory responses and so theoretically make the patients more susceptible to hypoglycaemia. Ultimately what matters is if the risk of hypoglycaemia outside the hospital is increased.

Professor Keen: Perhaps I could add a word to that.

Dr Viberti and I looked at a group of insulin-dependent diabetics and selected on no basis other than that they were available and prepared to take part in studies of beta adrenergic blockers on recovery from the hypoglycaemia. They were infused intravenously with insulin to the point of hypoglycaemia and then the insulin was stopped and the counter-regulatory response studied on one occasion after beta blockers, and on another occasion after placebo.

Of the patients that we studied, not nephropaths or neuropaths, just ordinary diabetics from the diabetic clinic, all showed counter-regulatory palsy. The blood glucose stayed down when the insulin was stopped, despite a prompt rise in fatty acid levels and other indicators of response.

The counter-regulatory response to hypoglycaemia in the average insulin-dependent diabetic is poor. One of the questions is can it improve? There is contradictory evidence of the effects of exposure to normalized levels of blood glucose, on recovery of the counter-regulatory response. But these are still very important areas of investigation if only because increasing numbers of patients will be subjected to intensified control.

The problem with counter-regulation seems to me to be an argument in favour of carefully metered administration of insulin by some such method as continuous subcutaneous insulin infusion, where at least one knows and can control the rate of insulin access to the system, rather than depositing two or three large doses of insulin a day under the skin. Absorption from day to day we know to be very variable. We need carefully constructed studies to compare the relative efficacy and hazards of the two approaches to tighter control.

Dr G Viberti (UK): I want to come back to the problem of hypoglycaemia in the patient with established diabetic nephropathy, especially in the light of pump treatment. The problem that Professor Berger raised is a very important one. We have been looking at this problem in our series of patients with nephropathy before they get to end-stage renal failure.

The problem of hypoglycaemia in a patient with established nephropathy is important whether treated by conventional treatment or by pump treatment. Such patients are more prone to hypoglycaemia. An added problem is that most of these patients do not feel their hypoglycaemia; they lose their warning symptoms. We have compared a group of renal failure patients on pumps with a matched group of patients on conventional treatment. There is no question that the nephropaths treated with the pump had better glycaemic control, but when we defined as hypoglycaemia a level of blood glucose below 3 mmol/l, what came out was that the patients treated by pump had three times as many hypoglycaemic values compared with the matched group treated by conventional injection therapy.

We have to weigh up advantages against disadvantages, but this is a serious problem in the patient with established nephropathy, and we should be aware of it.

What should we strive for? For normoglycaemia? Or should we accept average control which avoids the risk of hypoglycaemia?

Professor Tamborlane: These problems are problems that accompany targeting the glucose at a certain level. When we are striving for mean plasma glucose of 100 mg/dl and glycosylated haemoglobin values within the normal range, then universally there are problems with hypoglycaemia with whatever treatment. Fortunately in most of the patients from a clinical point of view it is relatively mild, but I do not think it is a pump versus injection issue. Our experience has been that the problems with hypoglycaemia occur more commonly with injections rather than with pump therapy – if we are shooting for the same target glycaemic goal. We are then faced with the risk benefit decision. The advantage is to try to individualize the risk of hypoglycaemia against the potential benefits. There are many patients who manage to sail through without major problems. But even in the Kroc collaborative trial a good 10% of values in the intensive or pump group were below 45 mg/dl. So it is a problem.

Professor Keen: It is anecdotal, but still worth presenting, that the sort of individual in whom we get the best comparison of tightest control possible with multiple injections versus pump is to be seen in the occasional doctor or medical student who is really doing his best to maintain himself in normoglycaemia. We have had experience of several of these, doctors who spend much of their time in near, or sometimes symptomatic hypoglycaemia at various times of the day because they really are trying to maintain normoglycaemia to prevent complications. We are struck by the improvement in well-being and lifestyle when those same people go on to continuous subcutaneous insulin infusion. They continue to maintain as close a control as they can over their glycaemia, find that they get equal or even better mean levels of glycaemia, and fewer episodes of hypoglycaemia. The over-conscientious normalizers, if we can call them that, do well in this comparison.

Professor Slama: I only partly agree with what has been said concerning the risk of hypoglycaemia in conventional therapy versus pump therapy. There is considerable difference, a striking and very important difference, between the two kinds of treatment. When a substantial dose of insulin is injected by syringe under the skin, this insulin will last at maximum 12 hours, and after that there is no more insulin. When hypoglycaemia occurs with a pump, the pump will run, run and run until the reservoir is empty, so if the patient lives alone, or is left alone, the potential risk of continuing hypoglycaemia is important in patients treated by pump and not in patients treated by injection.

Professor E Ritz (Germany): I should like to pursue Dr Viberti's argument and present a consideration which does not relate to pump versus subcutaneous infusion, the question of whether the subcutaneous resorption rate is altered in the uraemic patient. I have published, with Dr Andrassy, evidence that subcutaneous heparin absorption is altered in the uraemic patient. We certainly do need information on whether insulin absorption from subcutaneous depots is altered in the uraemic patient as well.

Professor Lameire: It is an important question. There was a recent paper in *Ann. Intern. Med.* showing that at different sites of injection in the body the absorption of insulin subcutaneously could be different.

A diabetologist should answer that.

Professor Keen: Professor Berger would certainly have something to say on the subject. There is little question but that if the patient takes a hot bath following the insulin injection, or gets into the sauna, he will get more insulin into the circulation faster. If he gives the insulin injection site a good massage, that too will accelerate the rate of insulin access to the circulation. We currently are looking at the effect of locally-injected prostaglandins to see if by actually inducing local vasodilation at the injection site we can sharpen up the rate of insulin access to the circulation.

So far as the patient in renal failure is concerned, we have no information ourselves, and I am not sure that anybody has looked specifically at this group to see if subcutaneous insulin absorption either by injection or from pump administration is different. I know of no information.

Dr A De Vecchi (Italy): When a patient has a subcutaneous or other continuous infusion device, does the insulin absorption change over time or not?

Professor Keen: Remarkably little. Dr Pickup just a few days ago showed - during his R. D. Lawrence Lecture - the data on about 90 diabetic patients treated with continuous subcutaneous insulin infusion looking at the rates of basal administration over the course of some months or years, and it was a straight line. It is quite extraordinary how little the dose changes.

Professor Tamborlane: Our data is not as pretty, but generally it is not a problem, although in individual patients who are having some local site problems where there is some inflammation and so forth, we have found some fluctuations in diabetic control accompany those.

We do not have nice insulin measurements, but it would seem likely that that was accompanied by some decreased absorption.

Professor Keen: And this does not take into consideration the question of pregnancy, or chronic infection, or many other stresses which may influence basal requirements. But under ordinary, unchallenged, normal conditions of life dose changes are very small.

Professor Lefebvre: We have a lot to learn about the pharmacokinetics of insulin. From our own experience with continuous subcutaneous insulin infusion, an interruption of an hour is sufficient to lower circulating free insulin.

Secondly, with all the conventional insulin therapies available, in our experience there is no intermediate insulin which covers 2–12 hours and no lente insulin which covers 24 hours. And this may explain all the difficulties we have in achieving control.

My next comment relates to the burden we put on the patients with these types of therapy. I have a very good friend in the United States who is a diabetic and who wears a pump. She is a nurse working in Dallas and I told her that for once I should like to imitate her, to wear a pump for a week, prick my fingers four or five times a day, and live the life of a diabetic. A year later she asked me whether I had done it. I said no. I would not do it for a day. I know that there are people in the audience who have tried the life of a diabetic for a week or so, or even two, and we have to consider that when we become involved with these processes.

I should also like to know whether there has been any study in which juvenile insulin-dependent diabetic patients have been treated from the time of diagnosis with continuous subcutaneous insulin infusion. What is very clear here is that in all these patients who have had diabetes for one, two, three or four years it improves control, but, for instance, retinopathy, is not very much influenced and can even worsen.

Professor Tamborlane: We have to be extremely cautious about that comment. Just as the anecdotal stories about vast improvements in retinopathy with control certainly appear to overstate, we have to be cautious not to take preliminary results over the short term in small numbers of patients to be the same as those for a larger number of patients over a longer term. Admittedly I think the outcome will be best if there is no established microvascular disease to start with, but I am still not totally sure that we might not have some beneficial effect on very early retinopathy. We have to be very cautious about this but there are some reports that the second year of follow up with tight control shows differences from the first year.

Professor Lefebvre: In the slide showing the regression line, with all the dots on the line or below the line, with on the line meaning no change and under the line aggravation, there is not a single dot above the line indicating improvement.

Professor Keen: That is right. We do not know how people on ordinary injections have been. They might have been right on the bottom line.

But to take up the point of the quality of life and how people get on with wearing pumps. It is unquestionably a damn nuisance. However, many feel that it is worthwhile. At the end of the Kroc Study that Professor Tamborlane and I have been involved in, patients who had been randomly allocated to the pump were offered the chance of continuing if they wanted to, and with few exceptions they decided they would rather stay on pump than go back on to conventional treatment. Furthermore, several of the people who had been allocated to the conventional treatment opted to go on pump. So that although Professor Lefebvre is right and it is a nuisance, it does carry certain advantages as well. It carries the advantage of flexibility, which is a very considerable one.

The diabetic who does not want to eat does not have to eat; he can run for a day without eating on basal, unboosted infusion if he must. And he can feel that he has the control of his diabetes much more clearly and understandably in his hand. That counts for a lot.

Professor Lameire: I was impressed as a nephrologist that Professor De Leeuw put so much emphasis on only 15% of the patients being able to maintain good glycaemic control under strict conventional therapy, and, secondly, on the problems of patient education. As nephrologists we know that we can teach patients a lot. We can teach them to dialyse themselves at home, which is technically much more complicated. We can teach them CAPD. But then the combination of teaching them dialysis, and self-monitoring of blood glucose, and pump infusion of insulin - does anybody have any idea of the complications of teaching that to patients all at once?

Professor De Leeuw: To answer the first question. The 130 patients we took were random diabetes patients. We finally got a selection, a spontaneous selection, of about 15%, which is the same figure as was mentioned, between 10–20%, for the currently available methods, who will prick their fingers every day and do everything that must be done.

A figure of 15% from our selection probably indicates the same patients who would do well with the pump. The patient who is given a pump is selected out by the clinician. It is not the patient who asks for the pump. The doctor selects him himself - generally. So there is a preselection done by the physician. In the conventional treatment group that was not the case.

Professor Tamborlane mentioned everything over 1, 2 and 3 years except bodyweight.

Professor Tamborlane: In some patients a transient increase in bodyweight is noted. Usually it goes back to normal. The Kroc Data, which are the best I know, showed no significant change in bodyweight. That was in a group of 35 patients put on pump treatment.

Some teenagers seem to gain a lot of weight. I think eating habits need to be reassessed. As Dr Gabbay pointed out, they stop losing all those calories that go to waste in the urine and so intake needs some reassessment.

To answer Professor Slama's question, I had some concerns about the comparison between subcutaneous and intravenous infusion in the data from Dr Esslinger's group. They showed significantly lower blood glucose values in the i.v. or intraperitoneal groups compared to the subcutaneous group. But the subcutaneous values they reported showed mean values of about 150 mg/dl. This is in contrast to most other people who report being able to maintain glucose values between 110 and 120 mg/dl, and that is almost exactly what was reported for the i.v. and the intraperitoneal routes.

Professor Slama: I am not qualified to answer for Dr Esslinger, who is not here.

May I add a comment on bodyweight. In my experience there is no increase in bodyweight in our patients. However for patients on pump the diet is more liberal, and it has been shown that when the diet is liberalized for the diabetic, he eats less than the conventionally treated diabetic patient. So probably under pump treatment he will eat less than when he was obliged to eat snacks and his three meals.

Professor Lameire: I would eat more! But what happens with the daily dose of insulin injected at the start when he is in good balance, and a year later? If I was a diabetic and I came regularly to Paris and I was wearing my pump, then I would visit a good restaurant each time, give myself a little push with my insulin, and probably at the end of the year I would need more insulin than at the beginning. What about these figures?

Professor Keen: It would depend on whether he became a fat diabetic at the end of the year, too.

Most of us are regulated by factors that we do not really understand. When we come to Paris we live it up, and when we get home again, I suspect the diabetic would pay his penance and press his button less. The proof of the pudding is in the eating. People may put on a little weight once they stop losing all their urinary sugar, but then they usually stop there. There is very little change either in the basal level or in boost doses of insulin over the course of the years.

Professor Slama: I would not be rich enough to become overweight in Paris!

Professor De Leeuw: In our group, who were on good conventional treatment, the mean insulin dose per kilogram of weight went up from 0.7 to 0.9 units/kg at the end of the three years - slowly, slowly but progressively, while maintaining the same degree of control.

Dr V Parsons (UK.): There is the impression that if insulin is given into the peritoneum and high into the abdomen, it is slightly better than giving it lower into the abdomen. Is a peritoneal dialysis catheter that fundamentally goes right down into the pelvis of the abdomen really the best way to give insulin? Should we be thinking either of putting two devices in, or of rerouting in some way the peritoneal catheter up into the higher abdomen? Is that really worthwhile, and are there scientific facts to back it up?

Professor Mirouze: We have the same results with the subcutaneous intraperitoneal catheter whether the catheter is in the lower or the upper part of the peritoneum. There is no difference.

Professor M Legrain: Is there anyone in the audience who has considerable experience of using pump and subcutaneous infusion among diabetics with severe renal insufficiency at the end stage of being dialysed, whether they are dialysed on haemodialysis, on CAPD or on intermittent peritoneal dialysis? In our experience, and I agree with Professor Viberti, the big change in blood glucose levels, rising and falling at a very fast rate, is a major problem in patients with end-stage renal failure, mainly patients on HD. It is better on CAPD. Right now I have seen no papers and heard nothing of importance to prove that patients with end-stage renal failure gain much benefit from tight control. It is quite possible, and we may perhaps avoid some late complications, but I would like to discuss that if possible.

Professor Lameire: The nephrologists will love the question, but it is the duty of the diabetologist to answer.

Professor Keen: All I would say is that something very curious does happen to carbohydrate metabolism and to insulin effect in the patient in chronic renal failure. This has been known for decades, and the mechanism remains very elusive; a tendency to both hypoglycaemia and to insulin resistance. The mechanisms of both of these have been looked at partially, but never fully worked out.

Dr Viberti: Professor Legrain asked for somebody having a large series. We do not have a large series. We have a number of patients which is very small at the moment who were on pump treatment before reaching end-stage renal failure. When they got to that stage, the problem of managing haemodialysis or CAPD and the pump is put to the patient and we ask the patients whether they would like to remain on the pump. As far as our limited experience goes, of those patients who go on CAPD, most opt to have their insulin put into the peritoneum. The glycaemic control achieved by that route is often better than the glycaemic control we have been able to achieve with pump treatment in the previous weeks or months.

I am sure it is a study which needs to be done, and I should like to see it done for insulin-treated transplanted patients. There are large prospective studies under way in Minneapolis and we are waiting for the results from that group with great expectations. But the experience is very limited indeed at the moment.

Professor Gabbay: I wanted to make two comments. First, we hardly ever see retinopathy in a patient who is pre-pubertal. Before the age of 17 I have seen only one person with proliferative retinopathy. Puberty is a very important determinant.

Secondly, with regard to Professor Keen's question about pumps in newly-diagnosed juvenile diabetic patients and how they would do in terms of complications, juvenile diabetics are not a homogeneous group. The older the patient is at diagnosis, the milder the disease and the easier it is to control. Most of the studies have been done in patients who develop their disease after the age of 15 or 16.

Thirdly, I have seen a very rare complication of the pump and I wonder if anyone else has seen it – a hypoglycaemic cataract that we just heard about.

People think that cataracts in diabetics occur only with hyperglycaemia, but hypoglycaemic cataracts can also occur. This particular patient kept her blood sugar in the 1950s most of the time and within 6 months of going on the pump developed a cataract.

Dr Bosi (Lyons): I should like to answer Professor Legrain's question on the use of the micropumps in haemodialysis patients. In Lyons, in Professor Traeger's clinic, we currently have four diabetic patients on haemodialysis treated by continuous subcutaneous insulin infusion. We were obliged to try the micropump treatment because of the problem of wide fluctuation of glycaemic values over 24 hours, which was a major problem. Although our experience is still limited, the impression is that the achievement of normoglycaemia is easier with the micropump, and the occurrence of hypoglycaemic episodes is less frequent with the micropump.

Professor F L Shapiro (USA): I am not quite sure I understand what is the target when one considers close glycaemic control in a patient who is far advanced with renal failure on dialysis, whose life is already exquisitely complex. There are many things one can do with usual approaches to intermittent use of insulin without complicating the picture more. When somebody has renal failure and requires dialysis, one is interested in control of the blood sugar so as to avoid tremendous shifts in weight. When they are hyperglycaemic they are thirsty, they drink more, the blood pressure goes up, and it is my strong bias that they die as a consequence of hypertension or complications thereof. They do not die from hyperglycaemia. They do not even have polyuria with hyperglycaemia.

The key problem is that people have been trying to use the intermediate and long-acting insulins as the predominant insulin in treating the patient with haemodialysis, getting a lot of blood sugars, because we cannot treat much else in those patients, and getting carried away by the laboratory results. By using regular insulin as the predominant insulin with a little bit of long-acting, they can be controlled clinically very effectively because we can watch their weight, they will tell us when they are thirsty, and particularly so in those very few patients in my experience who will cooperate and do self-monitoring at home when they already have the commitment of dialysis.

Professor Keen: Of course that is absolutely right. One has to temper justice with mercy. At the same time I should like to ask Professor Shapiro to recall that most of the studies that we have been involved in with tight control in patients in advancing renal failure have been controlled studies where we have looked to see whether we have been able to arrest or slow the rate of advance. I am sure he would have no objection to the use of tight control in that sort of situation.

I would argue, too, that in terms of management of the patient over the period of renal transplantation, that the better the metabolic status of the patient, perhaps the better the surgical outcome and the more comfortable the patient. But again one has to balance cost against benefit and one does not want to plunge the already unhappy patient into hypoglycaemia.

We yet have to see the effect of good control on the transplant over the course of the subsequent years, and that too has to be looked at carefully.

Session Four

MANAGEMENT OF THE DIABETIC IN RENAL FAILURE

(i) Medical and Surgical Care

Chairmen:
G. d'AMICO and T. KANGAS

(ii) Transplantation

Chairmen:
I. H. DE LEEUW and R. VAN SCHILFGAARDE

Introduction

Professor d'Amico: In earlier sessions we heard some good news and some bad news about the possibility of preventing the occurrence of diabetic nephropathy. The topic of this Session will be what to do when renal damage has already developed and renal failure has occurred.

In the intermediate stage between the development of renal damage and the final stage, requiring regular dialysis treatment, we can try to give our patients an acceptable quality of life, try, for instance, to avoid their becoming blind or having major cardiovascular metabolic complications. We can do even more. We can try to slow down the progression of renal damage if we are able to control hypertension.

This will be the topic for our first presentation, by Professor Ritz.

11
Genesis and management of hypertension in diabetic nephropathy

Ch. HASSLACHER, M. RAMBAUSEK, and E. RITZ

INTRODUCTION

There is little doubt that the treatment of hypertension in diabetic patients has to some extent been the Cinderella of diabetology. This is presumably because in the past diabetologists have been preoccupied with problems of metabolic control, and have disregarded minor blood pressure elevation in incipient stages of clinically overt glomerulopathy. Increasing evidence suggests that not only macroangiopathic sequelae, but also irreversible renal damage may be induced by such blood pressure elevation. The interrelation of systemic haemodynamics and glomerular damage has become one of the most fascinating recent developments, and one of the great challenges, in clinical diabetology.

EPIDEMIOLOGY OF HYPERTENSION IN DIABETICS

Although, in recent decades, an increased prevalence of hypertension in diabetic patients has been suspected[1], definite epidemiologic information has only recently been forthcoming. In a classical paper, Pell and D'Alonzo[2] examined almost 100 000 employees of Dupont Co. and found that the prevalence of hypertension was 54% greater among diabetics. Such increased prevalence was particularly striking in younger age groups. It could also be shown that over a 10 year period death rates among diabetics were higher than in the general population[3]. This was mostly accounted for by cardiovascular and renal disease; thus excess mortality was related to an hypertensive status. Such global assessment of both insulin-dependent (type I) and non-insulin-dependent (type II) diabetics may blur some important distinctions relevant for the pathogenesis of hypertension.

In a recent study, Fabre *et al*[4] reported on a series of 510 *type II diabetics*. 26 of the patients were hypertensive prior to diagnosis of diabetes; this may correspond to the expected prevalence of essential hypertension in an obese age-matched group. 30% developed hypertension after diagnosis, and such hypertension was more frequent in females and increased with advancing age. A highly significant correlation was found between hypertension on the one hand and proteinuria or reduced glomerular filtration rate (GFR) on the other hand.

Table 1 Prevalence of hypertension at various stages of nephropathy in 53 type I diabetics followed sequentially

	Hypertension
No albuminuria	6/28 = 21%
Intermittent albuminuria	15/28 = 54%
Persistent albuminuria	35/53 = 66%
Elevated S-creatinine	30/32 = 94%

Epidemiological features are somewhat different in *type I diabetes*. Table 1 shows our experience in the diabetes outpatient clinic. 53 type I diabetics were followed sequentially; 38 were admitted prior to onset of intermittent albuminuria and a further 25 after onset of persistent albuminuria. It is obvious that even prior to intermittent albuminuria, some individuals do have hypertension (RR> 160/95 mmHg on three separate occasions under resting conditions). The prevalence of hypertension may even be slightly higher than the 10.3% prevalence reported for 30–39 year old males and 2.7% for 30–39 year old females in a West German population in Munich[5]; this figure is in close agreement with our local prevalence rate of 10.5% (males 30–34 years) in Heidelberg (courtesy Dr Buchholtz).

Our limited experience would agree with the experience of others[6,7] that hypertension prior to development of proteinuria does not usually accelerate the development of nephropathy. There is, however, no doubt that there is a close temporal relationship between rising prevalence of hypertension and clinically overt nephropathy[8-11]. This is well illustrated by the progressive rise in the prevalence of hypertension with increasing severity of nephropathy in our patients. As shown in Table 1, once serum creatinine is elevated, more than 90% of patients with type I diabetes are hypertensive.

PATHOGENESIS OF HYPERTENSION IN DIABETES

Increased arterial blood pressure may be related to excessive body fluid volumes, increased activity of pressor systems, or a combination of both. In diabetes mellitus, evidence has been advanced which documents that both regulation of total body sodium and pressor activity are abnormal.

Weidmann and his collaborators[12–14] demonstrated increased *exchangeable body sodium*, higher by approximately 10%, in young, middle-aged and elderly diabetics with no elevation of serum creatinine. It is of note that plasma volume, factored for lean body mass, was not increased in parallel; it tended even to be slightly lower. Lower plasma volume may be related either to hypoalbuminaemia, to pressure-induced changes of fluid volume partitioning, or both. The mechanism of sodium retention is unknown. It may have been the consequence of incipient nephropathy, since proteinuria with no elevation of serum creatinine, as present in some of the patients studied[13] may well indicate renal damage and interfere with sodium excretion. On the other hand, sodium retention may have resulted, at least in some patients, from a hyperinsulinaemic state, as insulin in itself increases sodium transport across various transporting epithelia[15].

Although sympathetic nerve dysfunction, including baroreflex dysfunction, is common in longstanding diabetes mellitus[16], normal basal and stimulated *plasma noradrenaline* and adrenaline levels were observed in diabetic patients without advanced nephropathy[17] and in animals with experimental diabetes[18]. A subgroup of diabetics, however, had abnormally low plasma noradrenaline levels during orthostasis[17].

In parallel with normal plasma noradrenaline, basal *plasma renin* activity (PRA) was normal in the majority of diabetics[12,17] but in a substantial proportion (22%), subnormal PRA and/or aldosterone responses to posture were observed. Normal or suppressed PRA may explain the clinical finding that malignant hypertension is distinctly uncommon in longterm diabetes, and may also explain the propensity of diabetes to hyporeninaemic hypoaldosteronism.

However, Weidmann *et al*[13] found decreased threshold doses and pressor doses of noradrenaline or angiotensin II in hypertensive patients with diabetes mellitus, as compared to age-matched normal subjects. Such increased *pressor responsiveness*, which confirms previous observations of Christlieb[18] was reversible after 6 weeks of treatment with chlorthalidone (100 mg/day).

The reason for such increased vascular responsiveness has not been adequately defined. Intrinsic vascular smooth muscle contractility may be increased in sodium loaded vessel walls, although experimental work demonstrated diminished contractile responses of aortic smooth muscle of alloxan-diabetic rat aorta[19]. Alternatively, according to the concept of Folkow[20], altered vessel geometry resulting from vascular hypertrophy could give a greater increment of peripheral resistance for any given amount of fibre shortening[20]. This possibility must be seriously considered in view of work of Karlefors[21] who showed that the pressure response to exercise was significantly higher in diabetics of 5–14 years duration despite no elevation of resting systolic blood pressure. Intermittent stress-induced hypertension might well explain vascular hypertrophy and exaggerated pressor-induced blood pressure response in normotensive diabetics. This would not explain, however, altered threshold doses as found by Weidmann[13].

CONSEQUENCES OF HYPERTENSION IN DIABETES

The high prevalence of hypertension in diabetics[22] has been shown to be a major risk factor for cardiovascular death. In a recent prospective study[23], duration of diabetes and systolic pressure were statistically the most significant factors predicting *cardiovascular death*. The macroangiopathic circulatory consequences of arterial hypertension in diabetes have been recently reviewed[24].

One of the exciting developments in this area has been the recent recognition that *deterioration of renal function* in patients with diabetic glomerulosclerosis depends on the level of arterial blood presssure[25,26], although this has not been observed by all investigators[27-29]. This discrepancy may be the result of differences in blood pressure levels which tended to be somewhat lower in the latter studies. Our own experience is summarized in Table 2 and Figure 1. As shown in Table 2, elevation of serum creatinine above 1.4 mg/dl was observed in 60% of hypertensive type I diabetics with persistent proteinuria with a known duration of diabetes of 23 years, but only in 11% of non-hypertensive patients. The deleterious influence of hypertension on renal function in type I diabetics with persistent proteinuria is also evident from longitudinal data depicted in Figure 1. Two years after onset of persistent proteinuria, 50% of hypertensive, but none of the normotensive, diabetics had developed elevated creatinine. After 10 years, almost 100% of hypertensive, but only 28% of normotensive patients had developed elevated serum creatinine.

Table 2 Development of increased S-creatinine in 53 type I diabetics with persistent proteinuria

	Hypertension	*No hypertension*
Renal insufficiency	60% (21/35)	11% (2/18)
Median duration of diabetes	23 years	21 years

These observations gain considerable clinical importance because of the demonstration by Mogensen[26] (although only in a limited number of patients) of a beneficial effect of blood pressure lowering on the decay of renal function in type I diabetics. Confirmation of these results with regard to consistency and magnitude of the effect in larger series of patients is anxiously awaited. It is also unknown – but irrelevant for the management of diabetics – whether the effect is specific for diabetic glomerulosclerosis or more generally applicable to other glomerular diseases.

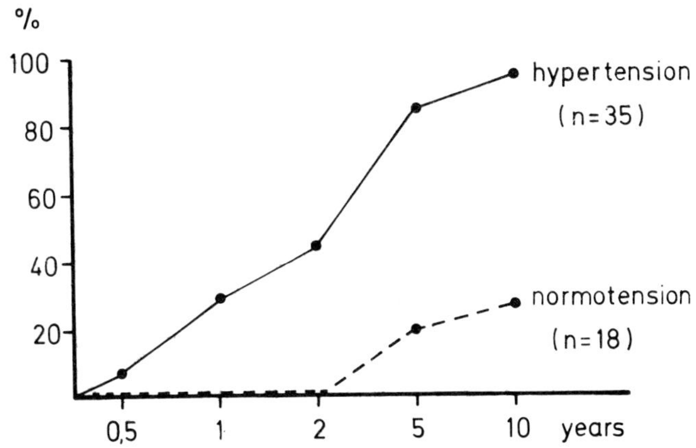

Figure 1 Interval between onset of persistent proteinuria and detection of elevated S-creatinine (> 1.4 mg/dl) in 53 Type I Diabetics

This observation[26] obviously raises two questions:

(1) What level of blood pressure must be attained to preserve renal function, and

(2) What is the mechanism by which preservation of renal function is brought about?

Although no data are available on critical blood pressure level and renal function, the findings of Knowler *et al*[30] on the evolution of retinal lesions in Pima Indians may be relevant. He found that the age-adjusted 6 year incidence of retinal lesions (exudates or haemorrhages) was higher in hypertensive individuals, as expected. However, it was also higher in individuals with blood pressure in the upper normal range (125–144 mmHg systolic) as opposed to individuals with blood pressure in the lower normal range (below 125 mmHg systolic). This raises the important question as to what level of blood pressure one should aim at. It may well be that normotension according to the WHO criteria is not good enough for the retina, and perhaps also for the kidneys, of a diabetic patient.

Recent experimental work[31,32] has provided a conceptual framework to explain why lowering of blood pressure in diabetic patients may preserve renal function. In streptozotocin diabetic Munich rats with moderate hyperglycaemia, Hostetter *et al*[32] found an increased single nephron glomerular filtration rate and glomerular plasma flow rate (Table 3). It is of note that afferent and efferent resistances were decreased. This would permit transmission of a greater fraction of systemic arterial pressure into the glomerular capillary bed. A conceptual schema by which one might explain the deleterious effect of hypertension, and the beneficial effect of its reversal, on glomerular filtration is shown in Figure 2. Transcapillary hydraulic pressure and single

Table 3 Glomerular filtration dynamics in experimental diabetes of the rat

	MAP (mmHg)	*Glomerular hydraulic pressure* (mmHg)	*P* *Transmembrane P.* (mmHg)	Q_A (nl/min)	R_A (10^{10}dynes sec^{-1} cm^{-5})	R_E (10^{10}dynes sec^{-1} cm^{-5})
Control ($n=8$)	103 ±4	47.5 ±1.2	35.2 ±1.3	142 ±11	3.0 ±0.3	2.1 ±0.2
Diabetes with moderate hyperglycaemia ($n=6$)	114 ±5	56.4 ±1.9	44.4* ±1.6	240* ±34	1.6* ±0.3	1.6* ±0.3

$\bar{x} \pm$ SEM
**p* 0.025 rsp. 0.005
reference 31

MAP = mean arterial pressure
Q_A = single glomerular plasma flow rate
R_A = afferent renal arteriolar resistance
R_E = efferent renal arteriolar resistance

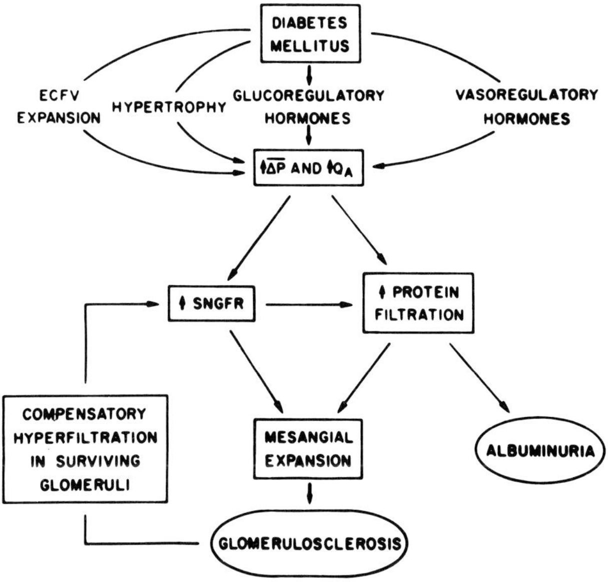

Figure 2 Schematic representation of mechanisms culminating in renal disease and failure in the diabetic

nephron plasma flow are known to be increased in early diabetes. Consequently this first results in an increased single nephron glomerular filtration, and an impaired permselectivity with increased protein filtration. This will lead to albuminuria and to overloading of the mesangium with protein and consecutive mesangial expansion. The resulting glomerulosclerosis will cause even more severe compensatory hyperfiltration in surviving glomeruli, adding an element of a self-perpetuating vicious circle to this mechanism, as in diabetic glomerulopathy following unilateral nephrectomy[33].

Such a schema could explain some clinical and experimental observations. Berkman and Rifkin[34] observed a fascinating case of a diabetic patient who showed unilateral nodular diabetic glomerulosclerosis with little evidence of glomerulosclerosis in an ischaemic kidney protected by renal artery stenosis. This is in line with observations of Mauer *et al*[35] in rats with alloxan-diabetes and coexisting Goldblatt hypertension. They showed aggravated glomerulosclerosis in the non-protected, and attenuated glomerulosclerosis in the ischaemic kidney protected from overperfusion by the presence of renal artery stenosis.

MANAGEMENT OF HYPERTENSION IN THE DIABETIC PATIENT

There is little argument that hypertension in the diabetic patient with *elevated serum creatinine* is exquisitely volume sensitive, more so than in other types of renal disease. In the extreme case of the diabetic patient on maintenance haemodialysis, volume control with ultrafiltration will permit normotension in the majority of patients. Table 4 summarizes our experience with 65 non-diabetic and 16 diabetic patients with end-stage renal failure on centre haemodialysis. Normotension (10 consecutive predialytic blood pressure measurements > 150 mmHg systolic; > 100 mmHg diastolic) could be achieved in all but 2 of the 16 diabetic patients. In no patient was predialytic blood pressure above 165 when the patient had achieved ideal 'dry weight'. It is of note, though, that 53% of the diabetic, but only 27.7% of the non-diabetic uraemic patients on dialysis required some antihypertensive medication. Antihypertensive medication was mostly needed because patients did not comply with fluid restriction, and/or because ultrafiltration was not tolerated as a consequence of autonomic polyneuropathy. The volume-sensitive character of hypertension is shown by the fact that in 11 of 14 patients who had occasional predialytic weight gain of >4 kg, predialytic blood pressure rose above 155 mmHg when the patient was overweight.

Table 4 Hypertension in dialysed patients (Centre Dialysis, Heidelberg)

		Non-Diabetic	*Diabetic*
Antihypertensive medication		18 (27.7%)	8 (50%)
No antihypertensive medication		47	8
Total		65	16
	At 'Dryweight'	Normotensive	14
		Hypertensive	2
	4 kg above* 'Dryweight'	Normotensive	3
		Hypertensive	11

* Only 14 diabetics had episodes of overhydration (⩾4 kg)

The main challenge, however, is antihypertensive treatment of the *diabetic patient prior to end-stage renal disease*. These problems have been recently discussed in several reviews[24,36-39]. Although few controlled trials have been reported to date[25,26] some clinical experience is available which allows us to rationally discuss advantages and disadvantages of the several antihypertensive drugs available. These are listed in Table 5.

A *diuretic* would seem to be a rational first choice, since increased exchangeable sodium and increased pressor responsiveness, reversible with chlorthalidone treatment, was noted in diabetic patients[13]. However, apart from the known generally adverse effects of diuretics, e.g. hyperuricaemia, hypokalaemia, impairment of lipid profile and impotence in the male, some specific problems have to be considered in the diabetic. These are primarily

Table 5 Antihypertensive drugs in diabetic patients

Diuretics	— thiazide (with reduced GFR furosemide)
β-Blockers	— β_1-selective
Vasodilators	— hydralazine — prazosin — minoxidil
Central sympathicoplegics	— α-methyldopa, clonidine
Captopril	

impaired metabolic control with a proneness to hyperosmolar or ketoacidotic coma in type II diabetics. Furthermore, particularly in patients with impaired baroreflex function[16], orthostatic hypotension may become very troublesome. This is particularly important in patients with impaired renal function in whom the more potent loop diuretics have to be used with the associated risk of hypovolaemia. Because of their increased responsiveness to sympathetic activity[14] *β-blockers* are a logical adjunct or alternative.

There has been much discussion on the safety of the use of β-blockers in diabetics. A recent controlled study on the use of the β-selective blocker metoprolol in hypertensive insulin-dependent diabetics demonstrated achievement of normotension with either metoprolol alone, or a combination with thiazides and hydralazin, in all patients with few side effects[40]. In the past, several arguments have been raised against the use of β-blockers. The islet has β_2-receptors and it has been argued that non-selective β-blockade will interfere with insulin release, but this is of negligible relevance in the type I diabetic on insulin. It has also been argued that recovery from hypoglycaemia will be delayed with β-blockade. In one study, Lager *et al*[41] showed no augmentation of hypoglycaemia but impaired late recovery after intravenous insulin in 7 diabetics on propranolol as compared with placebo or metoprolol, but the difference was not impressive. Hepatocytes have predominantly α-receptors. Consequently, catecholamine mediated hepatic glycogenolysis and gluconeogenesis is not affected to a major extent by β-blockade, although - depending on cortisol and thyroid status - some β-receptors may be present on hepatocytes. Glucagon mediated glucogenolysis would not be expected to be altered in any case. Non-selective β-blockers reduce muscular and splanchnic blood flow, and this may account for an impaired recovery from hypoglycaemia. Most importantly they interfere with release of gluconeogenic substrates, particularly lactate and glycerol, despite no change of counterregulating hormones.

It has also been argued that hypoglycaemia awareness is affected by β-blockers. Although the tachycardia response is certainly abolished with non-selective or selective β-blockers, the more important sweating response persists despite β-blockade. This was documented by Viberti *et al*[42] who demonstrated that sweating scores, 10 min after the plasma glucose nadir, were even increased in oxprenolol or metoprolol treated diabetics. Another consideration is hyperkalaemia upon administration of β-blockers in diabetics with hyporeninaemic hypoaldosteronism. Finally, a possible hypertensive reaction to hypoglycaemia must be considered with non-selective β-blockers. It is thought to result from unopposed α-vasoconstriction to adrenaline when β_2-vasodilatation is blocked. This is supported by the experience of Östman *et al*[43], who found a greater increase of systolic and diastolic blood pressures during insulin-induced hypoglycaemia when hypertensive type I diabetics received propranolol than when they received the β_1-selective blocker metoprolol. Consequently, one would predict that β_1-selective blockers can be used relatively safely in diabetics[25,26,40], and this is supported by the results of controlled studies[40].

In our experience, one complication of β-blockers which has not been widely commented upon, may be an impaired cardioacceleration and resting bradycardia in type II diabetics with latent or manifest sick sinus syndrome. In several of our patients, as a consequence of high blood pressure amplitude and impaired orthostatic cardioacceleration, blood pressure could not be controlled before a pacemaker was installed.

The concept of reduced renal arteriolar resistance and glomerular overperfusion[31,32] would suggest that on theoretical grounds *vasodilators* are deleterious in the diabetic patient. However, hydralazin has apparently been used successfully in hypertensive type I diabetics[25,26]. Prazosin may cause orthostatic hypotension, particularly in the diabetic patient with autonomic polyneuropathy. In our experience, the potent vasodilator minoxidil is quite effective, but poses major challenges because of the problems of fluid retention and hypertrichosis, the latter of which may be absolutely intolerable in women.

A final comment concerns the use of the recently introduced *converting enzyme inhibitors*, captopril, or in the future enalapril, for diabetic patients who do not tolerate or are resistant to triple therapy. Their use in diabetics may seem paradoxical because plasma renin is not elevated, and even tends to be low[17,18]. We have used captopril successfully, however, in several diabetic patients with resistant hypertension; Table 6 shows one example. A type I diabetic with adequate renal function and nephrotic range proteinuria showed poor control of blood pressure with β-blockers and a vasodilator when first seen in the outpatient clinic. A diuretic had not been given because of suspected gout. The patient was put on a diuretic and captopril which promptly normalized blood pressure (mean of 5 outpatient measurements under resting conditions). Because of ageusia, captopril was stopped by another physician. Hypertension promptly reappeared, only to normalize when captopril was reinstituted in reduced dosage and with zinc supplements. It is not surprising that converting enzyme inhibitors are effective in diabetics despite normal or low circulating renin. As discussed by Unger *et al*[44] the acute blood pressure fall, but not the delayed blood pressure response to captopril, is closely correlated with circulating plasma renin. Inhibition of circulating converting enzyme and blood pressure lowering effect of captopril can be clearly dissociated in several conditions. Finally, captopril has definite actions, which are not mediated by circulating converting enyzme, e.g. on presynaptic facilitation (presumably via local vascular wall renin–angiotensin) and on vascular wall prostaglandin metabolism etc.

Table 6 Use of captopril in a diabetic patient with resistant hypertension

Male born 1936	*Clinical signs*	*Treatment*	
1949	diabetes		
1977	constant proteinuria		
1979	constant hypertension		
1982, April	S-Creatinine 1.2 mg/dl Proteinuria 3.2 g/d		
	RR 200/100 mmHg ($\bar{x}$)	Metoprolol Nepresol	400 mg/d 50 mg/d
June	RR 145/80 mmHg	Captopril Chlortalidon	2 × 25 mg/d 100 mg/d
	Ageusia, Captopril stopped		
December	RR 180/100 mmHg	Nepresol Chlortalidon	50 mg/d 100 mg/d
1983, February	RR 145/80 mmHg	Captopril Chlortalidon	25 mg/d 100 mg/d

SUMMARY

Overwhelming epidemiological evidence identifies hypertension of the diabetic as a major risk factor for cardiovascular accidents and – in proteinuric patients with glomerulosclerosis – for deterioration of renal function. Such deterioration may be related to glomerular hyperfiltration as one major factor perpetuating renal damage.

Both sodium retention and increased pressor response to noradrenaline or angiotensin have been demonstrated in diabetic patients with hypertension. Consequently, the combination of a diuretic and a cardioselective β-blocker is the logical first line treatment of choice for diabetics. Various arguments against the use of β-blockers (impaired recovery from hypoglycaemia, unawareness of hypoglycaemia, pressor response to hypoglycaemia) do not hold, at least not for β_1-selective beta blockers, the safety of which has been demonstrated in controlled clinical studies.

In the patient resistant to triple therapy, i.e. a combination of diuretic, β-blocker and vasodilator, either minoxidil or captopril may be effective.

The diabetic patient with advanced renal failure is exquisitely volume sensitive. In the predialytic phase potent loop diuretics, or during dialysis ultrafiltration, will control hypertension in the majority of patients.

References

1. Major, S. G. (1929). Blood pressure in diabetes mellitus: a statistical study. *Arch. Intern. Med.*, **44**, 797
2. Pell, S. and D'Alonzo, C. A. (1967). Some aspects of hypertension in diabetes mellitus. *JAMA*, **202**, 104
3. Pell, S. and D'Alonzo, A. (1970). Factors associated with long-term survival of diabetics. *JAMA*, **214**, 1833
4. Fabre, J., Balant, L. P., Dayer, P. G., Fox, H. M. and Vernet, A. T. (1982). The kidney in maturity onset diabetes mellitus: a clinical study of 510 patients. *Kidney Int.*, **21**, 730
5. Stieber, J., Döring, A. and Keil, H. (1982). Häufigkeit, Bekanntheits- und Behandlungsgrad der Hypertonie in einer Großstadtbevölkerung. *Münchn. Med. Wschr.*, **124**, 747
6. Moss, A. J. (1962). Blood pressure in children with diabetes mellitus. *Pediatrics*, **30**, 932
7. Deckert, T. and Polsen, J. E. (1981). Diabetic nephropathy: fault or destiny? *Diabetologia*, **21**, 178
8. Christlieb, A. R., Warram, J. H., Krolewski, A. S., Busick, E. J., Ganda, O. M., Asmal, A. C., Soeldner, J. S. and Bradlwy, R. F. (1981). Hypertension: the major risk factor in juvenile onset insulin-dependent diabetes. *Diabetes*, **30**, 90
9. Parving, H. H., Andersen, A. R., Smidt, U. M., Oxenboll, B., Edsberg, B. and Sandahl Christiansen, J. (1983). Diabetic nephropathy and arterial hypertension. *Diabetologia*, **24**, 10
10. Christiansen, J. S., Gammelgaard, J., Frandsen, M. and Parving, H. H. (1981). A prospective study of glomerular filtration rate and arterial blood pressure in insulin-dependent diabetics with diabetic nephropathy. *Diabetologia*, **20**, 457
11. Mogensen, C. E. (1976). Renal function changes in diabetes. *Diabetes*, **25**, 872
12. de Châtel, R., Weidmann, P., Flammer, J., Ziegler, W. H., Beretta-Piccoli, E., Vetter, W. and Reubi, F. C. (1977). Sodium, renin, aldosterone, catecholamines and blood pressure in diabetes mellitus. *Kidney Int.*, **12**, 412
13. Weidmann, P., Beretta-Piccoli, C., Keusch, G., Gluck, Z., Mujagie, M., Grimm, M., Meier, A. and Ziegler, W. H. (1979). Sodium-volume factor, cardiovascular reactivity and hypotensive mechanism of diuretic therapy in mild hypertension associated with diabetes mellitus. *Am. J. Med.*, **67**, 779
14. Weidmann, P. (1980). Recent pathogenic aspects in essential hypertension and hypertension associated with diabetes mellitus. *Klin. Wschr.*, **58**, 1071
15. DeFronzo, R. A. (1981). The effect of insulin on renal sodium metabolism. A review with clinical implications. *Diabetologia*, **21**, 165
16. Olshan, A. R., O'Connor, D. T., Cohen, I. M., Mitas, J. A., Stone, R. A. (1983). Baroreflex dysfunction in patients with adult-onset diabetes and hypertension. *Am. J. Med.*, **74**, 233
17. Beretta-Piccoli, C., Weidmann, P., Ziegler, W., Glück, Z. and Keusch, G. (1976). Plasma catecholamines and renin in diabetes mellitus. *Klin. Wschr.*, **57**, 681
18. Christlieb, A. R. (1973). Diabetes and hypertensive vascular disease. Mechanisms and treatment. *Am. J. Cardiol.*, **32**, 592
19. Sullivan, S. and Sparks, H. V. (1979). Diminished contractile response of aortas from diabetic rabbits. *Am. J. Physiol.*, **236**, H301
20. Folkow, B. (1982). Physiological aspects of primary hypertension. *Physiol. Rev.*, **62**, 415
21. Karlefors, T. (1966). Haemodynamic studies in male diabetics. *Acta Med. Scand.*, **180** (Suppl.), 45

22. Janka, H.U., Standl, E., Bloss, G., Oberparleiter, F. and Mehnert, H. (1978). Zur Epidemiologie der Hypertonie bei Diabetikern. *Dtsch. Med. Wschr.*, **103**, 1549
23. Janka, H.U., Grünwald, P., Waldmann, G., Standl, E. and Mehnert, H. (1982). Five-year mortality of diabetic patients and associated cardiovascular risk factors: The Schwabing study on macroangiopathy in diabetes (SSMD). *Diabetologia,* **23**, 176
24. Drury, P.L. (1983). Diabetes and arterial hypertension. *Diabetologia,* **24**, 1
25. Mogensen, C.E. (1976). Progression of nephropathy in long-term diabetics with proteinuria and effect of initial anti-hypertensive treatment. *Scand. J. Clin. Lab. Invest.,* **36**, 384
26. Mogensen, C.E. (1982). Long-term antihypertensive treatment inhibiting progression of diabetic nephropathy. *Br. Med. J.,* **285**, 685
27. Jones, R.H., Hayakawa, H., Mackay, J.D., Parsons, V. and Watkins, J.J. (1979). Progression of diabetic nephropathy. *Lancet,* **i**, 1105
28. Parving, H.H., Schmidt, U.M., Frusberg, B., Bonnevie-Nielsen, V. and Anderson, A.R. (1981). A prospective study of glomerular filtration rate and arterial blood pressure in insulin dependent diabetics with diabetic nephropathy. *Diabetologia*, **20**, 457
29. Viberti, G.C., Bilous, R.W., Mackintosh, D. and Keen, H. (1983). Monitoring glomerular function in diabetic nephropathy. A prospective study. *Am. J. Med.*, **302**, 645
30. Knowler, W.C., Bennett, P.H. and Ballintine, E.J. (1980). Increased incidence of retinopathy in diabetics with elevated blood pressure. *N. Engl. J. Med.,* **302**, 645
31. Hostetter, Th.H., Rennke, H.G. and Brenner, B.M. (1982). The case for intrarenal hypertension in the initiation and progression of diabetic and other glomerulopathies. *Am. J. Med.,* **72**, 375
32. Hostetter, Th.H., Troy, J.L. and Brenner, B.M. (1981). Glomerular hemodynamics in experimental diabetes mellitus. *Kidney Int.,* **19**, 410
33. Steffes, M.W., Brown, D.M. and Mauer, M.S. (1978). Diabetic glomerulopathy following unilateral nephrectomy in the rat. *Diabetes,* **27**, 35
34. Berkman, J. and Rifkin, H. (1973). Unilateral nodular diabetic glomerulosclerosis (Kimmelstiel–Wilson) report of a case. *Metabolism,* **22**, 715
35. Mauer, S.M., Steffes, M.W., Azar, S., Kupcho Sandberg, S. and Brown, D.M. (1978). The effects of Goldblatt hypertension on development of the glomerular lesions of diabetes mellitus in the rat. *Diabetes,* **27**, 738
36. Christlieb, A.R. (1982). The hypertension of diabetes. *Diabet. Care,* **5**, 50
37. Passa, P. (1980). Le traitement de l'hypertension arterielle chez les diabétiques. *Diabet. Metab.,* **6**, 287
38. Waal-Manning, H.J. (1979). Can β-blockers be used in diabetic patients? *Drugs,* **17**, 157
39. Bengston, C. (1979). Impairment of glucose metabolism during treatment with antihypertensive drugs. *Acta Med. Scand. (Copenh.),* (Suppl.), **682**, 63
40. Kølendorf, K., Bonnevie-Nielsen, V. and Broch-Møller, B. (1982). A trial of metoprolol in hypertensive insulin-dependent diabetic patients. *Acta Med. Scand.,* **211**, 175
41. Lager, I., Blohmé, G. and Smith, U. (1979). Effect of cardioselective and non-selective β-blockade on the hypoglycaemic response in insulin-dependent diabetics. *Lancet,* **i**, 458
42. Viberti, G.C., Keen, H. and Bloom, S.R. (1980). Beta blockade and diabetes mellitus: effect of oxprenolol and metoprolol on the metabolic, cardiovascular, and hormonal response to insulin-induced hypoglycemia in normal subjects. *Metabolism,* **29**, 866
43. Östman, J., Arner, P., Haglund, K., Juhlin-Dannfelt, A., Nowak, J. and Wennlund, A. (1982). Effect of metoprolol and alprenolol on the metabolic, hormonal, and haemodynamic response to insulin-induced hypoglycaemia in hypertensive insulin-dependent diabetics. *Acta Med. Scand.,* **211**, 381
44. Unger, T., Ganten, D., Lang, R.L. (1983). Neue Aspekte zum antihypertensiven Mechanismus von Converting-Enzym Inhibitoren (In press)

12
Retinopathy in diabetic nephropathy (a preliminary report)

E. M. KOHNER and P. S. CHAHAL

INTRODUCTION

Nephropathy and retinopathy are two microvascular sequelae of longterm diabetes. There is undoubtedly some correlation between the two; most patients with severe retinopathy have renal involvement - at least on renal biopsy - and probably no patient with severe diabetic nephropathy will be free of retinopathy.

When looking at the relationship more closely the questions that have to be answered are: firstly, is the retinopathy of those who eventually die from or with diabetic renal failure different from retinopathy in other diabetic patients? Secondly, can retinopathy be arrested so that end-stage renal disease and its treatment will not lead to complete loss of vision in 40–60% of all eyes as it does at present?[1,2]

The aim of this preliminary report is to answer primarily the first question, although attempts will be made to answer the second, at least partially.

PATIENTS STUDIED

In order to answer the questions posed, we studied patients selected from almost 900 patients seen and followed at the diabetic retinopathy clinic at Hammersmith Hospital between 1965 and 1978, whose eye data was entered on computer. Some general information about the patients was also on computer; such as their date of birth, year of diabetes diagnosis and treatment. The patients were 'flagged' so that when they died their death certificates became available.

Three groups of patients were studied. The index population consisted of 43 patients (group 1) who died with or from end-stage diabetic renal disease. The computer matched these for sex, age and duration of diabetes with patients who died from conditions other than renal disease, group 2 (42 patients) and a group of patients still alive in 1980, group 3 (43 patients). Details of these patients is given in Table 1. This table demonstrates that the matching was very good, and as expected more patients in group 3 were followed for at least 5 years.

Table 1 Comparison of patient details

	Group 1	*Group 2*	*Group 3*
Total No	43	42	43
Males	26	26	26
Females	17	16	17
Age at diagnosis ± SD	24.7 ± 17.2	25.4 ± 17.4	24.7 ± 17.2
(range)	(3–58)	(4–58)	(3–59)
Followed 5 y or more	15(4)*	16	25
Followed 3–4 y	16	14	12
Followed 1–2 y	10	10	2
Followed 1 y	1	2	4

( )* = For at least last 3 years not followed at Hammersmith Hospital

Entry characteristics

Eye findings at entry

The eye findings at entry are shown in Tables 2, 3 and 4. These demonstrate that there are more patients with mild background retinopathy among those alive than those who died. More patients in group 2 had pituitary ablation than

Table 2 Retinopathy grade in worst treatable eye

	Group 1	*Group 2*	*Group 3*
No retinopathy	0	0	1
Mild background retinopathy	8	9	16
Maculopathy	7	4	4
Proliferative retinopathy (florid)	28(3)	29(6)	22(3)

in the other groups. The three groups were comparable in visual acuity of their better eye, but those in group 3 had better visual acuity in their worse eye than the other 2 groups; this was expected as more patients in group 3 had mild background retinopathy.

Table 3 Treatment for diabetic retinopathy

	Group 1	*Group 2*	*Group 3*
No specific treatment	11	14	13
Pituitary ablation	8	21	6
Photocoagulation	24	4	24

There were 35 eyes with disc new vessels at entry in group 1, 37 in group 2 and 30 in group 3. These differences were not significant. Considerably more group 1 and group 2 eyes had peripheral new vessels at entry (50 and 51 respectively) than eyes in group 3 (34) ($\chi^2 = < 0.01$). Cotton wool spots were present in 22 group 1 patients, 10 in group 2 and 14 in group 3; i.e. significantly more patients in the renal failure group had cotton wool spots ($\chi^2 = < 0.05$).

Table 4 Vision characteristics at entry

	Group 1	*Group 2*	*Group 3*
Worse eye			
$^6/_6$ - $^6/_{12}$	17	13	29
$^6/_{18}$ - $^6/_{36}$	15	14	17
$^6/_{60}$ and worse	11	15	6
Better eye			
$^6/_6$ - $^6/_{12}$	36	33	42
$^6/_{18}$ - $^6/_{36}$	7	7	1
$^6/_{60}$ and worse	0	2	0

Medical data at entry

At entry patients in group 1 had a significantly higher mean serum urea concentration of 10.7 ± 6.7 mmol/l than either group 2 (6.8 ± 1.7) or group 3 (6.5 ± 1.8) with $p < 0.01$. There were 34 patients in group 1, 24 in group 2 and 16 in group 3 in whom serum urea was above 6.5 mmol/l at the time they were first seen (Table 5.). Since creatinine was not available until 1975, this parameter was not analysed. Proteinuria was present in 21 patients in group 1 at entry, 11 in group 2 and 6 in group 3. Systolic and diastolic blood pressures (BP) are shown in Table 6a. This shows that those who later died of renal failure had higher systolic pressure than the other two groups, but the diastolic pressures were similar.

Table 5 Serum urea levels

Time	*Group 1 (mean ± SD)*	*Group 2 (mean ± SD)*	*Group 3 (mean ± SD)*
Initial	10.7 ± 6.7* (34/40)	6.7 ± 1.7 (24/41)	6.5 ± 1.8 (16/37)
3 y	15.4 ± 7.7* (28/30)	8.1 ± 3.5 (23/30)	6.9 ± 2.5 (17/36)
5 y	17.6 ± 8.2* (13/13)	9.3 ± 6.9 (12/19)	6.7 ± 1.6 (11/21)

( ) = Number with serum urea over 6.5 mmol/l, only those in whom data was available included

* = $p < 0.01$ compared with other two groups

Changes seen during the follow-up period

Eye changes

Visual acuity deteriorated in both the worse and the better eye, so that after 5 y of follow-up only 6 eyes in group 1 had 6/6–6/12 vision, 5 in group 2 and 17 in group 3, this difference being significant ($\chi^2 < 0.05$). Blindness (6/60 or worse vision) was more common in groups 1 and 2 than in group 3 (10 and 11 respectively, compared to 4 in group 3).

Cotton wool spots disappeared in all groups so that by 3 y only occasional eyes had this abnormality. It is well known that the natural history of cotton wool spots is gradual disappearance after 12 months[3], and since many of the patients had pituitary ablation or photocoagulation new lesions were not expected to form.

The progression of new vessels in the three groups was also similar. Thus in group 1, out of the 24 eyes with disc new vessels at entry, only 5 still had some after 3 years. By 5 years only 4 eyes still had some disc new vessels but all were greatly reduced. Similar improvement with treatment was seen in the other groups.

The response of peripheral new vessels to treatment was also spectacular and comparable in the 3 groups. Out of 42 eyes with peripheral new vessels in group 1, only 3 still had gradable vessels, and 5 became unassessable at 5 years. In group 2, 40 eyes had new vessels initially, 7 still had some at 5 years, and 4 eyes could no longer be assessed. In group 3 there were 26 with peripheral new vessels, 6 still had some at 5 years, while 2 became unassessable. None of these

Table 6a Blood pressure at entry

	Group 1	*Group 2*	*Group 3*
Systolic mean ± SD	157.4 ± 32* (21/42)	147.4 ± 31 (11/41)	199.3 ± 30 (16/41)
Diastolic mean ± SD	94.6 ± 17 (28/42)	89.4 ± 15 (24/41)	89.4 ± 14 (18/41)

( ) = number out of total with systolic blood pressure over 160 mmHg or diastolic pressure over 90 mmHg

* = $p < 0.05$

differences were significant, indicating that all three groups responded well to treatment, especially as the new vessels still present were mostly inactive.

Medical changes

The blood urea rose significantly in group 1 patients and by 5 years all 13 still alive in whom data is available, had raised urea. In group 2 there was also a rise, while group 3 showed little change (Table 5).

Proteinuria was commonest in the nephropathy group, but even in this group there were 3 in whom no proteinuria was noted throughout their follow-up at Hammersmith Hospital. In group 2 there were 26 such patients and in group 3, 25 had no proteinuria at any yearly examination.

The systolic and diastolic BP rose during the follow-up period in all 3 groups (Table 6b). This was in spite of the fact that all patients with pressures over 160/90 had treatment, and the aim of the treatment was to keep the BP below that level. It is noteworthy that by 5 years the systolic BP rose in groups 2 and 3 to the level of group 1 at entry.

Table 6b Blood pressure at 5 y

	Group 1	*Group 2*	*Group 3*
Systolic mean ± SD	162.3 ± 32 (6/13)	152.3 ± 27 (6/18)	154.5 ± 29 (11/22)
Diastolic mean ± SD	97.3 ± 14* (12/13)	91.7 ± 16 (9/18)	91.6 ± 13 (13/22)

Annotation as in Table 6a

COMMENTS

The data reported in this preliminary communication indicate that patients who die with renal failure do not differ significantly in retinopathy from those who die of any other cause. However, in patients who die there are more with more severe, sight threatening retinopathy than among those who stay alive.

This confirms the observation of Davis *et al*[4] who observed that proliferative retinopathy is associated with high mortality rate; the cumulative 5 year mortality in his patients was 50%.

Other reports[1,2] show that many patients with end-stage renal disease go blind. The observation in our study was that patients with impaired renal function also respond to treatment, indeed the treatment effects are similar to those found in patients without significant diabetic renal disease. The only patients whose retinopathy deteriorated badly were those in whom no treatment was given before the development of renal failure.

These findings emphasize the importance of screening patients for retinopathy before there is established renal disease. Photocoagulation at this early stage is effective and vision can then be maintained during management of end-stage renal disease, greatly improving the quality of life for these patients.

References

1. L'Esperance, F. A., Friedman, E. A. and Mondschein, L. G. (1983). Long term retention of vision following panretinal photocoagulation in diabetics. In Friedman, E. A. and L'Esperance, F. A. (eds.). *Diabetic Renal-Retinal Syndrome*. Vol. 2, pp. 285–300 (New York: Grune and Stratton)
2. Ramsay, R. C., Knobloch, W. H., Cantrill, H. L., Comty, Ch.M., Najarian, J. S. and Goetz, F. C. (1983). Visual states in transplanted and dialysised diabetic patients. In Friedman, E. A. and L'Esperance, F. A. (eds.). *Diabetic Renal-Retinal Syndrome*. Vol. 2, pp. 427–436 (New York: Grune and Stratton)
3. Kohner, E. M., Dollery, C. T. and Bulpitt, C. (1969). Cotton wool spots in diabetic retinopathy. *Diabetes,* **18**, 691
4. Davis, M. D., Hiller, R., Magli, G. L., Podger, M. J., Ederer, F., Harris, W. A., Long, J. W. and Haug, G. A. (1979). Prognosis for life in patients with diabetes in relation to severity of retinopathy. *Trans. Am. Ophthal. Soc.,* **77**, 144

13
Diabetic nephropathy: metabolic management of the patient with chronic renal failure

J. P. WAUTERS

INTRODUCTION

The rehabilitation observed in diabetic patients once end-stage renal failure has been reached is very poor, since less than one patient out of 4 treated by haemodialysis can have any physical activity beyond caring for himself[1]. This poor rehabilitation is usually not related to inadequate application of dialysis or transplantation, but generally results from multi-organ damage induced before the stage of terminal uraemia has been reached. This is illustrated in the list of complications observed among the 20 diabetic patients seen in our unit at the time of end-stage renal disease (Table 1). At present there is no doubt that control of hypertension and management of retinopathy can prevent part of those complications[2,3]. There is also strong circumstantial evidence that improved metabolic control can be beneficial[4].

Table 1 Complications in diabetics at time of ESRD

Complication	*No. patients*
Hypertension	17
Severe autonomic dysfunction	14
Severe retinopathy	10
blindness	5
Ischaemic heart disease	8
Peripheral vascular disease	6
amputation	4

$n = 20$
Type I 15
Mean age 52 y (20–70)

I would like to focus here on those metabolic problems which could be improved clinically by a more adequate control.

GLYCAEMIC CONTROL

The controversy between those believing in glycaemic control able to prevent or arrest multi-organ damage and those who believe that hereditary or other toxic factors are more important in the appearance of those lesions is still continuing[5], although the arguments for improved control are overwhelming[6].

The risk of hypo- and hyperglycaemia in those patients is relatively high, particularly once patients have been admitted to the hospital. In the series of Comty *et al*[7] the number of metabolic problems, which accounted for 14% of the reasons for admission, dramatically increased once the patients had been admitted. In the hospital 24% of the patients developed severe hyperglycaemia (> 350 mg/dl), 12% developed hypoglycaemia and 11% malnutrition[7]. Due to reduced carbohydrate intake and probably prolonged insulin halflife, the requirements for insulin are usually reduced when renal failure progresses. Once haemodialysis is started, the doses of insulin have generally to be doubled. A more stable control can be obtained with two daily injections of a mixture of regular and NPH insulin. Since the glucose-free dialysate we had previously been using, led to hypoglycaemic episodes and increased disequilibrium syndrome in diabetics, it has now been replaced for those patients by a 200 mg/dl concentration. Moreover, glucose-free dialysate leads to increased gluconeogenesis and amino acid losses[8].

In Continuous Ambulatory Peritoneal Dialysis (CAPD) patients, hyperglycaemia on the contrary is most often seen when hypertonic solutions are used. A much better glycaemic control can be obtained by the administration of insulin via the intraperitoneal catheter instead of subcutaneously[9].

One more reason to obtain a good glycaemic control is to reduce thirst, and thus decrease fluid overload and consecutive heart failure and hypertension in those patients.

In diabetics with renal failure the risk of keto-acidosis seems less common than the risk of hyperosmolar non-ketotic coma with hyperglycaemia[10].

PROTEIN AND CALORIC INTAKE

The glomerular hyperfiltration theory proposed by Brenner has shed some new light also on the pathogenesis of diabetic glomerulosclerosis[11]. In a group of rats submitted to partial nephrectomy it was possible, after 7 and 14 days of dietary protein reduction, to prevent the progression of renal failure, and to decrease the level of proteinuria. Some clinical observations have confirmed the benefits of modified diets during renal failure[12,13]. Barsotti *et al* have shown that the introduction of a diet of approximately $0.2\,g\,kg^{-1}\,d^{-1}$ of protein with essential amino acids (EAA) and keto-analogues (KA) supplements instead of $0.5\,g\,kg^{-1}\,d^{-1}$, without any other changes in therapy or diet, resulted in a stabilization or improvement of renal function[14]. The progression of the renal failure following a predictable pattern which had been shown in non-diabetics has also been confirmed for diabetic patients by Jones *et al*[15]. Correction of hypertension can modify the slope of those regression lines[2], but it remains to be demonstrated that in diabetic patients modifications of protein and caloric intake may, in addition to the euglycaemia effect, modify those slopes.

To be successful those diets need caloric intakes of 25–35 $kcal\,kg^{-1}\,d^{-1}$ usually given as carbohydrates. It is very difficult to convince diabetic patients to adjust themselves to large amounts of carbohydrate intake when they have been told for so many years to adhere strictly to a reduced carbohydrate diet. Our current practice is to recommend the following diet in diabetics with advanced renal failure:

30 kcal/kg body weight
1 g/kg of protein, with compensation for urinary losses (g per g)
carbohydrate 200–250 g/d
fat, polyunsaturated fats are recommended
restriction in K to less than 70 mEq/day, since diabetics are particularly prone to hyperkalaemia
restriction in phosphate, sodium and fiuid following the usual principles for non-diabetic patients

The risk of developing malnutrition is particularly high in diabetic patients with uraemia, since gluconeogenesis rather than protein synthesis will occur with inadequate diabetic control. During episodes of acute illness, the use of intravenous hyperalimentation seems warranted in order to avoid large losses of body mass[16].

LIPID ABNORMALITIES

The lipid abnormalities observed in uraemic diabetics are the same as in non-diabetics: the predominant lipoprotein pattern is the type IV phenotype according to Frederickson[17]. Those patients have shown an increase in the triglyceride contents of very low density lipoproteins (VLDL) and low density lipoproteins (LDL) and decrease in the high density lipoprotein (HDL) cholesterol[18]. Once haemodialysis is started in diabetic patients, cholesterol levels do not change but triglyceride levels increase[7]. When CAPD is applied in non-diabetic patients, cholesterol and triglycerides levels increase dramatically[19]. In diabetics on CAPD however, conflicting results have been reported[19,20]. In some patients the addition of insulin, intraperitoneally, allowed the reduction of serum triglyceride levels[20].

In patients with normal renal function the euglycaemia obtained through a portable insulin infusion pump can correct fasting serum cholesterol, triglycerides and free fatty acids levels after 7 and 14 days of therapy[21]. Drugs such as clofibrate are effective, but their use in patients with renal failure and often with hypoalbuminia has proven to be difficult. Diet, charcoal intake and physical exercise are also able to reduce the lipid abnormalities[18,22]. The longterm benefit of the correction of those anomalies is not definitely proven.

OSTEODYSTROPHY

It is often believed that there are no differences in renal osteodystrophy between diabetics and non-diabetics with renal failure, but in fact patients with diabetes may well have less problems with bone disease than other uraemic patients. Vincenti *et al* have shown that, on chronic haemodialysis, diabetics have, despite a lower calcaemia, lower parathyroid hormone (PTH) levels than non-diabetics; in addition they also have better skeletal scintigraphic scores and, after transplantation, less avascular necrosis[23]. Those observations could not be attributed to different durations of renal disease, levels of magnesaemia, vitamin D or phosphate-binders administration. Pabico *et al* confirmed these lower PTH levels despite comparable Ca, Mg and P levels; they attributed the lower PTH levels to vascular impairment in the parathyroid glands[24].

When we compared our groups of 10 diabetics treated with CAPD and 10 with haemodialysis, we did not observe any significant difference at 6 and 12 months in the evolution of Ca, P, alkaline phosphatase and also radiologic lesions (Table 2). These observations do not exclude bone problems in diabetic patients. One of our stable chronically haemodialysed diabetic patients recently developed, during a 7 month period, 5 spontaneous fractures of the hip. This was due to osteomalacia unresponsive to vitamin D, and not attributable to Al intoxication.

Table 2 Diabetic nephropathy – osteodystrophy

	Months	*CAPD* (n = 10)	*HD* (n = 10)
Ca mmol/l	0	2.13 ± 0.25	2.09 ± 0.31
	6	2.34 ± 0.23	2.34 ± 0.18
	12	2.40 ± 0.29	2.37 ± 0.08
P mmol/l	0	2.1 ± 0.8	2.4 ± 1.5
	6	1.7 ± 0.9	1.4 ± 0.7
	12	1.5 ± 0.6	1.4 ± 0.5
Alkaline Phosphatase IU/l	0	40 ± 14	41 ± 13
	6	35 ± 12	46 ± 15
	12	33 ± 16	38 ± 16

Mean ± SD

Once substitutive therapy is started, the hypercalcaemia often observed at the end of an haemodialysis session should be avoided, since the subsequent decrease is a potent stimulus for PTH secretion[25]. During CAPD however enough Ca should be added to the dialysate: the increase in the hyperparathyroidism observed in some CAPD patients was probably related to a negative Ca balance[26]. In one series of diabetics treated with CAPD there was, after a mean of 10 months, a slight increase in serum alkaline phosphatase but no change in PTH *N*-terminal and *C*-terminal levels[27]. de Fremont and Fournier observed, after 6 and 12 months of CAPD, a decrease in PTH *N*- and *C*-terminal levels and a regression of hyperparathyroidism, but those patients received routinely 3 g/d of Ca carbonate orally; since vitamin D depletion occurred after 12 months, they recommend systematic Vitamin D prescription[28].

The principles of management of renal osteodystrophy recommended for non-diabetic patients should also be applied to diabetic patients. The following points appear important:

(1) Treatment should be started early.

(2) Normalization of phosphataemia should be checked frequently, since diabetics seem to be prone to hypophosphataemia favoured by episodes of reduced food intake due to gastrointestinal disturbances; this hypophosphataemia probably explains most of the hypercalcaemic episodes which occur in diabetic patients.

(3) Vitamin D substitutes should be added routinely if there is no contra-indication to this therapy.

ANAEMIA

Shideman *et al* observed that diabetic patients were more anaemic than non-diabetics when haemodialysis was initiated[29]. We did not observe such a difference. During haemodialysis an increase of 1.5 g/dl in haemoglobin levels during a 4 month period was reported by White *et al*[30]. This is comparable to non-diabetics. In the patients treated with CAPD, the classical improvement in the haemoglobin and haematocrit levels has also been observed for diabetic patients.[9]. In our series, however, we did not observe a difference in the

Table 3 Diabetic nephropathy – anaemia

	Months	*CAPD* (n = 10)	*HD* (n = 10)
Haematocrit	0	25 ± 5	25 ± 3
Vol %	6	31 ± 3	27 ± 5
	12	30 ± 5	29 ± 5

Mean ± SD

evolution of haematocrit levels at 6 and 12 months between the diabetics treated with CAPD or haemodialysis (Table 3). It may be postulated, however, that in the longterm the splenic sequestration which has been found systematically in our 11 most anaemic haemodialysis patients – and which Bommer *et al* have related to silicone deposits – will not be observed in CAPD patients[31,32].

CONCLUSIONS

(1) The poor rehabilitation observed in diabetics with end-stage renal failure is generally due to previously induced multi-organ damage.

(2) Control of hypertension and management of retinopathy are no longer discussed methods to improve longterm rehabilitation.

(3) Improved metabolic control appears to be able to:
 reduce the morbidity related to wide glycaemic fluctuations
 slow the progression of renal failure
 provide adequate nutrition
 correct lipid abnormalities
 improve renal osteodystrophy.

(4) Those goals can be attained only by a team approach.

(5) Longterm controlled studies are needed to exactly establish those advantages, and define 'improved metabolic control'.

References

1. Gutman, R. A., Stead, W. W. and Robinson, R. R. (1981). Physical activity and employment status of patients on maintenance dialysis. *N. Engl. J. Med.*, **304**, 309
2. Mogensen, C. E. (1982). Long-term antihypertensive treatment inhibiting progression of diabetic nephropathy. *Br. Med. J.*, **285**, 685
3. L'Esperance, F. A., Jr., James, W. A., Friedman, E. A., Feinroth, M. V. and Mondschein, L. G. (1982). Long term retention of vision following vitrectomy in diabetic patients. In Friedman, E. A. and L'Esperance, F. A. Jr. (eds.). *Diabetic Renal-Retinal Syndrome*, pp. 277–283. (New York: Grune & Stratton)
4. Cahill, G. F. (1982). Will euglycemia prevent vasculopathy? In Friedman, E. A. and L'Esperance, F. A., Jr. (eds). *Diabetic Renal-Retinal Syndrome,* pp. 529–535. (New York: Grune & Stratton)
5. Siperstein, M. D., Foster, D. W., Knowles, H. C. Jr., Levine, R., Madison, L. L. and Roth, J. (1977). Control of blood glucose and diabetic vascular disease. *N. Engl. J. Med.*, **18**, 1060
6. Friedman, E. A. (1982). Diabetic nephropathy. Strategies in prevention and management. *Kidney Int.*, **21**, 780
7. Comty, C. M., Leonard, A. N. and Shapiro, F. L. (1974). Nutritional and metabolic problems in the dialyzed patient with diabetes mellitus. *Kidney Int.*, **6**, (Suppl.) S51
8. Aviram, A., Peters, J. H. and Gulyassy, P. F. (1971). Dialysance of amino acids and related substances. *Nephron,* **8**, 440
9. Rottembourg, J., El Shahat, Y., Agrafiotis, A., Thuillier, Y., de Groc F., Jacobs, C. and Legrain, M. (1983). Continuous ambulatory peritoneal dialysis in insulin-dependent diabetic patients: A 40-month experience. *Kidney Int.*, **23**, 40
10. Uribarri, J., Alveranga, D. and Carroll, H. J. (1983). Water, electrolyte, and acid-base abnormalities in diabetes mellitus. *Diabet. Nephrop.*, **2**, 34

11. Brenner, B.M., Meyer, T.W. and Hostetter, T.H. (1982). Dietary protein intake and the progressive nature of kidney disease: The role of hemodynamically mediated glomerular injury in the pathogenesis of progressive glomerular sclerosis in aging, renal ablation, and intrinsic renal disease. *N. Engl. J. Med.*, **307**, 652
12. Giordano, C. (1982). Protein restriction in chronic renal failure. *Kidney Int.*, **22**, 401
13. Maschio, G., Oldrizzi, L., Tessitore, N., d'Angelo, A., Valvo, E., Lupo, A., Loschiavo, C., Fabris, A., Gammaro, L., Rugiu, C. and Panzetta, G. (1982). Effects of dietary protein and phosphorus restriction on the progression of early renal failure. *Kidney Int.*, **22**, 371
14. Barsotti, G., Guiducci, A., Ciardella, F. and Giovannetti, S. (1981). Effects on renal function of a low-nitrogen diet supplemented with essential amino acids and ketoanalogues and of hemodialysis and free protein supply in patients with chronic renal failure. *Nephron*, **27**, 113
15. Jones, R.H., Hayakawa, H., Mackay, J.D., Parsons, V. and Watkins, P.J. (1979). Progression of diabetic nephropathy. *Lancet*, **i**, 1105
16. Batist, G., Bistrian, B.R., Kaldany, A., Phinney, S., Busick, E.J., Miller, D.G. and D'Elia, J.A. (1981). Intravenous total parenteral nutrition in diabetic renal failure. *Nephron*, **28**, 244
17. Brunzell, J.D., Albers, J.J. and Haas, L.D. (1977). Prevalence of serum lipid abnormalities in chronic hemodialysis. *Metabolism*, **26**, 903
18. Chan, M.K., Varghese, Z. and Moorhead, J.F. (1981). Lipid abnormalities in uremia, dialysis, and transplantation. *Kidney Int.*, **19**, 625
19. Khanna, R., Breckenridge, C., Roncari, D., Digenis, G. and Oreopoulos, D.G. (1983). Lipid abnormalities in patients undergoing continuous ambulatory peritoneal dialysis. *Perit. Dial. Bull.*, **3**, (suppl.) S13
20. Moncrief, J.W., Pyle, W.K., Simon, P. and Popovich, R.P. (1981). Hypertriglyceridemia, diabetes mellitus, and insulin administration in patients undergoing continuous ambulatory peritoneal dialysis. In Moncrief, J.W. and Popovich, R.P. (eds.). *CAPD Update. Continuous Ambulatory Peritoneal Dialysis*, pp. 143–165. (New York Masson)
21. Tamborlane, W.V., Sherwin, R.S., Genel, M. and Felig, P. (1979). Restoration of normal lipid and aminoacid metabolism in diabetic patients treated with a portable insulin-infusion pump. *Lancet*, **i**, 1258
22. Manis, T., Zeig, S., Feinstein, E.I., Lum, G. and Friedman, E.A. (1979). Oral sorbents in uremia and diabetes; charcoal-induced hypolipidemia. *Trans. Am. Soc. Artif. Intern. Organs*, xxv, 19
23. Vincenti, F., Hattner, R., Amend, W.J. Jr., Feduska, N.J., Duca, R.M. and Salvatierra, O. Jr. (1981). Decreased secondary hyperparathyroidism in diabetic patients receiving hemodialysis. *JAMA*, **245**, 930
24. Pabico, R.C., Rivero, A.J., McKenna, B.A. and Freeman, R.B. (1982). Parathyroid hormone (PTH) in patients with diabetes mellitus and end-stage renal disease (ESRD) on chronic hemodialysis (CHD). In *Abstracts XIXth Congress of the European Dialysis and Transplant Association*, p. 106, Madrid
25. Burckhardt, P. and Wauters, J.P. (1979). Acute plasma parathormone fluctuations induced by varying calcium dialysate during chronic hemodialysis. *Kidney Int.*, **15**, 583
26. Delmez, J.A., Slatopolsky, E., Martin, K.J., Gearing, B.N. and Harter, H.R. (1982). Minerals, vitamin D, parathyroid hormone in continuous ambulatory peritoneal dialysis. *Kidney Int.*, **21**, 862
27. Llach, F. (1983). Metabolic bone disease in the CAPD patient. *Periton. Dial. Bull.*, **3**, (suppl.) S24
28. de Fremont, J.F., Bataille, P., Morinière, P., Kaczmareck, P., Fievet, P. and Fournier, A. (1981). Metabolic tolerance of continuous ambulatory peritoneal dialysis. In Gahl, G.M., Kessel, M. and Nolph, K.D. (eds.). *Advances in Peritoneal Dialysis*, pp. 446–448. (Amsterdam: Excerpta Medica)
29. Shideman, J.R., Buselmeier, T.J. and Kjellstrand, C.M. (1976). Complications in insulin-dependent patients accepted for renal transplantation. *Arch. Intern. Med.*, **136**, 1126
30. White, N., Snowden, S.A., Parsons, V., Sheldon, J. and Bewick, M. (1973). The management of terminal renal failure in diabetic patients by regular dialysis therapy. *Nephron*, **11**, 261

31. Wauters, J.P., Biollaz, J., Delaloy-Bischof, A., and Delaloye, B. (1980). Facteurs aggravant l'anémie en hémodialyse chronique: destruction exagérée ou pertes? *Schweiz. Med. Wschr.*, **110**, 1888
32. Bommer, J., Waldherr, R. and Ritz, E. (1981). Silicone filings in macrophages of viscera: An iatrogenic complication of hemodialysis. In Robinson, B.H.B., Hawkins, J.B. and Davison, A.M. (eds.). *Proceedings of The European Dialysis and Transplant Association*. Vol. 18, pp. 731–735. (London: Pitman)

Open discussion

Professor Ritz: There is no doubt from the DRS Study that laser coagulation is efficacious and beneficial. I was struck with the observation of one patient who after laser coagulation had progressive vaso-occlusion of the retina. A colleague in Essen confirmed similar observations. I am very much concerned about this possibility and would ask whether this is related to the laser coagulation or is part of the spontaneous course of the retinopathy?

Dr Kohner: Probably it is the natural course of retinopathy. It is very difficult to be absolutely sure of this. When roughly half of the retina, or sometimes even more, is destroyed, there is no doubt that there is reduction of blood flow, and certainly peripheral occlusion is very common. But then there is no peripheral retina so there is no need for blood flow.

But I think it is a natural history of the disease, and certainly neither pituitary ablation nor photocoagulation affects the large vessel disease in the eye.

Professor E A Friedman (USA): There is a danger when trying to separate diabetics who have died from kidney failure from those who have not died from kidney failure of not recognizing that some of those classed as not dying from kidney failure have in fact been deceased from that cause.

In the UK, Dr Parsons has reported that nephrologists tend to under-recognize deaths from kidney failure in patients whom they cannot treat, and since diabetics in renal failure are generally not treated in the UK, many of the deaths attributed to other causes may in fact, as in Dr Kohner's Group 2, have been deaths from uraemia. I would wish to be convinced that the two groups were really different.

Dr Kohner: Very few were azotaemic. There were some azotaemics. I knew all these patients myself and in the patients who died, we went through their case notes very carefully. Since 1976 we have also had creatinine levels.

Blood urea is not the best estimate of what happens to these patients' renal condition, because if they are hyperglycaemic and dehydrated, their blood urea will rise, so creatinine is a much better estimate of renal function.

I am not saying that those in Group 2 had no renal involvement. I am saying that they had no significant renal failure.

Professor Friedman: I shall leave that until I read the paper. But, what is significant may be that which caused a heart attack or a stroke.

Now, to Dr Wauters. I think that he has identified a very important syndrome which we have also seen in the patient with the multiple pelvic fractures without cause. We had one femoral neck fracture in a patient who did not respond to Vitamin D and appeared to be osteomalacic. We treated that patient with electromagnetic irradiation, as has been used at Columbia, an electrical field therapy, and it healed without need for pinning. I wanted to ask about the outcome for Dr Wauters' patient. I think he said with four separate fractures of the pelvis. It would be fascinating to get it reported because I believe it is a relatively unrecognized syndrome in the ureamic diabetic.

Dr Wauters: I believe the syndrome has been described in non-diabetics and I do not think it is specific for diabetes. But, the evolution of this patient was really dramatic. All the orthopaedists recommended that we should put the patient on bed rest for several weeks. The patient died two weeks before the Symposium and we did not try the treatment Professor Friedman described.

Professor M Leski (Switzerland): What was the level of PTH? If it is a *C*-terminal assay, one could ask if it is secretion or redistribution.

Dr Wauters: The assay used was an *N*-terminal assay, so it is not a question of fragments accumulating.

Dr G Viberti (UK): Professor Ritz postulated that elevation of systemic blood pressure could lead to increased GFR. Have we any data on whether patients with early idiopathic hypertension have got high GFRs?

My second question is, if they have, can Professor Ritz speculate on the possible determinants of the high GFR in idiopathic hypertension?

Professor Ritz: This is very pertinent. Actually, the only evidence in support of the hypothesis is the experimental study of Hostetter & Brenner. I do not feel that essential hypertension is the proper control to look at. The proper control for an analogous mechanism is the animal with some other type of a problem. Indeed, in a basement membrane glomerulonephritis when there is an impairment of K_f of hydraulic permeability, what one does see is an increase in filtration pressure, in hydraulic pressure, vasodilatation with a decrease of afferent arteriolar resistance and glomerular hypertension despite systemic normotension. And there is good indirect evidence that the same thing happens in patients with glomerulonephritis.

We have described patients with IgA glomerulonephritis whom we had biopsied at a time when they were normotensive, and they already had lesions in the afferent arterioles, without immune deposits. It was only two or three years subsequently that they developed systemic hypertension.

That is the best evidence I can present that normotension or hypertension in the presence of a glomerular problem will lead to glomerular hypertension.

The flaw in the argument is that in essential hypertension there is no primary glomerular problem.

Professor d'Amico: If Dr Wauters believes in the Brenner theory, there is no doubt that we should restrict the amount of protein in diabetic diets. What would he recommend as the amount of protein per kilo in patients with severe renal insufficiency or renal failure, and how in this case, if proteins are reduced, can the patient have an adequate caloric intake?

Perhaps, too, Professor Ritz would discuss his policies on this.

Dr Wauters: Brenner's theory is very stimulating and needs additional clinical support before it can be applied to all patients. For diabetics it is too early to say. These patients are prone to malnutrition, and at this time it is too early to recommend restricting protein to < 1 g/kg. Similarly with renal failure.

Professor d'Amico: Would Professor Ritz agree?

Professor Ritz: Irrespective of my own convictions, my patients do what they like. Germans, who once had the reputation of being over-obedient to authority, now do not respect any medical authority at all.

Dr G A Cinotti (Italy): What is Professor Ritz's experience of orthostatic hypotension during antihypertensive treatment in diabetic patients?

Secondly, in view of the known tendency of the hyporeninaemic–hypoaldosteronism of diabetic patients, could the use of captopril and other inhibitors of the converting enzyme be a problem in these patients?

Professor Ritz: In response to the first question, the worst medical problem one encounters in a hypertensive patient is proneness to orthostatic hypotension. Frankly there is no ideal solution. Instruction as to proper lifestyle is very helpful but will certainly not eliminate hypotensive episodes.

There is some experimental work going on based on pharmacodynamic considerations that yohombine is efficacious in such patients, and there has been preliminary information from Essen on this, but it would certainly be premature to recommend it as a general procedure.

On the second question, regarding captopril. The reported incidence of hyperkalaemia in patients treated with captopril was very low. The reason is probably the following. If captopril is used as monotherapy, the risk would probably be very high. But captopril as a monotherapy is only able to eliminate hypertension in 20% of those patients who had been resistant to triple therapy in a series of over 100 patients that we published. Since we use high doses of frusemide, we have at the same time wiped out the risk of hyperkalaemia, at least in my view, and in fact I have not seen it in our diabetic patients. It is certainly something to watch for, but it is partially eliminated by the concomitant administration of frusemide.

Dr R Khanna (Canada): Has Professor Ritz got any experience of captopril used in non-dialysis patients with residual kidney function. During treatment with captopril, kidney function will gradually reduce. How does Professor Ritz account for this?

Professor Ritz: Predictably, yes. I would anticipate that it would go down. Whenever there is high intrarenal angiotensin activity, there must be a fall in GFR. This was observed three years ago in various transplantation centres, when kidneys which had been ischaemic and vasospastic from a rejection crisis became acutely oliguric after the administration of captopril. There was a flurry of reports recently in *N. Engl. J. Med.* and *Ann. Intern. Med.*

The reason for it is the following. The kidney has two different autoregulatory processes. One is responsible for plasma flow, and this is largely unrelated to renin. The second is responsible for autoregulation of glomerular filtration rate. Angiotensin 2 is responsible for the latter aspect. If angiotensin is taken out in a kidney which depends on angiotension 2 for maintaining GFR, there is bound to be a fall in GFR when captopril is administered.

Dr Khanna: Even in the absence of renal artery stenosis.

Professor Ritz: Certainly yes. There was a fascinating report at the last annual meeting of the American Society of Nephrology where in isolated perfused afferent and efferent renal arterioles, dose response curves to angiotensin were established. There was a difference by a factor of 100 in the angiotensin sensitivity of the efferent over the afferent ateriole. It was quite obvious that efferent vasoconstriction to maintain glomerular filtration rate is probably one of the major intrarenal actions of angiotensin, in the presence or in the absence of renal artery stenosis.

Dr Wauters: Concerning the fall in glomerular filtration rate, we had the impression that clinically this lasted approximately for 15 days. Would Professor Ritz agree with this early fall in GFR and recovery afterwards when the hypertension is corrected?

Professor Ritz: In transplanted patients?

Dr Wauters: No. In patients with renal failure.

Professor Ritz: I was less courageous than Dr Wauters was. I stopped captopril when GFR came down.

Dr Wauters: On the problem of hyperkalaemia we have had experience with captopril of some 15 patients now on dialysis. It has been a problem in one of our patients where we had to increase the exchange resins. But in the other patients we did not see any problem.

Professor J Simoes (Portugal): Professor Ritz compared total exchangeable sodium in hypertensive diabetics and normals. How does total exchangeable sodium compare between diabetic hypertensives and idiopathic hypertensives?

Professor Ritz: I wish I had done that study. Peter Weidmann, in Berne, reported it in *Kidney International* in 1977. But I can answer the question to the extent that measurements of exchangeable sodium have been performed in quite a number of laboratories in essential hypertension, in incipient hypertension and in borderline hypertension to prove or disprove the hypothesis of low renin hypertension being due to volume expansion, and there is unanimity that there is no expansion of the exchangeable sodium in the neutral phase of hypertension.

Interestingly, there is an expanded extracellular and a total sodium space in advanced hypertension, and this may explain why aged hypertensive patients are sensitive to diuretics, whereas the juvenile incipient hypertensive is less sensitive.

Peter Weidmann's data show a marginal increase in patients in whom he was not able to exclude – to my satisfaction – a renal problem. That is probably the explanation for his data. In essential hypertension, although he did not compare it, there is no increase of exchangeable sodium.

Professor M Legrain (France): If we can go back to nutritional requirements, I should like to be sure that the speakers and the experts in the audience would agree on the fact that our advice to patients with diabetes plus end-stage renal failure should be that they receive adequate caloric intake, according to their activity, and that they should get half that caloric intake from carbohydrate. They should ingest 1 g/kg bodyweight of protein, and the remaining rations should be given as lipids.

Are there people against this?

Professor d'Amico: I am a little bit against. We have to reduce protein. There is sufficient evidence to cut the protein and to increase the carbohydrate intake. We must drop it to 0.7–0.8 g/kg protein in severe renal failure, if we believe that a high-protein diet is dangerous for severe renal damage. If it is true in the normal uraemic patient, then it is even more so in diabetic patients.

Professor Ritz: I would strongly disagree, and for the following reasons. P. Degoulet, from data from the French Diaphane Registry (*Nephron* (1982), **31,** 103) clearly showed that malnutrition in dialysed patients is a most important predictor of cerebrovascular catastrophe. Epidemiological data from Japan support this; that the more malnourished the patient and the lower the protein, the greater the risk of cerebrovascular accident at any given level of hypertension. There is evidence on this from the stroke-prone strain of the SH rat. When given a low-protein diet, it will have more severe and earlier cerebral haemorrhage than if it has adequate nutritional status.

I am aware of a study – unpublished – of Dr Klinkman in East Germany where, because of restriction of facilities, they had their patients prior to haemodialysis on severe protein restriction. I was told, although I did not read the data, that those who had severe protein restriction had higher cardiovascular mortality during dialysis than those who had less restriction.

I think the balance of evidence is strongly in favour of adequate nutritional status.

Professor d'Amico: And does good nutritional status require a protein intake of at least 1 g/kg? Surely 40 g protein is enough for a patient of average weight?

Professor Ritz: I think there are national differences. German patients are heavier, and national dietary habits are different. One thing that must be given very careful consideration is the hypercatabolic state of uraemia. In uraemia, for any given dietary intake of protein there would be less growth in the experimental rat - as Dr Mehls and I published. If the patient is maintained at 40 g protein, that is a very narrow margin of safety. The slightest infection, the slightest catabolic stress will throw the patient severely out of balance.

Professor E A Friedman (USA): There may be some confusion. I thought Professor Legrain asked about the azotaemic diabetic. For that patient protein restriction to 40 g, plus the amount lost in a nephrotic urinary excretion produces a metabolic balance as shown by J. Kopple. To my knowledge, the only metabolic balance studies of various protein diets in pre-dialysis patients were done by Dr J. Kopple.

Secondly, Dr Ritz responded about dialysis patients. I agree with Dr Ritz that a 40 g protein diet in a patient already on dialysis may be insufficient to maintain nutrition. So let us be specific. The predialysis diabetic should have some degree of protein restriction. Right now the religion, not the fact, says 40 g plus the amount lost in the urine. The dialysis diabetic may be badly nourished even with as much as 1 g/kg, and there we have yet to have a proper balance study to answer the question with precision.

Dr Wauters: I agree.

Professor Ritz: May I respond briefly. If Professor Friedman is referring to the 1973 paper of J. Kopple and J. Coburn, looking this paper through very carefully, with the 20 g diet they had catastrophic compliance and negative nitrogen balance. With the 40 g diet they still had a high rate of non-compliance, and only in those patients who stuck to the diet did they achieve balance. But, J. Kopple was very careful to point out that plasma in a sero-balance does not mean that the patient is in equilibrium, because of various artefacts related to the technique. The risk of protein depletion with respect to future complications on dialysis outweighs any delay in the deterioration of renal function.

We are talking about a condition, as Dr Mogensen showed, where the monthly rate of progression is 1 ml/minute GFR, so whether he is dialysed four weeks earlier or six weeks earlier does not matter if future life expectancy is endangered from cardiovascular risk on dialysis.

Professor Friedman: Would Professor Ritz concur that what he is emphatically presenting is his religious belief and not a factual statement?

Professor Ritz: OK.

Professor d'Amico: It is time to break . . .

14
Selection principles and outcome of renal transplantation in diabetics

H. BRYNGER, O. LARSSON, P. O. ATTMAN, B. FRISK, M. LUNDBERG, M. MULEC and L. SANDBERG

INTRODUCTION

The renal transplant programme in Gothenburg, Sweden started in 1965, and developed into a routine procedure for treatment of end-stage renal disease in the beginning of the 1970s. In 1972 diabetic patients were also included into the programme, but on a limited scale up to 1976. During this period 21 patients were grafted. However, since 1977 the number of diabetic patients with renal failure accepted for treatment has steadily increased and today constitute almost 30% of all primary grafts performed in our centre, thus the second most frequent cause of end-stage renal failure in our programme. We have previously reported on our experiences[1-5]. The present study deals with the results up to June 1982 in 100 consecutive patients.

PATIENTS AND METHODS

Between December 1972 and June 1982 100 diabetic patients received a total of 121 renal transplants. Ninety-four of the patients had juvenile onset diabetes, i.e. onset of disease prior to 24 years of age, and four patients had concomitant renal disease besides the diabetic nephropathy contributing to end-stage renal failure. All patients were insulin dependent, i.e. type I diabetes. The patients were divided into two periods, 1972–1976 (period I, 21 patients) and 1977–1982 (period II, 79 patients). During the latter period the selection and treatment has been uniform, while the first period could be described as a period of trial and error. During period II, 72 patients with juvenile onset diabetes without concomitant renal disease were grafted, 36 with kidneys from living related donors (LRD) and 36 with kidneys from cadaveric origin (CD).

During period II, 168 non-diabetic patients aged between 20 and 54 years served as controls. Of these 36 received LRD kidneys from donors sharing one HLA-haplotype with the recipient and 132 patients received primary cadaveric kidneys.

Selection principles

During the first period selection principles varied considerably, while during the second period quite uniform general selection principles have been applied. Most of the patients have been referred to our unit for medical evaluation in a preuraemic state with serum-creatinine levels corresponding to 200–300 μmol/l. Only patients with the following conditions have been considered unsuitable for transplantation:

(1) Cardiac decompensation in spite of adequate treatment of hypertension and oedema

(2) Advanced neuropathy in combination with trophic ulcers

(3) Peripheral vascular disease with imminent or established gangrene

A stabilized postamputation situation has not precluded transplantation.

Timing of transplantation

During period I, the majority of patients were transplanted before dialysis had been instituted, while during period II 60/79 patients were treated with dialysis before transplantation, but generally the time on dialysis was short and exceeded 1 year in six patients only (Table 1). Of the dialysed patients the majority were treated with haemodialysis, three patients received Intraperitoneal Dialysis (IPD) and six patients Continuous Ambulatory Peritoneal Dialysis (CAPD).

Table 1 Timing of transplantation in diabetes

	1972–76	*1977–82*
Dialysis	5	60
Creatinine >1000	4	3
Creatinine <1000	12	16
Total	21	79

Tissue typing, matching and transfusion policy

During period II the possibility of a living related donor was thoroughly investigated in all potential transplant candidates. In most cases kidneys from parental origin were used, only seven siblings provided kidneys. Of the siblings only three shared two haplotypes with the recipient while the remaining four together with all the parents shared one haplotype. In cadaver kidney transplantation HLA- A and B typing was performed, but the matching principles were not very strict, the only rule was to avoid two mismatches within the HLA-B locus. During the same period a deliberate transfusion policy was followed; previously non-transfused recipients were given two units of leukocyte-poor blood as preparation before transplantation, both in LRD- and CD transplantation[6]. Out of 72 juvenile onset diabetics 40 were transfused according to this protocol while 30 patients had been transfused earlier from medical reasons.

A standardized, uniform immunosuppressive treatment was used in all patients based on prednisolone and azathioprine only. Prednisolone was given at an initial dosage of 3 mg/kg body weight, and quickly tapered to 0.5 and 0.3 mg/kg body weight after 6 weeks and 3 months, respectively. Antirejection therapy was based on bolus doses of methyl-prednisolone using a 3 day course with 0.5, 0.25 and 0.25 g. The total dose of methyl-prednisolone given, seldom exceeded 3 g.

RESULTS

The overall actuarial patient survival in the two periods is accounted for in Table 2. As can be seen a significant improvement of patient survival occurred in the second period.

Table 2 Patient survival in 1972–76 (period I) and 1977–82 (period II)

	1 year	*2 years*	*3 years*
Period I[(a)] ($n = 21$)	62	52	48
Period II[(a)] ($n = 79$)	85	76	76

(a) Period I *vs* period II $p < 0.05$

In Table 3 patient and graft survival is given for the 72 juvenile diabetics without concomitant renal disease and for non-diabetic controls. In both categories of patients, living related donors kidneys give the best results both regarding patient and graft survival. However, this difference is especially striking regarding graft survival in diabetics where 3 year survival of CD grafts of 37% depicts the difficulties with immunosuppression in this category of patients. However, the patient survival was much better with 70% at 3 years which has enabled us to regraft a number of these patients. Thus, the present overall situation is that of the 100 patients consecutively receiving primary grafts 31 are dead, and consequently 69 alive. Of these 69 patients 64 are alive with a functioning graft and only five are maintained on dialysis.

Table 3 Patient and graft survival in juvenile diabetics and non-diabetic controls, period II (%)

			Patient survival (y)			Graft survival (y)		
			1	2	3	1	2	3
Diabetics	LRD	(36)	91	82	79	79	79	79
	CD	(36)	79	70	70	48	37	37
Non-diabetic	LRD	(36)	97	97	97	92	88	88
	CD	(132)	91	84	77	70	64	56

LRD = Living related donor
CD = Cadaveric donor
No. of transplants given in parenthesis

The causes of death during period II for diabetics and non-diabetic controls are given in Table 4. As can be seen the main causes are distributed quite similarly in both these groups, with a slightly higher incidence of infectious causes of death among diabetics. It should be pointed out, however, that the majority of both diabetic and non-diabetic patients died with poor graft function or on dialysis after graft failure.

Table 4 Causes of death, 1977–82

	Juvenile onset diabetics (n = 72)	*Non-diabetics* (n = 168)
Cardiovascular	4 (29%)	10 (40%)
Cerebrovascular	2 (14%)	2 (8%)
Pulmonary embolism	1 (7%)	2 (8%)
Infections	5 (36%)	6 (24%)
Other	2 (14%)	5 (20%)
Total	14	25

The main cause of graft loss in both diabetics and the non-diabetics controls was rejection. Among the diabetics two grafts had to be acutely removed because of anastomosis bleeding due to arteritis. It should also be pointed out that two of the LRD grafts failed with a histological and clinical picture of *de novo* glomerulonephritis without evidence of rejection.

COMMENTS

The satisfying results of renal transplantation in diabetic recipients in Gothenburg since 1977 could be ascribed to the extensive use of living related donors. Both patient and graft survival in patients receiving such kidneys has been very gratifying. On the other hand, the primary cadaver transplants have not been at all that successful, however, the patient survival has been acceptable, which has enabled us to perform a number of successful regrafts in these patients improving the overall graft survival considerably.

The selection and monitoring of the patients up to the moment of transplantation, which has been very uniform during the last period has been of utmost importance for the outcome of transplantation. This is further stressed by the fact that even after a failure of a cadaveric graft, the patient has been in many cases a suitable candidate for another transplantation. Finally, it should be mentioned that renal transplantation in diabetic recipients has evolved into a routine procedure which today has an undisputed place in active treatment for end-stage renal disease in our country.

References

1. Larsson, O., Brynger, H., Bengtsson, U., Ewald, J. and Gelin, L.-E. (1976). Kidney transplantation in patients with diabetes nephropathy. *Scand. J. Urol.*, **105** (Suppl.) 38
2. Ewald, J., Larsson, O., Brynger, H. and Bengtsson, U. (1977). Factors influencing the prognosis in diabetic patients accepted for renal transplantation. *Scand. J. Urol. Nephrol.*, **114** (Suppl.) 42
3. Larsson, O. and Brynger, H. (1980). Transplantation in patients with diabetic nephropathy. *Acta Endocrin.*, **113** (Suppl.) 238
4. Brynger, H. and Larsson, O. (1982). 10 years experience of renal transplantation in diabetic patients. In Küss R. and Legrain, M. (eds.). *Séminaires d'uronéphrologie,* 127. (Pitié-Salpetriêrè: Masson)
5. Larsson, O., Attman, P.-O., Blohmé, H. and Brynger, H. (1982). Transplantation in patients with diabetic nephropathy: A 10 year experience. *Transplant. Proc.*, **14**, 30
6. Frisk, B., Brynger, H. and Sandberg, L. (1982). Two random transfusions before primary renal transplantation - four years' experience from a single center. *Transplant. Proc.*, **14**, 386

Discussant

J. JERVELL

Dr Jervell (Norway): First, I should like to congratulate the Gothenburg Group on their very good results, especially in cadaver transplants, both in diabetics and in non-diabetics. I am not sure we can quite copy those results, but I should like to confirm that there is very little difference in survival between diabetics and non-diabetics, whether donor kidneys or cadaver kidneys are used. We should no longer be treating our diabetics as second-class citizens when it comes to transplantation.

In Norway, population 4 million, diabetics represented 19% of all transplants in the period under review; 4.1 diabetics per million inhabitants per year. Perhaps more surprising, in the younger age group, 25–40 years old, diabetics represented 40% of all transplantations. If we had an upper age limit of 45 and did not transplant diabetics we should be transplanting very few patients indeed.

The high number of diabetics transplanted in Scandinavia may not only be due to an active policy but also to a high incidence of juvenile diabetes; incidence being about 200 per million children per year in Sweden and Finland and slightly lower in Norway and in Denmark. I do not know the exact figures for Great Britain and Holland but I have been told about 10. Perhaps if we do 20% diabetics, then Holland should do 10% – if they are not much better at managing diabetes and thus preventing nephropathy. In Norway, therefore, there should be 125 new diabetic children each year, and 20 of these, and some of those that get diabetes at an older age, will end up with renal transplantation.

As to diabetic management during transplantation, the insulin dose is more than doubled due to renal tissue being present, better appetite and prednisolone. Even after 9 months the insulin dose is right up. In acute rejection treated with prednisolone treatment, dosage has to be increased. We do not use pumps or any infusion. We use the ordinary two or three times daily insulin, take blood sugar four times daily, and adjust the dose daily, automatically increasing the dose in cases of rejection. We never attain normoglycaemia, but we approach it sometimes in some patients.

We are hesitant in teaching these patients home glucose monitoring because of the considerable tendency to necrosis of the fingers and toes. If they go on pricking themselves 4–8 times daily, we might make the situation worse, so in some patients we advise against it.

Cyclosporin will perhaps make diabetic management for this group of patients easier because they need less prednisolone and there are fewer rejections on cyclosporin. So far we have transplanted ten diabetics using cyclosporin and it is our impression that they do much better.

As for rehabilitation, in patients with functioning grafts at 1 year 10% are in institutions, usually with cerebral atrophy. More than 50% are considered able to work, although not everybody can get work and their pensions may be too high for motivation. The main problems in rehabilitation are blindness and peripheral circulatory disturbances.

Data on transplantation are usually presented as a patient or graft survival curve. A vision survival curve shows that patients coming to transplantation with reading vision following a successful transplant usually maintain their ability to read. This is perhaps one indication for transplanting diabetics early, before there is rapid progression in retinopathy.

Renal transplantation in the Scandinavian countries, at least in Norway, has now become for diabetics a self-perpetuating benign circle, because the transplanted diabetic patients are very active in the patient associations, both in the renal patient associations and in the diabetic associations, seeing to it that they are treated like everybody else and not like second-class citizens.

15
Human segmental pancreatic transplantation for the treatment of insulin-dependent diabetes

J. TRAEGER, J. M. DUBERNARD, E. BOSI, A. SECCHI, A. GELET, S. EL YAFI, J. L. TOURAINE, A. E. PONTIROLI and G. POZZA

INTRODUCTION

The correction of the metabolic abnormalities of insulin-dependent diabetes depends on the ability of reproducing, by means of an appropriate replacing therapy, the insulin secretion which has been lost because of the disease.

The pancreatic beta cell, with its capability of self-regulation and of responsiveness to the whole humoral signals, represents the ideal means for the insulin restoration.

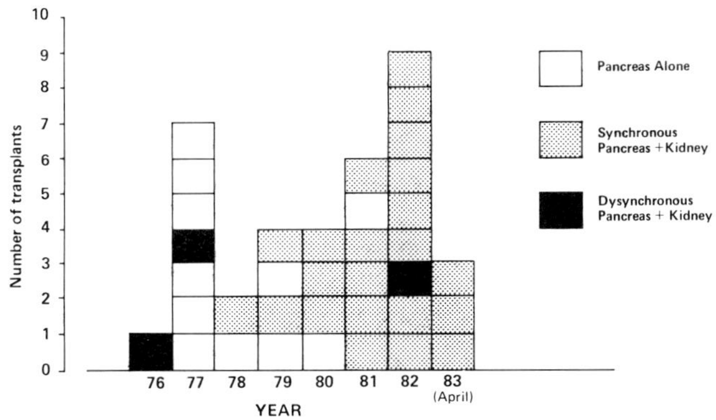

Figure 1 Number of pancreatic transplants performed at the Herriot Hospital of Lyon according to year and techniques

The attempts at transplantation of either pancreas or islets in humans have been difficult because of technical and immunological problems[1]. Only in the late 1970s, the development of new and safer surgical techniques for the segmental graft, led to a revival of interest for the clinical applications of pancreas transplantation[2]. At the Herriot Hospital of Lyon, the first pancreatic transplant was performed in October 1976. Between then and March 1983, 36 pancreatic transplants were performed in 34 diabetic patients using the same technique of segmental graft with handling of the pancreatic exocrine secretion by polymer injection (Figure 1). Some clinical and endocrinological aspects of our experience are reported herein.

PATIENTS AND TECHNIQUES

Patients

The 34 patients were all insulin-dependent diabetic patients, aged 35.1 ± 8.7 years with a duration of diabetes of 20.6 ± 6.2 years (mean ± SD). All the patients were affected by severe degenerative diabetic complications, six of them being completely blind at the time of transplantation. Diabetic nephropathy was present at a preuraemic degree in six recipients of single pancreatic transplants; all the others were affected by end-stage renal failure and they were maintained in haemo- (27 cases) or peritoneal (1 case) dialysis. Donors were heart-beating cadavers selected for ABO compatibilities and negative cross-matches.

Surgical technique

The segmental transplant technique, with suppression of the exocrine secretion by neoprene injection into the pancreatic ductal system, was employed overall, without significant differences from its original description[2]. Briefly, the pancreatic segment, including the body and the tail, is removed from the donor: a variable amount (3–8 ml) of neoprene, a liquid synthetic rubber which solidifies at contact with the pancreatic juice, is then injected in the Wirsung duct, leading to an extended fibrosis of the exocrine parenchyma, but preserving the islet tissue.

The segmental graft is then placed in the iliac fossa of the recipient and vascularized by anastomosis to iliac artery and vein.

When a kidney transplant is also performed, the renal graft is placed in the opposite iliac fossa.

In 11 cases pancreas was transplanted alone, in 2 cases it preceded and in 1 case it followed a kidney transplant; in 22 cases pancreas and kidney were transplanted simultaneously (Figure 1).

Immunosuppression

The recipients of pancreas allografts were treated with azathioprine, prednisone and anti-lymphocyte-globulins (ALG) in 22 cases, with cyclosporin A (CyA) and ALG plus prednisone in case of rejection episodes in 8 cases, and with CyA after an initial period of conventional treatment in 6 cases.

RESULTS

The survival rate of the 34 patients undergoing primary pancreatic transplantation was 75% at 6 months, 65% at 1 year and 49% at 2 years. The overall survival rate of the 36 pancreatic transplants was 49% at 3 months at 6 months, 21% at 1 year and 13% at 2 years. Different survival rates were obtained according to the different transplant techniques and immunosuppressive treatments employed.

Single pancreatic transplant series

Of the 13 single pancreatic transplants, only two survived more than 3 months, allowing the patients to receive a kidney allograft a second time.

The causes of failure were immediate or near-immediate vascular thrombosis in four cases, vascular thrombosis or rejection in two cases, rejection in four cases, and a death from cardiac failure in one case.

Of the two patients who received a renal graft after pancreas, one returned to insulin therapy 9 months after pancreatic transplantation because of chronic rejection, the other died of meningitis 11 months after pancreatic transplantation with both pancreas and kidney functioning.

The only pancreas transplanted after kidney was a second graft after pancreatic failure of a primary simultaneous double transplant, with kidney still functioning; the patient remained insulin-independent for 4 months, until the resumption of insulin therapy was necessary because of a recurrence of hyperglycaemia due to rejection.

In this series, only two patients received CyA as part of immunosuppressive treatment.

Simultaneous kidney plus pancreas transplant series

The survival rates obtained with the 22 simultaneous double grafts are shown in Figure 2. The patient survival was 70, 64 and 48 per cent at 6 months, 1 and 2 years, respectively. The renal graft survival was 81, 59, 47 and 30 per cent at 3

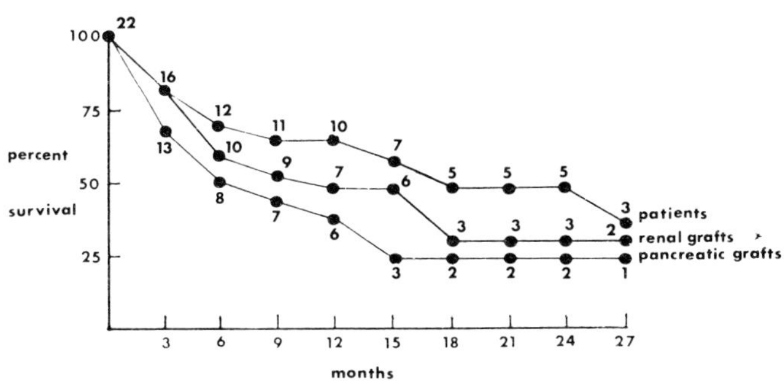

Figure 2 Actuarial rates of survival of patients, renal grafts and pancreatic grafts in 22 simultaneous kidney plus pancreas transplants in insulin-dependent diabetic recipients

and 6 months, 1 and 2 years, respectively. The pancreatic graft survival was 67, 50, 38 and 24 per cent at 3 and 6 months, 1 and 2 years, respectively.

Seven of the 22 transplants performed failed within 3 months from transplantation; in two cases the pancreatic function was compromised by a partial or total venous thrombosis which occurred in the immediate post-operative period. In two patients pancreatic failure occurred during the third month after transplantation, presumably due to rejection. Three patients died with pancreatic grafts functioning: one of mesenteric infarction, one of disseminated intravascular coagulation consequent to irreversible kidney rejection, and one of a lymphoproliferative syndrome.

Twelve pancreatic transplants survived more than 3 months: in five of them rejection occurred and insulin therapy was resumed 4, 5, 11, 12 and 14 months after transplantation; four patients died with functioning pancreatic grafts, one of myocardial infarction at 3 months and 2 weeks, one of lymphoproliferative syndrome at 5 months, one of cerebral vascular accident at 7 months and one of chronic hepatitis at 29 months.

Seven patients have currently (15 April, 1983) functioning renal and pancreatic transplants and are insulin-independent 1, 1, 3, 4, 12, 17 and 24 months after transplantation.

Two patients preserved the renal grafts after pancreatic failure, which are currently functioning 9 and 31 months after transplantation.

The introduction of CyA improved the longterm pancreatic graft survival, attaining the 30% at 2 years.

CONTROL OF DIABETES AND ENDOCRINE FUNCTION

The successful cases of pancreatic transplantation led to the correction of the clinical signs of diabetes (hyperglycaemia, glycosuria, ketosis, etc) and restored the insulin-independence within few days from the transplantation.

A substantial normoglycaemia with normalization of the glycosylated haemoglobin values was rapidly achieved and maintained over the whole duration of the pancreatic function.

In some cases, insulin therapy had to be temporarily resumed in concomitance with acute steroid treatments for rejection episodes, and it was discontinued as the steroid doses were reduced.

The investigation of endocrine function by means of the acute provocative tests, oral glucose tolerance test (OGTT) and arginine infusion, showed that the pancreatic grafts preserved the capability of responsiveness to glucose and non-glucose dependent stimulations.

Some differences were observed according to the presence of the steroids in the immunosuppressive regimen. Indeed, after OGTT the steroid-treated transplant patients showed a degree of glucose tolerance slightly impaired in comparison with the steroid-free subjects treated by CyA alone, with similar glycaemic values at fasting (92.9 ± 10.0 *vs* 80.0 ± 2.8 mg/dl, respectively), but significantly more elevated at 180 min (161.6 ± 23.9 *vs* 122.0 ± 3.7 mg/dl, respectively) (mean ± SEM) (Figure 3). On the contrary, the type of immunosuppressive treatment did not affect the insulin response to the arginine infusion, with comparable profiles for the steroid-treated and the steroid-free patients (Figure 4).

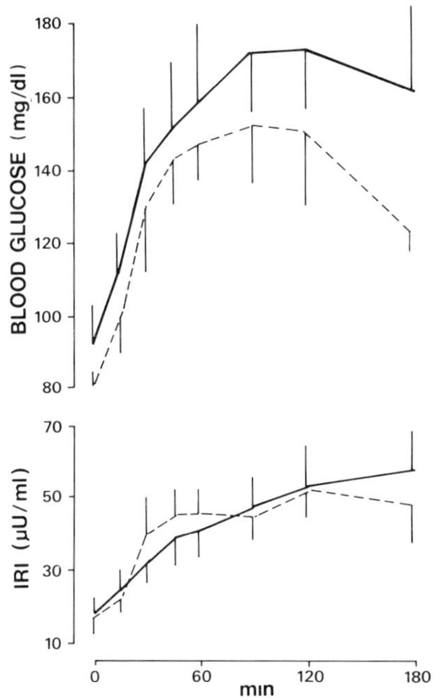

Figure 3 Glucose and insulin (IRI) response to oral glucose tolerance test (75 g p.o.) in 8 steroid-treated (———) and in 4 steroid-free CyA-treated (-----) pancreatic transplant patients (mean ± SEM)

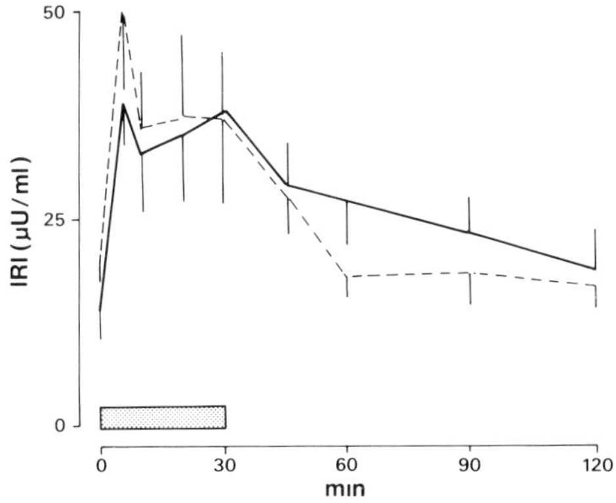

Figure 4 Insulin (IRI) response to i.v. arginine infusion in 3 steroid-free CyA-treated (-----) and in 6 steroid-treated (———) pancreatic transplant patients (mean ± SEM)

DIABETIC COMPLICATIONS

Neuropathy

Improvement or disappearance of some clinical neuropathic symptoms (paresthesias, pain, weakness, loss or impairment of vibration and cutaneous sense) were observed in most of the cases. At least three patients who were unable to walk before transplantation, recovered the capacity of deambulation within some weeks after successful pancreatic transplantation. An increase of the muscular mass was observed in all the patients with a pancreatic function longer than 3 months. However, the electromyographic studies performed in five patients showed only minimal variations of the single nerve motor conduction velocities (Figure 5).

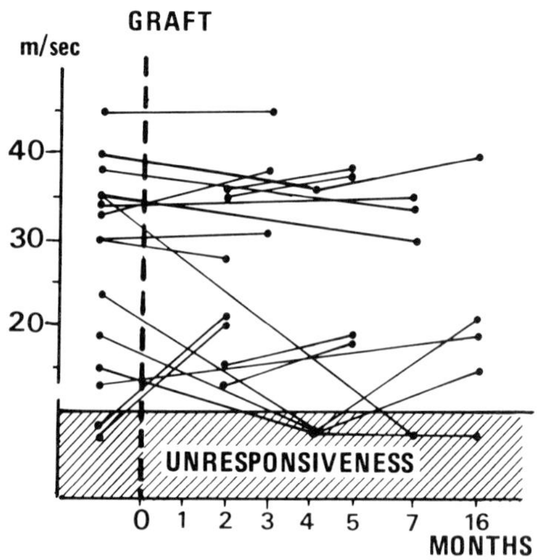

Figure 5 Single motor nerve conduction velocity in 5 pancreatic transplant patients

Retinopathy

In some successful transplants a moderate improvement of the visual acuity rapidly occurred after transplantation. Retinography and fluoroangiography could never show a regression of the retinal lesions, but no evidences of progression were detected throughout the duration of the pancreatic function, and the retinopathy in the non-blind patients appeared on the whole stabilized.

DISCUSSION

After the early unsatisfactory attempts, the re-evaluation of pancreas transplantation as an eventual approach for the management of end-stage insulin-dependent diabetes mellitus, was made possible by the availability of new grafting techniques, which made the surgical procedure safer and simpler than previously[1,2].

At present, the success rate of pancreas transplantation, although still below those of kidney and liver, has improved and this procedure could be advised for a larger number of patients. Until now, the most employed technique has been that of segmental pancreatic graft with duct occlusion by injection of polymers[3]. Although the more physiological technique of pancreatico-enteric anastomosis has recently been reconsidered with preliminary encouraging results[4], we prefer to continue with the polymer (i.e. neoprene) technique; indeed this procedure, which was developed in our laboratory, has been validated by experimental studies and by many longterm transplant survivals in our own, as in other, clinical series.

More than one reason suggests performing pancreatic transplantation in diabetic patients in association with a kidney transplant: the first advantage is that, in such patients, immunosuppression is obligatory, and therefore the pancreatic transplantation does not increase the related risks.

Moreover, the success rate of pancreatic graft has resulted in an increase when a kidney graft was associated; in our series of 13 single pancreatic transplants, only 2 survived more than 3 months, while all the longterm survived pancreatic transplants belonged to the pancreatico-renal series. One explanation could be that the chronic renal failure and the haemodialytic treatment prior to transplantation induce an immunodeficiency which can contribute to a decrease in the host responsiveness. Furthermore, for reasons still unclear, the kidney has a tendency to be rejected before the pancreas, and the monitoring of plasma creatinine can also be useful in preventing pancreatic rejection by an adequate treatment of renal rejection. This peculiar timing of rejection for kidney and pancreas has recently been confirmed by experimental studies[5].

In our experience, the causes of pancreatic failure were due to technical, vascular and immunological reasons or to the death of the patients.

In the 11 single pancreatic transplant series an immediate or near-immediate vascular thrombosis occurred in four cases (36%); in two cases (18%) it was not possible to ascribe the cause of the failure to a vascular thrombosis or to a rejection; four transplants (36%) were presumably rejected. In one case (9%) the cause of the failure was the death of the patient.

In the 25 pancreatico-renal transplants, synchronous and disynchronous, the vascular thrombosis accounted for 2 failures (12%) the rejection for 8 cases (44%) and the death of the patient for 8 cases (44%).

The introduction of CyA improved the pancreatic graft survival at 1 and 2 years, but did not succeed in reducing the rate of the early failures. Because of our still limited experience and of the uncertainty about the causes of many graft failures, a correct estimation of the capability of CyA in preventing pancreatic rejection is not yet possible. However, a further motivation for the use of CyA in pancreatic transplantation rises from the necessity in such patients of abolishing, or at least reducing, the diabetogenic effect of the steroid treatment[6]. A previous report[7] and the data here presented, indicate a more satisfactory glucose tolerance in the patients treated by CyA alone.

The accumulation of evidence of the hyperglycaemia as the main factor responsible for the development of microangiopathy in diabetic patients[8], emphasizes the importance of the metabolic correction as a means for preventing such severe and invalidating complications. The restoration of an endogenous self-regulating source of insulin secretion obtained by pancreas transplantation theoretically offers the best chance for achieving this goal. This hypothesis cannot yet be validated by our experience, the cases of longterm survival being still limited, and the degree of diabetic complications already being at an irreversible stage at the time of transplantation. However the rapid normalization of the glycosylated haemoglobin values occurring after a successful graft is consistent with a correction of the metabolic abnormalities of diabetes, which can account for the stabilization of retinopathy and neuropathy observed in the successful transplant patients. In addition, the association of pancreas to kidney transplantation, would prevent the relapse of glomerular lesions on the renal graft, as supported by many experimental data[9].

In conclusion, pancreatic transplantation appears, at present, a simple and safe surgical procedure which represents a concrete alternative approach for the treatment of end-stage insulin-dependent diabetes, validated by many longterm graft functioning survivals. A clarification of the immunological events occurring after this heterotopic graft as well as a further improvement of the transplant techniques are needed in order to make this procedure proposable to a larger number of patients. At present, the association of kidney and pancreatic transplants seems to offer more chances of success than the transplantation of the pancreas alone. The metabolic control, obtained after successful pancreatic transplants, is a promising tool for the prevention of the degenerative diabetic complications which with the improvement of immunosuppressive therapy will allow a graft transplantation earlier in the course of the disease.

References

1. Sutherland, D. E. R. (1981). Pancreas and islets transplantation. II, Clinical trials. *Diabetologia,* **20,** 435
2. Dubernard, J. M., Traeger, J., Neyra, P., Touraine, J. L., Tranchant, D. and Blanc-Brunat, N. (1978). A new method of preparation of segmental pancreatic grafts for transplantation. Trials in dogs and in man. *Surgery,* **84,** 633
3. Sutherland, D. E. R. (1983). Current status of pancreas transplantation: Registry statistics and an overview. *Transplant. Proc.,* **15,** 1303
4. Groth, C. G., Collste, H., Lundgren, G., Wilczek, H., Klintmalm, G., Ringden, O., Gunnarsson, R. and Ostman, J. (1982). Successful outcome of segmental human pancreatic transplantation with enteric exocrine diversion after modifications in technique. *Lancet,* **ii,** 522
5. Severyn, W., Olson, L., Miller, J., Kyriakides, G., Rabinovitch, A., Flaa, C. and Mintz, D. (1982). Studies on the survival of simultaneous canine renal and segmental pancreatic allografts. *Transplantation,* **33,** 606

6. Pozza, G., Traeger, J., Dubernard, J.M., Secchi, A., Pontiroli, A.E., Bosi, E., Malik, M.C., Ruitton, A. and Blanc, N. (1983). Endocrine responses of type I (insulin-dependent) diabetic patients following successful pancreas transplantation. *Diabetologia*, **24**, 244
7. Traeger, J., Dubernard, J.M., Pozza, G., Bosi, E., Secchi, A., Pontiroli, A.E., Touraine, J.L., Betuel, H., El Yafi, S., Da Ponte, F., Cantarovich, D., Diab, N., Cardozo, C., Martin, X., Kamel, G. and Gelet, A. (1983). Influence of immunosuppressive therapy on the endocrine function of segmental pancreatic allografts. *Transplant Proc.*, **15**, 1326
8. Tchobroutsky, G. (1978). Relation of diabetic control to development of microvascular complications. *Diabetologia,* **15**, 143
9. Mauer, S.M., Steffes, M.W. and Brown, D.M. (1981). The kidney in diabetes. *Am. J. Med.,* **70**, 603

Open discussion

Dr Van Schilfgaarde: Pancreatic transplantation should, if successful, be viewed as the ideal therapy, since if successful it should allow for complete and normal control of diabetes mellitus. Obviously it should be done by transplanting islets. Regrettably, so far none of the clinical efforts in islet transplantation has been successful. It may be that there is some new development in Australia and St Louis, where some very promising experiments are in progress on islet tissue culture but it seems to be generally felt that this type of therapy will not be clinically applicable for the coming few years.

So, there is the alternative of transplanting endocrine and exocrine tissue, with the obvious drawback that something has to be done about the exocrine secretions. That is the reason why until 1977 all experiences were disastrous. Patients had to endure many complications, nearly all of them as a consequence of exocrine secretion or our efforts to do something about it. It is beyond doubt that the Lyons Group, with Professors Traeger and Dubernard, has given an enormous positive impetus to the revival of pancreatic transplantation, and Professor Traeger illustrated this quantitatively for us. However, besides this there has also been an enormous amount of disappointment.

Open duct technique has been applied a few times; the technique by which pancreatic juices are permitted to drain freely into the peritoneal cavity. The duct ligation has been applied only twice. Duct obliteration is the Lyons technique, now taken over by many others. The Roux en Y procedure is a technique which has reappeared since many people became disappointed in the long run with duct obliteration technique. The number of technical failures – failures on the basis of some kind of technical problem, were 50% in the open group but only 8%, which is very low, in the duct obliteration group, and 31% in the Roux en Y procedure. This confirms that the duct obliteration technique is safe and reliable. However, if we look at the technical success, we find that eventually 56% of those who have been duct obliterated cease to function, as compared with only 8% in the Roux en Y procedure. However, the follow up period was much longer in the duct obliteration group as compared with that in the Roux en Y procedure.

Much the same is to be seen in worldwide experience where by far the largest group has been duct obliterated. What we might conclude from these data is that duct obliteration is safe, but that it might not be the best technique in terms of function. It has at least induced many to try again with other techniques which might preserve the normal architecture of the pancreas.

We feel very strongly that if one wants to apply some kind of aggressive therapy like organ transplantation in diabetics, one should try to use the safest technique, namely the technique invented by the Lyons researchers. On the basis of these conflicting data we have tried to start an experimental programme in a dog model, using autografts, in which we have tried to concentrate on the long-term effects, since many of the data are short-term effects after three months, or long-term effects, but not very detailed studies. We are trying to work on long-term experiments and to remain with them for at least one year following operation, to try to find the answers to a number of metabolic and technical questions in the absence of immunosuppression, in an autografted model.

16
Duct obliteration in segmental pancreatic transplantation – longterm effects on endocrine function and histology in dogs

R. VAN SCHILFGAARDE, H. G. GOOSZEN, F. T. BOSMAN and M. FRÖLICH

INTRODUCTION

Clinical pancreatic transplantation has gained renewed interest during the last few years, but the success rate is still relatively low. Of the total of 163 pancreas transplants performed in 154 patients during the 5 year period between July 1, 1977 and June 30, 1982, only 37 (23%) were functioning on August 1, 1982, for 2 to 49 months. Although low, these results are much better than those obtained during the preceding $10\frac{1}{2}$ years from December 16, 1966 until June 30, 1977, since during that period 60 pancreas transplants were performed of which only 3 functioned for at least 1 year[1]. There is no doubt that the major impetus to this renewed interest and improved success rate originated from the Lyon group, who introduced the technique of duct obliteration for ablation of exocrine secretions in segmental pancreatic transplantation[2]. Until 1977, the surgical management of exocrine secretions had been attempted by means of ductligation, duct-ureterostomy or various modifications of Roux-en-Y pancreatico-jejunostomy. But during the following years, duct obliteration was applied in 68% of all cases, and this modified surgical approach was accompanied by an unmistakable reduction in mortality. While before 1977 overall mortality after pancreas transplantation had been 73%, and early or procedure-related mortality was 52%[3], during the following years these percentages were 31% and 18%, respectively. In addition, the surgical approach of duct obliteration was associated with technical failure in only 8% of grafts, whereas during the same time period technical failure was observed in 31% of grafts with a Roux-en-Y pancreatico-jejunostomy, and even more often if ductligation or free drainage had been applied. However, these encouraging results of duct obliteration as a surgical approach were not associated with better graft function nor graft survival when compared to other surgical techniques[1].

We have applied a dog model (beagles weighing 9–16 kg) in order to investigate whether the effects of duct obliteration were restricted to the exocrine pancreatic tissue. Here we report some of our results pertinent to the topic of clinical segmental pancreatic transplantation as reviewed by the Lyon group elsewhere in this volume. These results were obtained in two types of experiments. The first type consisted of removal of the right lobe of the pancreas, after which the ductal system of the left lobe was injected with 0.2–0.5 ml of duct obliterating material. In the second type of experiment, the duct-injected left lobe was autografted to the iliac fossa using the surgical technique as previously described[4]. Serial relaparotomies were performed at different intervals up to 15 months after duct obliteration, in order to obtain tissue specimens for histological (haematoxylin and eosin staining) and immunocytochemical (indirect peroxidase labelled antibody method for the detection of insulin, glucagon, somatostatin and pancreatic polypeptide) examinations. Prior to each relaparotomy, intravenous glucose tolerance tests were performed, results of which were expressed in K-values and peak values of insulin response curves.

In this report we restrict ourselves to results obtained in those dogs which were injected with neoprene[2] and randomly selected for longterm evaluation (*in situ* duct obliteration: 6 dogs, segmental autograft: 4 dogs). These results were similar to those obtained in identical experiments performed with other duct obliterants like polyisoprene[5] and prolamine[6].

ENDOCRINE FUNCTION AFTER DUCT OBLITERATION

Duct obliteration of the left lobe in combination with removal of the right lobe was invariably associated with a significant reduction in glucose tolerance. As early as 1 month after duct obliteration, the mean K-value was 1.4 ± 0.4 and the mean insulin peak value was $23 \pm 6\,\mu$U/ml plasma. This represents a considerable reduction when compared to normal findings in unmodified beagles ($n = 20$), in which the mean K-value is 3.1 ± 0.5 and the mean insulin peak value $61 \pm 18\,\mu$U/ml plasma.

The decrease in glucose tolerance appeared to be completed within the first month after duct obliteration, since no further deterioration was observed throughout the longterm observation period of 15 months. At that time, the mean K-value was 1.2 ± 0.4 and the mean insulin peak value $26 \pm 7\,\mu$U/ml plasma. Fasting blood glucose levels remained within the normal range.

Next, we tested 4 dogs at 9 months after autotransplantation of duct obliterated left pancreatic segments. The mean K-value was 2.1 ± 0.5 and the mean insulin peak value fell within the normal range (58 ± 33 μU/ml plasma). Thus, changing from portal to caval venous drainage appears to be associated with a relative amelioration of glucose tolerance if a duct obliterated left pancreatic segment is the only source of insulin.

MORPHOLOGY OF EXOCRINE AND ENDOCRINE TISSUE AFTER DUCT OBLITERATION

Both qualitative and quantitative morphological studies were performed on biopsies obtained from duct obliterated left pancreatic segments.

At 1 month after duct obliteration, almost complete atrophy of exocrine tissue was observed in all pancreases, which largely consisted of loose fibrous tissue with scattered mononuclear cells, acinar remnants and endocrine elements. The inflammatory response had usually disappeared at 3 months after duct obliteration and the fibrous tissue had become more dense and less cellular. As evidenced by immunocytochemical staining, islet architecture was severely disturbed in all instances. Sometimes, the dispersed endocrine cells tended to rearrange in islet-like clusters at 12 months after duct obliteration.

Quantitative studies showed that after 3 months exocrine tissues had completely disappeared and had been replaced by fibrous interstitial tissue, while the relative volume of endocrine tissue had been maintained. Immunocytochemical evaluation did not reveal significant changes in the number of β, α, δ and PP-producing cells when their relative amounts at 12 months after duct obliteration were quantitatively compared to those in unmodified left pancreatic segments.

CONCLUDING REMARKS

The first finding of our studies is that the effects of duct obliteration are not restricted to the exocrine pancreas, since both glucose tolerance and islet morphology were shown to be severely affected by duct obliteration, irrespective of the type of obliterant used. In the first report on duct-obliteration of left pancreatic segments, blood glucose levels and islet histology were found to be normal[2]. However, in that study details of glucose tolerance tests were not reported and only routine histology but no immunocytochemical analysis was performed. Our findings corroborate those of others[7] who found islets after duct obliteration to be distorted and broken up into small cell groups. The same investigators explained the decrease in glucose tolerance to be caused by a quantitative reduction in functioning islet mass induced by surgical removal of the right pancreatic segment[8]. However, we have demonstrated in experiments to be reported elsewhere[9] that hemi-pancreatectomy as such is only of minor, if any, importance in causing reduced glucose tolerance after duct obliteration.

The second finding of our studies is that the effects of duct obliteration are brought about during the first month after injection of the obliterant. After that time, glucose tolerance was shown to have stabilized, and changes in relative quantities of different types of islet cells were not observed up to 12 months.

The most commonly favoured hypothesis holds that the severe fibrosis invariably observed after duct obliteration is responsible for partial or complete loss of endocrine function. However, this hypothesis is not corroborated by our finding that neither glucose tolerance nor the relative amounts of endocrine cells change significantly as of 1 month after duct obliteration, while the originally loose fibrous tissue starts to become more dense just at that time. Neither is it corroborated by our previous finding that the arterial blood flow (a reduction of which could, conceivably, be the mediating mechanism in reducing endocrine function) is not significantly influenced by duct obliteration as such, or by the fibrosis resulting from duct obliteration[10], nor by the fact that heavily fibrotic pancreatic segments have been shown to be capable of allowing a more than threefold increase in blood flow[11].

It appears more likely that the active inflammatory reaction occurring early after duct obliteration is the predominant cause of reduced glucose tolerance. This inflammatory response is not restricted to acinar tissue, but goes accompanied by severe destruction of islet architecture. Normal islet architecture has been argued to be a prerequisite for normal islet function[12]. We cannot exclude the possibility that the inflammatory reaction induced by duct obliteration exerts, in addition, a degenerative effect on islet cells, which may represent a second pathway for reducing the glucose tolerance.

Finally, we found that.duct obliterated pancreatic segments were compatible with a far less disturbed glucose tolerance if they were autografted onto the systemic circulation and thus draining into the caval venous bloodstream, as compared to the severely disturbed glucose tolerance if venous drainage was into the portal venous bloodstream. Caval venous drainage is uniformly applied in clinical segmental pancreas transplantation, after which a nearly normal glucose tolerance can be achieved[13,14]. It remains to be elucidated, however, whether such an artificially achieved 'nearly normal' glucose tolerance also implies that the regulation of glucose metabolism is sufficiently normal in order to effectuate the basic goal of pancreatic transplantation, which is the reduction and, ultimately, the prevention of the complications of diabetes mellitus.

ACKNOWLEDGEMENT

This study was supported by grant No. C 80-269 of the Dutch Kidney Foundation.

References

1. Sutherland, D. E. R. (1983). Current status of pancreas transplantation: Registry statistics and an overview. *Transplant. Proc.,* **15,** 1303
2. Dubernard, J. M., Traeger, J., Neyra, P., Touraine, J. L., Tranchant, D. and Blanc-Brunat, N. (1978). A new method of preparation of segmental pancreatic grafts for transplantation: Trials in dogs and in man. *Surgery,* **84,** 633
3. Sutherland, D. E. R., Goetz, F. C. and Najarian, J. S. (1981). Review of world's experience with pancreas and islet transplantation and results of intraperitoneal segmental pancreas transplantation from related and cadaver donors at Minnesota. *Transplant. Proc.,* **13,** 291
4. Van Schilfgaarde, R., Gooszen, H. G., Overbosch, E. H. and Terpstra, J. L. (1983). Arterial blood supply of the left lobe of the canine pancreas. I. Anatomic variations relevant to segmental transplantation. *Surgery,* **93,** 545
5. McMaster, P., Calne, R. Y., Gibby, O. M. and Evans, D. B. (1980). Pancreatic transplantation in man. *Transplant. Proc.,* **12,** (Suppl. 2), 58
6. Land, W., Gebhardt, Ch., Gall, F. P., Weitz, M., Gokel, M. J. and Stolte, M. (1980). Pancreatic duct obstruction with prolamine solution. *Transplant. Proc.,* **12,** (Suppl. 2), 72
7. Baumgartner, D., Sutherland, D. E. R., Heil, J., Kyriakides, G. K. and Najarian, J. S. (1981). Long-term canine segmental pancreas transplants with the duct left open, neoprene-injected duct, and pancreaticoureterostomy: A comparative study. *Transplant. Proc.,* **13,** 812
8. Baumgartner, D., Sutherland, D., Heil, J., Hustad, J. and Najarian, J. (1980). Effect of systemic venous drainage and denervation of the pancreas on glucose tolerance (GT) after partial pancreatectomy in dogs. *Diabetes,* **29,** (Suppl. 2), 73
9. Gooszen, H. G., Van Schilfgaarde, R., Bosman, F. T., Frölich, M. and Van der Burg, M. P. M. (1983). A comparison betwen the effect of reduction if islet mass and duct obliteration on endocrine function. *Transplant. Proc.,* (In press)
10. Gooszen, H. G., Van Schilfgaarde, R. and Terpstra, J. L. (1983). Arterial blood supply of the left lobe of the canine pancreas. II. Electromagnetic flow measurements. *Surgery,* **93,** 549
11. Van Schilfgaarde, R. and Gooszen, H. G. (1983). The persisting capability for vasodilatation in duct-occluded canine pancreatic segments. *Horm. Metab. Res.,* **Suppl. 13,** 12
12. Orci, L., Malaisse-Lagae, F., Ravazolla, M., Rouiller, D., Renold, A. E., Perrelet, A. and Unger, R. H. (1975). A morphological basis for intercellular communication between A and B cells in the endocrine pancreas. *J. Clin. Invest.,* **58,** 1066
13. Sutherland, D. E. R., Goetz, F. C., Elick, B. A. and Najarian, J. S. (1982). Experience with 49 segmental pancreas transplants in 45 diabetic patients. *Transplantation,* **34,** 330
14. Traeger, J., Dubernard, J. M., Pozza, G., Bosi, E., Secchi, A., Pontirolli, A. E., Touraine, J. L., Betuel, H., El Yafi, S., Da Ponte, F., Cantarovich, D., Diab, N., Cardozo, C., Martin, X., Kamel, G. and Gelet, A. (1983). Influence of immunosuppressive therapy on the endocrine function of segmental pancreatic allografts. *Transplant. Proc.,* **15,** 1326

Open discussion

Professor N Lameire (Belgium): I was very impressed with the excellent results on transplantation in diabetics in Sweden and Norway. Seeing these results, we need not worry about the recipients of the grafts. However, I do worry about the donors. We see a very high incidence of diabetes in these countries, yet they use living related donors, and they do the only manoeuvre that strictly haemodynamically mimics what happens in the early stages of diabetes – they remove a kidney, forcing the other kidney to vasodilate and to hyperfilter. I wonder what will happen in a few years' time, when some of the donors become really diabetic having only a single kidney.

Professor Brynger: Only 7 of the 40 donors we used were young people. The others had a median age of 60. None of the donors had any signs of diabetes. In all cases where we used siblings of approximately the same age, we performed glucose tolerance tests, and it is mandatory that these are totally normal and beyond doubt. We are aware of the situation that we could run into, but using proven non-diabetic individuals aged > 60 I do not think we shall hurt them.

Dr Jervell: I have no hesitation in using parents. But, we have seen diabetes developing in one donor – HLA identical – and this made us think. We are following this patient particularly to study the hyperperfusion too.

We are now discussing our policy of using HLA-identical siblings because they are the most likely to develop Type I diabetes. I do not think they can be ruled out by normal glucose tolerance since this is an immunological process which might not have started at the point when they are used but could well start the next week or the next year.

So, we shall have to live with this.

Professor Brynger: Going on the data from Minneapolis where they used live donors for pancreatic transplantation, they told us that nothing will happen if the donor at the time of donation is 20 years older than the sibling was at the time when the diabetes started. If this is true, it will be true even in

Gothenburg, Sweden, where in fact very few sibling donors were used.

Professor M Legrain (France): I was quite happy with Professor Brynger's overall results, but a little disturbed about the proportion of deaths among patients on haemodialysis. I believe that when there is trouble with the transplant, transplant patients are being lost and there is a high death rate for different reasons – because of immunosuppressive drugs, corticosteroids and so forth. If treatment could be stopped earlier and the patients put back on haemodialysis or peritoneal dialysis, then death could be avoided. I was surprised that the late bad results show many deaths and few patients alive on HD or PD. Am I right from the data?

Professor Brynger: I am not quite sure. A number of these patients have been re-transplanted. The philosophy behind it is that if a diabetic patient runs into trouble, we remove the graft, put him back on dialysis, and after six months or so we take him on for another transplant.

I fully agree that a poorly functioning graft is not the best situation. If the graft functions well, then patient survival is very good. The trouble is when graft function is poor. In recent years the mortality due to over-treatment has been extremely low.

Dr Jervell: The impressive fact about the Gothenburg material is the high rate of patient survival in spite of fairly low graft survival in cadaver kidneys.

Dr Van Schilfgaarde: There are contraindications, cardiac decompensation and hypertension in spite of treatment, advanced neuropathy or peripheral vascular complications leading to amputations. I feel that these will always be contraindications. Could Professor Brynger turn it around and could he indicate how, as a matter of policy, the diabetic patient differs from the non-diabetic patient with renal insufficiency?

Professor Brynger: Very little as a matter of fact. If we have a patient with a huge heart we know that a transplant would be very likely to kill him, whether or not he is diabetic. The special considerations are the macroangiopathy problems we meet with occasionally. Today this happens very seldom probably because those patients are not referred to us.

What was not mentioned are the possible problems with gastrointestinal autonomic neuropathy. In a few cases the patients have been unable to feed themselves. They vomit all the time and we end up with total disaster. This kind of patient is contraindicated.

Different kinds of peripheral ulcers are also contraindications when in that situation, but those patients can be treated. They can have amputations and then later, if everything is all right, they are fully transplantable again. But the cardiac situation and severe gastrointestinal problems due to neuroregulatory disease which is irreversible – I think we should not touch those patients in the name of humanity.

Dr J Michael (UK): Recognizing, as Professor Traeger said, the difficulty in interpreting survival statistics on small numbers, we in Birmingham in the last two years have done nine combined segmental and renal transplants, and at present, of those that have been followed for at least a year, we have got a 50% pancreas survival and a 70% kidney survival; all were cadaveric, with duct injection and using clyclosporin as the means of immunosuppression.

I was interested in the Panel's view of the future role of pancreatic transplantation.

Professor Traeger: It is too early to answer the question. If islet transplantation someday succeeds as a means of correcting diabetes, with no problems, and there are some hopes of that, then there will be no place for vascularized pancreatic transplantation. If islet transplantation is not possible in the future, then there may be some value in the use of pancreatic transplantation.

As I said at the end of my paper, we are making progress. We are at the stage that kidney transplants had reached some twenty years ago.

In our own group how could we improve the results? We could select our patients. Until now we have made no selection. We have grafted all patients who come in, even in a really late stage of the disease, and I showed the complications. If among the twenty double transplantations which I showed on one slide only five had been lost due to rejection, which is very difficult to reverse, we would now have 15 living patients with functioning grafts. We counted the others as non-functioning grafts, but they died of other things. With better selection of patients – as Professor Brynger is doing; he is transplanting kidneys only in patients who do not have very severe complications – we may hope for better results. And if 60–70% of the Birmingham grafts are functioning, they are showing a good result. Unless islet grafts function in the future, this is the only way to get real correction of glucose metabolism, preventing – not reducing, but preventing the development of degenerative complications.

There is hope of gathering indications for our patients from elsewhere. For instance, the Minneapolis Group is working with quite a different type of patient and doing another job. They have a lot of kidney transplant diabetic patients, who were transplanted several years ago, and they are now putting pancreatic grafts into them to try to prevent degenerative complications. The results seem to be better because they are treating patients who are not in the end-stage of the disease. The future should bring indications from these trials.

Dr Michael: If I can come back, and perhaps play the devil's advocate. Is there any point in pursuing, or persisting with a technique designed to prevent the development of complications when we all know they exist in 90% of our patients at the time when we start? Is this technique likely to be applicable to the group that we ought to be aiming for, i.e., the early diabetic, before they develop these complications?

Professor Traeger: Given the current state of the technique, we must not think of grafting insulin-dependent diabetic patients with only slight or early degenerative complications. But we can take patients who already have degenerative complications, patients who have quite marked involvement, with polyneuritis for example. We may not expect to reverse this, but we may hope - and of this I am quite sure - to stabilize complications at this stage, which is short of the final stage and I think that is important.

Dr Van Schilfgaarde: Of course we cannot prevent what is already there. On the other hand, it must be nice for a patient who has been on insulin therapy for a long time to be off insulin - in terms of psychology, too. That in itself, irrespective of costs, might be worthwhile. If we say that the main purpose should be preventive, I agree completely. A wider application of pancreatic transplantations should wait until we have better answers to the many questions which we put to ourselves. These questions are not only technical, but also immunological. There is a need for much more understanding than we have at this point in time.

In my view that is the future.

Dr B Wikstrom (Sweden): Both cyclosporin A and ALG are reported to be associated with the development of malignancies and the combination of the two agents seems dangerous. Professor Traeger mentioned two cases of lymphoproliferative problems. What does he think of the risks?

Professor Traeger: The risks are high. We were very interested in avoiding the use of corticosteroids in diabetics so we tried out a protocol associating ALG and cyclosporin - these two drugs only. We treated some kidney transplanted patients too. We treated 60 patients who received either concomitantly or successively ALG and cyclosporin A.

Of these 60 patients we saw an abnormal peak of immunoglobulin appear in 32 cases. It was of no great consequence in most of them, but we lost six patients from acute lymphoproliferative lymphoma.

So, let me give a warning. Before using such powerful drugs together, cyclosporin and ALG, one must be very careful. This is why for now we have stopped using cyclosporin A, while we wait for an answer from the next batch of cyclosporin studies, and we do not know what protocol we shall be choosing in the future.

It may be possible to use ALG in not too high a dose, with cyclosporin several months after using ALG. But to use both drugs at the same time, as was said before by the Cardiac Group in Stanford, may give rise to trouble. The two drugs together are dangerous.

The use of the two drugs in itself may not be sufficient. It may take something more to cause acute lymphoma in these patients. We are looking for some kind of a virus that may be responsible for the lymphoma in the patients treated with the two immunosuppressives simultaneously.

Professor E A Friedman (USA): Professor Traeger has talked of late and early. Might it not be better to talk of late and very late? If we review the natural history of the histopathology of the type I diabetic patient, by four to six years after onset of insulin dependence there is severe vasculopathy, thickening of the glomerular basement membrane. By eight to ten years there is nodular and diffuse intercapillary glomerular sclerosis. At this time the physiologist still measures a super-normal glomerular filtration rate.

In diabetics receiving kidneys from non-diabetics, by the third year there is a return of glomerulopathy. By the fifth to sixth year it is very severe. So when it is proposed to move to what might be viewed as early, 12–14 years instead of 17–20 years, that early is still very late. We must remember that there is a strong dissociation between function and histopathology in the diabetic patient, and so when we would intervene, say at a creatinine of 2–3 mg/dl, and call that early, it is still very late.

Dr R Bouillon (Belgium): Have the Scandinavian Group seen a big difference in diabetes control in their transplanted patients, and has that affected the survival of the patients. Has it had any relation with the biopsy of the kidneys when the patients have died?

Professor Brynger: Even in Gothenburg we have problems with glucose management of the transplantation. We, or our diabetologists, find it extremely difficult, much as Dr Jervell reported. But I would not say that a single patient died from it. We have also seen – to confirm what Professor Friedman said – that after two years the transplanted kidney already shows histopathological changes.

Dr Jervell: They are much easier to control once the post-operative phase and rejection treatment are over, and it is certainly much easier to handle diabetics on haemodialysis. We follow the haemoglobin A_1 in these patients for what they may be worth, and they are generally better than the average insulin-dependent diabetic after three months.

Dr Bouillon: Is there a difference in the survival rate?

Dr Jervell: I do not know.

Professor Brynger: I do not think so. There are a lot who are really badly controlled, but who survive quite well – so far.

Dr Reach (France): The basal response of the islets – the transplant islets – to an i.v. glucose load is fairly good, but when the patient receives steroids his response falls. Am I right? Surely it is a bit surprising. Usually steroids will increase the insulin response. Does that not mean that the islet mass is much reduced?

Professor Traeger: In the abnormalities we have seen, we think that abnormal cell mass is a major factor. Dr Bosi is the man to answer the question.

Dr E Bosi (France): We have no clear explanation. Our patient population on different immunosuppressive schedules is still limited. Indeed, fasting hyper-insulaemia is more frequent in steroid-treated pancreatic transplant patients than in those not receiving steroids. It is surprising and we have no explanation, but the patterns of insulin release after actute stimulation are more satisfactory when the patient only receives cyclosporin A. We draw that conclusion only on the basis of four or five patients so we cannot definitively conclude that physiology of acute insulin release is better on cyclosporin A. In addition, this observation goes against the opinion of the Stockholm Group, that cyclosporin A impairs glucose tolerance. We have exactly the opposite impression. So we shall have to look into it further.

Dr Van Schilfgaarde: As a final comment, to contribute further to the confusion, we performed autografts in six dogs and treated them for one year with prednisolone and azathioprine. In the autograft model, our functional data after one year were identical to those not treated with any type of immunosuppression. So I hope nobody understands any of it any more!

Session Five

MANAGEMENT OF THE DIABETIC IN RENAL FAILURE

(iii) Dialysis

Chairmen:
G. PICCOLI and L. PUERTAS VARGAS

17
Haemodialysis in diabetic patients

F. L. SHAPIRO

ABSTRACT

Since 1966, the Regional Kidney Disease Program located at Hennepin County Medical Center in Minneapolis has provided dialysis care to over 1600 patients. Of the 378 diabetic patients treated during this interval, 349 received haemodialysis. Haemodialysis patient survival in diabetics and non-diabetics has improved progressively during this 17 year interval and has been particularly impressive since 1976. The death rate in Type I diabetics remains at 2.5–3 times that of similar aged non-diabetics, and approximates to non-diabetics 30 years older. Currently, Type I diabetics under age 61 undergoing haemodialysis have a first year survival of 85% and a 3 year survival of 65%. The survival rate of Type II diabetic haemodialysis patients is similar to that of Type I even though Type IIs average 22 years older. In Type I diabetics, age at onset of dialysis treatments has little effect on survival until 61 years or older, unlike results in non-diabetic patients, where age at onset of therapy does influence expected survival.

Vascular disease is responsible for most of the deaths occurring in diabetic patients undergoing haemodialysis. The most impressive recent results compared to early experiences with Type I diabetics has been the relatively stable vision in Type I patients undergoing regular dialysis since 1976. Visual stability compares favourably to results in Type I patients receiving renal transplants. Amputation rates have remained low in diabetic dialysis patients. Rehabilitation is poor in diabetic dialysis patients.

INTRODUCTION

Since 1966, the Regional Kidney Disease Program (RKDP) in Minneapolis has provided regular dialysis care to 378 diabetic patients. Our early experience treating these patients was discouraging[1]. There was an excessively high mortality and a high incidence of blindness, hospital inpatient complications and psychosocial problems. During the past several years there has been an impressive improvement in both the survival and the rates of development of blindness in diabetic patients treated with haemodialysis[2,3].

The proportion of new patients entering the RKDP programme who are diabetic has increased in recent years. During 1981 and 1982, 33% of our new patients were diabetic. Other programmes in the United States have also observed an increase in the proportion of their new patients who are diabetic, and the usual quoted proportion of new patients entering dialysis who are diabetic is in the range of 25%.

This report will discuss selected aspects and results of our experience in treating diabetic patients with haemodialysis.

DIABETES AND URAEMIA

As diabetic patients become uraemic several medical manifestations of their disease may change. Hypertension which begins shortly after the onset of proteinuria worsens related to fluid retention. This is also associated with rapid progression of diabetic retinopathy. The level of proteinuria may decrease but usually remains in the 2–10 g/day range. Insulin sensitivity manifested by frequent hypoglycaemic episodes or slowly decreasing insulin requirements is typical. Peripheral neuropathy may become incapacitating and visceral neuropathy, manifested as orthostatic hypotension, neurogenic bladder dysfunction and impotency is apparent by the time the patient's serum creatinine exceeds 5 mg/dl. Neuropathic ulcers may develop and gastrointestinal tract problems occur. However, diabetic diarrhoea has not been a common complication in these patients.

Patients with diabetes mellitus develop uraemic symptoms, particularly nausea, vomiting and anorexia, and manifest the anaemia of uraemia earlier in the course of renal failure than do patients with other forms of chronic renal insufficiency. We have found that when assessing the appropriateness of uraemic symptoms versus renal function in diabetic patients that the creatinine clearance of the diabetic should be divided by two (or the serum creatinine doubled) before comparing it clinically to what one would expect in non-diabetic patients.

HAEMODIALYSIS IN DIABETIC PATIENTS

The observations and data presented in this section are derived from the RKDP experience of treating a total of 236 Type I and 142 Type II diabetics accepted for regular dialysis therapy from 1966 through June 1982. The patient status as of December 31, 1982, was utilized as a closing date for the analysis. Therefore, all patients had a minimum dialysis exposure of 6 months, unless they died or were withdrawn alive during their first 6 months of regular dialysis. Although Type II diabetic patients are sometimes referred to as non-insulin dependent, most of them usually require insulin for adequate control of blood glucose.

The clinical characteristics of the diabetic patients treated during the 17 year interval are listed in Table 1. The proportion of Type I diabetics who were blind at the initiation of dialysis was 41%. Fifty-nine per cent of the Type I patients and 37% of the Type II patients are male. The modalities of therapy received

Table 1 Diabetic dialysis patients 1966–1982

	Type I	*Type II*
Number of patients	236	142
Males	140 (59%)	53 (37%)
Females	96 (41%)	89 (63%)
Mean age (y)	41.7	62.8
Age range (y)	21–77	25–84
Duration of diabetes (y)	22.4	12.8
Range (y)	2–48	0–48
Number 15 + y	214 (91%)	56 (39%)
Retinopathy	*227 (96%)	88 (62%)
Blind	84 (36%)	15 (11%)

* 6 of 9 without retinopathy were over 50 years of age

by these patients are listed in Table 2. Haemodialysis was used in 327 patients while 29 received either intermittent or continuous ambulatory peritoneal dialysis. Twenty-two patients received both haemo- and peritoneal dialysis at different times.

Table 2 Diabetic treatment modalities

	Haemo	*Haemo + Perit.*	*Perit*	*Total*
Type I	208	12	16	236
Type II	119	10	13	142
TOTAL	327	22	29	378

The most difficult problem in the preparation of the patient for haemodialysis is the establishment of adequate blood access. If the patient has suitable vessels for the creation of a simple arteriovenous fistula, this is undoubtedly the most successful form of access. Unfortunately, the success rate of establishing a patent simple fistula and having it develop adequately for use is low in diabetic patients. External cannula survival time is poor and complication rates are high in diabetics so that we employ Scribner type cannulae or subclavian catheters only for temporary use until an adequate internal access has been created. We have relied predominantly on bovine carotid artery grafts until recently when we have also utilized the Hemasite access devices to achieve effective access in diabetic patients. These forms of access, once successfully established, have compared favourably with our access results in non-diabetic patients, except for the rare occurrence of ischaemic contractures in diabetics which, on occasion, have necessitated the surgical reduction of the graft or vessel to diminish the blood flow rate. Of the diabetic patients receiving haemodialysis in December 1982, 45% had grafts, 44% had fistulae and 5% had Hemasite accesses.

During the stabilization period which may last 4–6 weeks, several clinical and metabolic changes take place in the diabetic patients. They usually complain of increased weakness and malaise compared to their pre-dialysis state. This begins to improve about the third week of dialysis. Vomiting without associated nausea occurs commonly, and is secondary to delayed gastric emptying. This problem usually is resolved within 6 weeks.

Insulin requirements vary significantly during the stabilization interval depending on the patient's appetite, food intake, incidence of vomiting, physical activity and associated medical complications. By the end of the stabilization period the patients usually require the same total doses of insulin that they did prior to developing renal insufficiency. We attempt to achieve blood glucose control in the 100–200 mg/dl range, because high blood glucose causes excessive thirst and, therefore, excessive interdialytic weight gain. When dialysis is initiated we convert the patient to a standard diabetic type of diet programme consisting of three equal meals and two snacks. We recommend 30–35 calories/kg body weight which should contain 1 g of high biological protein and 0.5 g of low biological value protein/kg body weight, and 70 mEq potassium and 4 g sodium daily. Our recommended daily fluid allowance is 500 ml and we ignore the urine output unless the patients lose weight and become hypovolaemic between dialyses.

We utilize combined treatment with neutral protamine Hagedorn (NPH) and regular insulin administered twice daily with slightly more than half being administered in the morning hours, and the remainder in the late afternoon. We recommend 3–5 units of regular insulin per unit of NPH when they are administered simultaneously, because the duration of action of the regular insulin is prolonged both in renal failure and when it is mixed with NPH insulin. Until acceptable blood glucose control is achieved, we encourage the patients to perform self-monitoring at home, and to supplement themselves with small doses of regular insulin on the basis of the observed results. On this regimen, peak blood glucose levels occur in the morning hours and late in the afternoon.

We recommend glucose be included in dialysate in the concentration of 150–200 mg/dl. Haemodialysis is a catabolic event in all patients, as reflected by the increase in certain serum ketone bodies during the dialysis procedure.

This is particularly true in diabetics, and studies have demonstrated that glucose in the dialysate minimizes the rise of ketone bodies compared to glucose free dialysate[4].

The high incidence and extent of orthostatic hypotension complicates the process of establishing the patient's optimum dry weight. Antihypertensive drugs compound this problem so they should be avoided if possible. We have been able to achieve normalization of the patient's blood pressure with clinically acceptable levels of orthostatic fall in over 90% of the diabetic patients without resorting to antihypertensive drugs by gradually reducing the patient's weight over several weeks of dialysis by progressive ultrafiltration. We utilize a dialysate sodium concentration of at least 140 mEq/l. If the patient's blood pressure falls during dialysis before optimum ultrafiltration has been achieved, we frequently administer 3% saline rather than normal saline to expand the intravascular volume maintaining blood pressure and decreasing the intracellular volume. When an optimum body weight has been achieved, patients may notice an improvement in their visual acuity because of the loss of previously present retinal oedema. They may have minimal residual pedal oedema at this time.

We encourage patients to increase their physical activity level to tolerance. We also stress that they maintain their usual foot and skin care and visit an ophthalmologist regularly. Photocoagulation has been used with increasing frequency in recent times to minimize the progression of the retinopathy.

RESULTS

The cumulative survival in the combined diabetic group is compared to that of non-diabetics during the 17 year interval in Figure 1. Although the non-diabetics on the average are slightly older, the death rate in the diabetics is considerably higher than non-diabetics. This Figure includes both haemodialysis and peritoneal dialysis experience. The remainder of the cumulative survival data includes only patients on haemodialysis.

The dramatic improvement in survival rates of Type I diabetics under 61 years of age commencing haemodialysis during three consecutive time intervals is illustrated in Figure 2. The average age of the patients has remained constant, while the death rate has dropped from 36.2 to 13.3 deaths per 1000 patient treatment months. The first year survival has increased to 85% while the third year survival is 65%. Similar data are presented in Table 3 depicting the deaths per 1000 patient treatment months for different age groups during the three time intervals. There has been a steady decline in the death rate in all groups and, during the most recent interval, the death rates for the groups aged 31–45 and 46–60 are similar, while those under 31 are surviving better. The Type I patients over 61 years of age continue to have a very high death rate.

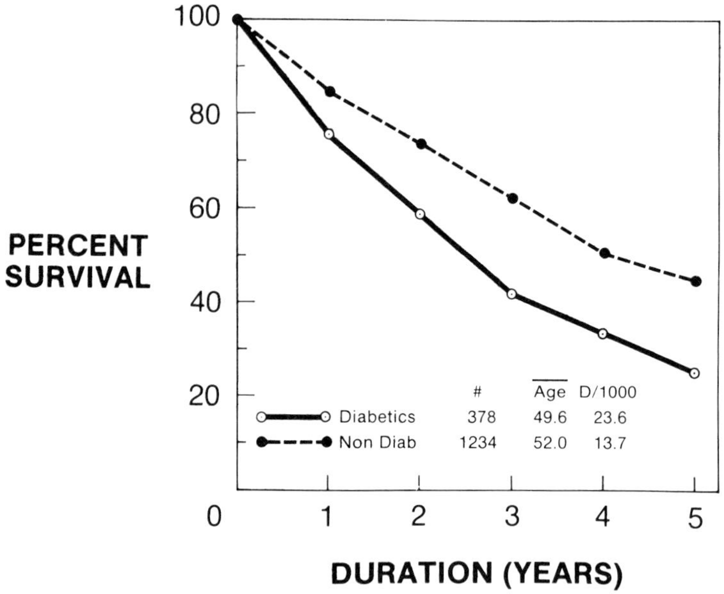

Figure 1 Cumulative survival, diabetic *vs* non-diabetic patients, 1966–1982

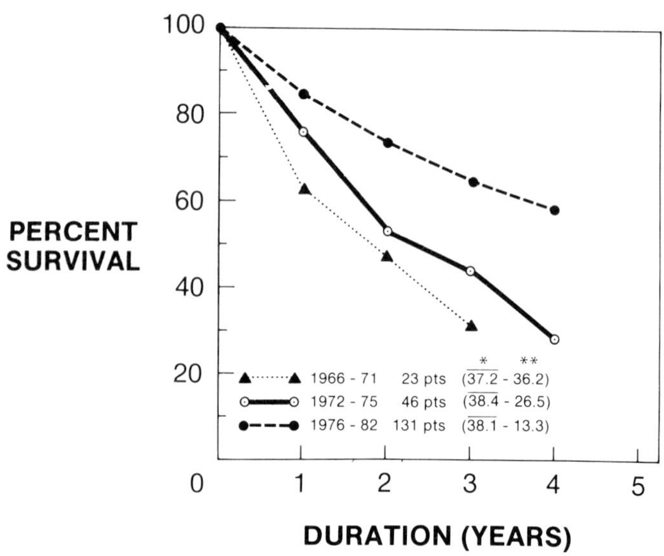

Figure 2 Cumulative survival, diabetics under 61 years commencing haemodialysis 1966–71 *vs* 1972–75 *vs* 1976–82

Table 3 Type I diabetic haemodialysis deaths per 1000 patient treatment months: different time intervals and age

Age	*1966–71*	*1972–75*	*1976–82*
<31	43	37	9
31–45	30	21	14
46–60	59	22	15
61+	—	108	44
All ages	36 (23)	30 (50)	18 (148)

( ) = number patients

Similar improvement in results has occurred in the Type II diabetic patients during the two most recent time intervals (Figure 3). The 1976–82 group of patients is slightly older but has a death rate that is 50% lower. The improvement in survival rates with time had not been restricted to diabetic patients. Figure 4 illustrates the changes in the survival rates during the three time intervals in non-diabetic patients under 61 years of age. The 5 year survival rate for these patients is now 78%. The death rate has dropped from 14.8 to 4.5 deaths per 1000 patient treatment months. The death rates for the periods 1972–75 and 1976–82 are compared for three groups of patients in Table 4. The mortality rate has decreased by 50% in all three groups. In non-diabetics, the death rate of patients 46–60 years of age is thrice that of patients

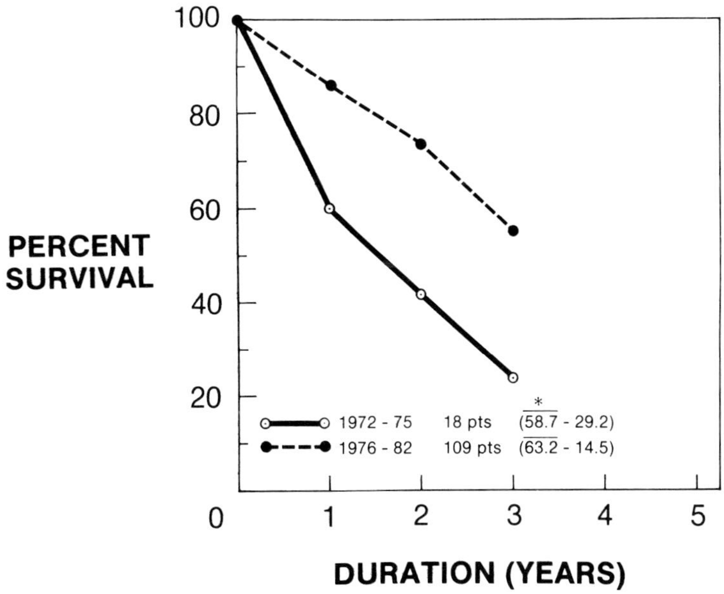

Figure 3 Cumulative survival, type II diabetics commencing haemodialysis 1972–75 *vs* 1976–82

under 46 years of age (6.8 *vs* 2.3 deaths per 1000 patient treatment months). The effect of age is not apparent in the diabetic population until their age exceeds 61 years.

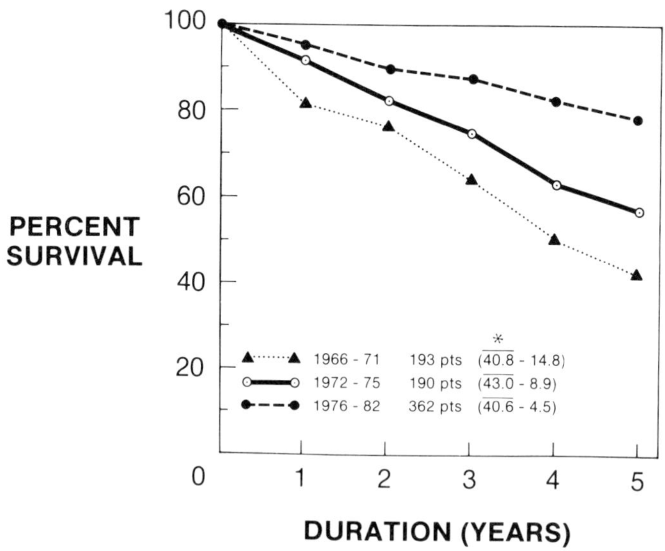

Figure 4 Cumulative survival, non diabetics under 61 years commencing haemodialysis 1966–71 *vs* 1972–75 *vs* 1976–82

Table 4 Comparative deaths per 1000 patient treatment months

	1972–75		*1976–82*	
	Death Rate	*No Patients*	*Death Rate*	*No Patients*
Type I diabetics <61 y	26.5	23	13.3	131
Type II diabetics	29.2	18	14.5	109
Non-diabetics <61 y	8.9	190	4.5	362

Table 5 Renal function at dialysis initiation in diabetics – 1966–71, 1972–75, *vs*. 1976–82

	Serum Creatinine (mg/dl)	*Creatinine Clearance* (ml/min)
Type I		
1966–71	11.2	5.6
1972–75	12.7	4.8
1976–82	9.3	5.8
Type II		
1972–75	12.0	3.2
1976–82	9.8	5.3

The level of renal function in diabetic patients when dialysis was initiated for the three time intervals is tabulated in Table 5. Patients commencing dialysis after 1976 have had slightly better renal function than those initiated prior to that time. However, the small difference in renal function does not explain the observed longterm improvement in survival.

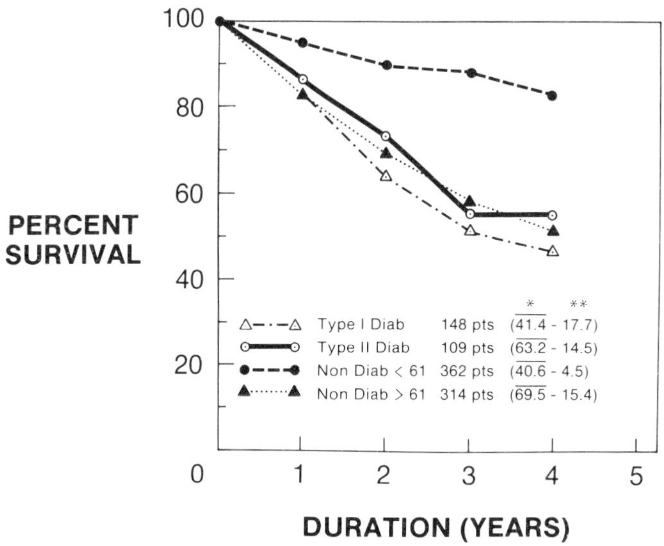

Figure 5 Cumulative survival, type I diabetics *vs* type II diabetics *vs* non diabetics over and under 61 years, 1976–1982 haemodialysis

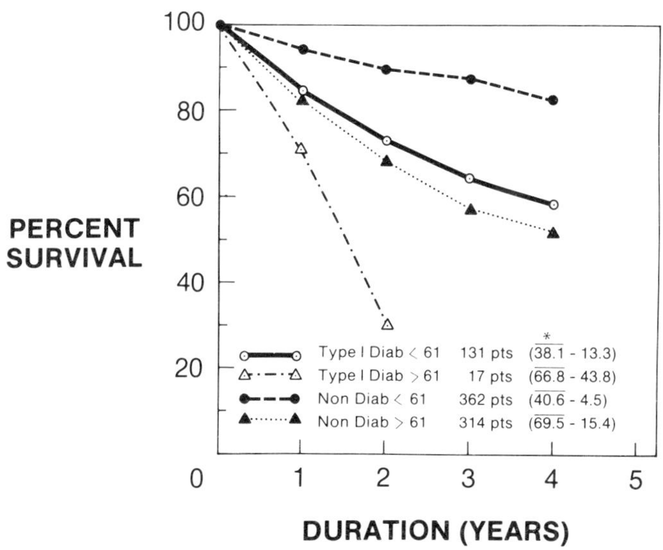

Figure 6 Cumulative survival, type I diabetics over and under 61 years *vs* non diabetics over and under 61 years, 1976–82 haemodialysis

The cumulative survival during the past 7 years of non-diabetic patients under 61 is compared to Type I and II diabetics and non-diabetics over 61 in Figure 5. The survival rates of the diabetics and non-diabetics over 61 are quite similar, even though there are considerable differences in age. As illustrated in Figure 6, Type I diabetics under 61 years have a death rate similar to non-diabetics over 61 years of age, even though the average age of the diabetics is much less than that of the non-diabetics (the difference being greater than 30 years).

The cause of death of diabetic patients entering haemodialysis since 1976 is listed in Table 6. Cardiac and cerebrovascular events account for 59% of the deaths in diabetic dialysis patients. Uraemia, resulting from discontinuation of dialysis, caused 14% of the total deaths. Although sepsis was responsible for almost 27% of the late deaths, it accounts for less than 10% of total deaths.

Table 6 Cause of death in diabetic haemodialysis patients initiated since 1976

	Under 24 months		*Over 24 months*		*Total*	
	No	*(%)*	*No*	*(%)*	*No*	*(%)*
Cardiac	29	(54)	5	(36)	34	(50)
CVA	5	(9)	1	(7)	6	(9)
Uraemia	9	(17)	—		9	(14)
Sepsis	1	(2)	5	(36)	6	(9)
Hyperkalaemia	3	(6)	—		3	(5)
Cancer	3	(6)	—		3	(5)
Miscellaneous	4	(7)	3	(21)	7	(11)
Total	54		14		68	

The inpatient complication rate for diabetics is compared to non-diabetics since 1976 in Table 7. The diabetics require similar hospitalization time compared to non-diabetics.

Table 7 Inpatient complication rate 1976–1982

	No Patients	*Mean Age*	*Days Treatment months*
Type I Diabetics	148	41.4	1.58
Type II Diabetics	109	63.1	1.67
Non-Diabetics	676	54.0	1.72

There has been a dramatic improvement in the rate of visual loss during recent years in Type I patients (Table 8). The overall rate of the development of blindness is now 12%; however, the rate has fallen from 44% in the 1966–71 group to 3% in patients initiated since 1976. Three patients who had no useful vision when dialysis was initiated have regained useful vision. Several other patients regained some useful vision transiently. Of the eyes with useful vision at the initiation of dialysis, 5% have become blind due to retinal disease in those patients commencing dialysis since 1976. These results continue to compare favourably with published results in insulin-dependent diabetics receiving renal transplants[5].

Table 8 Type I diabetic dialysis patient blindness

Initial Status *Last Status*	*1966–71*	*1972–75*	*1976–82*	*Total*
NB⟶NB	6	24	65	95
NB⟶UB	1	1	6	8
NB⟶BB	4	4	2	10
UB⟶UB	2	7	22	31
UB⟶BB	3	4	1	8
BB⟶BB	7	10	64	81
BB⟶NB	—	—	2	2
BB⟶UB	—	—	1	1
Total	23	50	163	236
Average months of treatment per patient	22.8	24.2	15.6	17.5
Patients ⟶B	7 (44%)	8 (20%)	3 (3%)	18 (12%)
Eyes ⟶B/Eyes at Risk	2/27 (44%)	13/69 (19%)	11/169 (5%)	36/265 (14%)

NB = Not blind
UB = Unilaterally blind
BB = Bilaterally blind

The amputation experience in diabetics undergoing dialysis therapy is presented in Table 9. The rate continues to be quite low compared to the post-transplant experience in these patients. Rehabilitation in diabetic haemodialysis patients is very limited and disappointing.

Table 9 Diabetic dialysis patient amputations 1966–1982

	5	Above knee (vascular)
	16	Below knee (vascular)
	4	Fingers (vascular)
	1	Fingers (osteomyelitis)
	6	Toes (vascular)
	3	Toes (osteomyelitis)
Total no. amputations	35	

25 Patients
378 patients treated for 596 treatment years

DISCUSSION

During the past 7 years, an impressive improvement in haemodialysis patient survival rates of both diabetics and non-diabetics has occurred. The explanation for this improvement is not obvious.

Initiating dialysis at slightly higher levels of renal function does not appear to be a major factor as the data on renal function status at the time of dialysis initiation show only a modest change, whereas the improvement in survival rates has been sizable and sustained. The utilization of more peritoneal dialysis as a modality of therapy could also have influenced the haemodialysis results, because the peritoneal patients have been, for the most part, medically less stable. However, when the peritoneal and haemodialysis data are combined, there is little change in the survival rates compared to haemodialysis alone as the number of patients treated with peritoneal dialysis is relatively small.

There have been several technical changes in the dialysis procedure which may have influenced survival rates. We currently use higher sodium levels in the dialysate (140 mEq/l) which permits better tolerance of ultrafiltration and, therefore, more effective blood pressure control without the use of anti-hypertensive agents in the large majority of patients. The duration of dialysis treatments has been reduced to between 4–5 hours by utilizing more efficient dialysers. Also, more emphasis has been placed on adequate nutritional status of the patient, and this may have contributed to improved survival.

It is interesting that with the overall improvement in survival of both diabetics and non-diabetics, the Type I diabetic patients continue to die at a rate similar to non-diabetics who are 30 years older. This finding is unchanged from our earlier analysis[2,3].

The relative stability of vision in the Type I diabetic patients continues to be one of the more encouraging aspects of recent results utilizing haemodialysis therapy in these patients. As with the improvement in survival rates, the underlying factors responsible for this improvement are unclear. In recent years, our patients have received more intensive ophthalmological care with greater use of panretinal photocoagulation. In addition, there has been increased emphasis on diabetic control, utilizing both diet and multiple insulin injections. Normalization of blood pressure undoubtedly is a major factor contributing to these results. Heparinization regimen is unchanged and is the same as for non-diabetics.

Diabetic dialysis patients have a lower incidence of amputation than diabetic patients who have successful renal transplants. At this time, we still recommend transplantation to our diabetic patients, emphasizing that there is no urgency and the first year mortality rate in transplantation exceeds that of dialysis; however, the longterm survival rates favour transplantation. Although the amputation rate is high in the transplanted diabetic patients, and steroid complications are not infrequent, the patients' assessment of the quality of their life after successful transplantation continues to be superior to that on dialysis. We, therefore, recommend that transplantation be the treatment of choice, when medically appropriate.

References

1. Leonard, A., Comty, C. M., Raij, L., *et al.* (1973). The natural history of regularly dialyzed diabetics. *Trans. Am. Soc. Artif. Intern. Organs.,* **19,** 282
2. Shapiro, F. L. and Comty, C. M. (1979). Hemodialysis in diabetics - 1979 Update. In Friedman, E. A. and L'Esperance, F. A. Jr., (eds.). *Diabetic Renal–Retinal Syndrome.* pp. 333 (New York: Grune and Stratton)
3. Shapiro, F. L. and Comty, C. M. (1982). Hemodialysis in diabetics - 1981 Update. In Friedman, E. A. and L'Esperance, F. A. Jr., (eds.). *Diabetic Renal–Retinal Syndrome. Prevention and Management.* pp. 309 (New York: Grune and Stratton)
4. Wathen, R., Keshaviah, P., Hommeyer, P., *et al.* (1977). Role of dialysate glucose in preventing gluconeogenesis during hemodialysis. *Trans. Am. Soc. Artif. Intern. Organs,* **23,** 393
5. Peters, C., Sutherland, D. E. R., Simmons, R. L., *et al.* (1981). Patient and graft survival in amputated *vs* non-amputated diabetic primary renal allograft recipients. *Transplantation,* **32,** 498

Discussant

V. PARSONS

Dr Parsons (UK): To follow Professor Shapiro is virtually impossible and we are full of admiration. I ought not to be a discussant. I ought to be an admirer.

Nevertheless, I am here to wave a small British flag to say that we are trying to treat diabetes in the United Kingdom, despite what Eli Friedman might say.

In King's College Hospital Renal Unit we have seen 92 patients with diabetes and renal failure. I want to make an appeal that when we talk about the sort of patients we are accepting, that we have some sort of categorization. If we were talking about carcinoma of the breast or some other malignant disease, we would have Grade 1, 2, 3, 4 and 5. Professor Brynger from Sweden at least told us that he rejected people with big hearts and with severe neuropathy, and those that had severe vascular disease. Professor Shapiro was not quite so definite about how all his patients got to Minneapolis and how many patients were left behind, and this is a point we must stress in future discussion.

My revered senior, Frank Parsons, always says we must add to our success rates all those patients we did not treat, so that from the success rate is subtracted those who were not welcomed to the Unit. We have welcomed virtually every diabetic who has been sent to us, but of those 92 there were 10 whom we turned down. In other words, there are something like 10% of patients whom we feel are totally untreatable.

The other interesting point is that we believe that diabetics get nephritis, maybe even more than the normal population. So hidden in there are people with good eyes whose diabetes and renal failure are discordant; that is it has come on with a nephritic rather than a nephrotic episode.

We have treated very few patients with pure haemodialysis but twice as many with peritoneal dialysis. So here we find immediately a difference in British practice, that we treat few patients wholly with haemodialysis for a period of time – and even six of those slipped through to renal transplantation. In our unit the majority go straight to transplantation without going through a haemodialysis phase.

We had six patients on maintenance haemodialysis out of this number, and the majority of them died of cerebrovascular, cardiovascular and septic incidents.

We have tried to plot things slightly differently than they do in Minneapolis. By the end of 1983 we hope to have taken on a total of 600 patients in one fairly small renal unit in one part of South-East England. The number of patients who are transplanted are rising with the total. This is the dominant form of treatment in our unit. The patients who are unable to be transplanted, and therefore kept on dialysis, is slowly rising too, but rather like Minneapolis – perhaps we are five years behind – we are now beginning to see an increasing number of patients who refuse to die.

A few words about access. I quite agree that access is a very difficult thing in patients with diabetes. We do do vascular studies with the biomedical engineers to look at the blood flow in the vessels concerned. Usually we end up with an anticubital fistula. We use quite a lot of prostacycline in patients on dialysis with very severe impairment of the peripheral circulation of hands or feet.

Peritoneal dialysis is our chosen form of treatment. Most of these are offered transplantation. At the moment we have only two maintained on peritoneal dialysis.

Transplantation, though, is only limited by the rate at which the donor kidneys present.

In the future, with cyclosporin, which we have just begun to use, and none of the patients I have discussed had cyclosporin – we expect to see an improvement in the survival rate from transplantation and we shall be able then to offer this preferred form of treatment to patients who at the moment are struggling on haemodialysis.

Finally, like Professor Shapiro we do give the opportunity to the patients and their relatives to withdraw from treatment. In this group there are three patients where the patients themselves and the relatives felt that dialysis no longer offered them a quality of life that they wished to pursue. When we talk about the rejection of patients our attitude is to accept every one for treatment, to give the treatment of choice, whether it be peritoneal dialysis or haemodialysis, a three months' chance, and then to ask the patient whether despite having a big heart, or an amputated leg, or neuropathy, he or she wishes to continue the treatment.

This is what we have tried to do at King's. We hope one day to slowly emulate Minneapolis.

18
Home intermittent peritoneal dialysis in the treatment of end-stage diabetic nephropathy: 1982 update

C. MION, A. SLINGENEYER, B. CANAUD, R. OULÈS, B. BRANGER, G. CHONG and G. MOURAD

INTRODUCTION

Since February 1974, all diabetics with end-stage renal disease referred to us have been treated by home peritoneal dialysis. Until September 1978, intermittent peritoneal dialysis (IPD) was the only available technique. Later on, continuous ambulatory peritoneal dialysis (CAPD) was developed and offered to all patients including diabetics. Surprisingly, many of the latter preferred to continue with IPD, a technique to which they were well accustomed, that suited their life style and was accompanied by low morbidity. Therefore, IPD has remained one of the main treatment modalities for diabetics with end-stage nephropathy in our programme.

This report, updating previous publications[1,2], summarizes our experience with this dialysis technique. Special emphasis will be given to some nutritional aspects, the outcome of diabetic retinopathy and neuropathy, the incidence of peritoneal infection and long term survival of the patients.

PATIENTS AND METHODS

Classification of diabetes mellitus

To evaluate adequately the results obtained with various treatment modalities in end-stage diabetic nephropathy, it is of importance to identify the type of diabetes mellitus (DM) in each patient studied in a given series[3]. Accordingly, our patients were separated into two subgroups following the World Health Organization (WHO) recommendations[4]: Type I (insulin dependent, juvenile onset) DM was characterized by proneness to ketosis, onset before 30 years of age, a delay after onset of less than 2 years before starting insulin treatment and the absence of obesity; Type II (non-insulin dependent, maturity onset) DM was characterized by onset after age 30, delay before starting insulin treatment of more than 2 years after diagnosis, and the presence of obesity. In view of the practical difficulties in classifying some patients, we decided to identify two subgroups among Type II diabetics: Type II A included the patients who were receiving insulin at the time of referral, and Type II B included those patients who were not treated with insulin when they reached end-stage renal failure.

Patients

From February 1974 to 30 November 1982, 58 diabetics were admitted on IPD. There were 19 Type I diabetics (8 males, 11 females; mean age ± SD: 33.7 ± 5 years) and 39 Type II diabetics (22 males, 17 females; mean age: 61.2 ± 7.8 years). The two subgroups of Type II patients were constituted as follows: Type II A, 10 patients, Type II B, 29 patients; there was no significant age difference between these two subgroups (60.5 ± 6.0 versus 62.0 ± 8.4 years in Type II A and Type II B respectively).

Table 1 describes the cardiovascular complications noted in the patients before initiation of IPD. Congestive cardiac failure, cardiac arrhythmias and prior cerebrovascular accidents were more frequently observed among Type II than Type I diabetics. Peripheral vascular disease (including distal ischaemic necrosis of lower limb) and left ventricular hypertrophy on the electrocardiogram had the same prevalence in both Type I and Type II patients.

Creatinine clearance at the start of treatment had a mean value of 4.1 ± 2.6 ml/min (range 2 to 8 ml/min).

Table 1 Cardiovascular status of 48 diabetics before starting home intermittent peritoneal dialysis (IPD)

	Type I		*Type II*			
			Receiving insulin		*Without insulin*	
	n	(%)		(%)		(%)
Number of patients	19		10		29	
Myocardial infarction	1	(5)	1	(10)	3	(10)
Angina	3	(15)	1	(10)	8	(26)
Congestive cardiac failure	1	(5)	3	(30)	15	(50)
EKG abnormalities						
Arrhythmias	2	(10)	5	(50)	18	(60)
Left ventricular hypertrophy	13	(65)	6	(60)	19	(63)
Ischaemia	7	(35)	3	(30)	20	(66)
Cerebrovascular accident	1	(5)	3	(30)	9	(30)
Symptomatic peripheral vascular disease	4	(20)	3	(30)	9	(30)
Lower limb gangrene	6	(30)	5	(50)	9	(30)
Vascular calcifications	16	(80)	9	(90)	22	(73)

Dialysis techniques

In all patients, the peritoneal access was a double cuff 'chronic' Tenckhoff catheter, implanted surgically according to our technique[5].

The programme was exclusively developed in the home. The patient and his/her helper were trained for a period of 6 to 8 weeks in a special unit (Clinique du Mas de Rochet, 34170 Castelnau-l-Lez) independent of the home haemodialysis training centre. Two types of equipment were available, both permitting closed circuit delivery of the dialysis fluid. The first apparatus was an automatic cycler (Etablissements Villevieille, 5, rue François Perier, 34000 Montpellier), using commercially available sterile apyrogenic dialysis solutions in 10-l plastic containers (Laboratoires Dubernard Hospital, 5 Quai de Bacalan, 33000 Bordeaux). These containers could be connected in series to form a single reservoir for each IPD session as described elsewhere[6]. The other equipment was a peritoneal dialysis system (PDS 300, Physiocontrol, Redmond, WA, USA; ABG SEMCA, Villa Thoreton, 75015 Paris) using reverse osmosis (RO) treated water and adequate concentrates to prepare continuous dialysis solutions with a wide range of sodium and dextrose concentrations[7].

The composition of commercial dialysis solutions was the following (in mmol/l): Na 130, K 0 to 2, Cl 95, acetate 35, Ca 1.75, Mg 0.75, glucose 82.5 or 220. The final electrolyte composition of dialysate produced by RO machines was similar when an electrolyte–dextrose concentrate was used, giving a glucose concentration of 82.5 mmol/l. The final dextrose concentration could be increased up to 247.5 mmol/l by the addition of a 50% dextrose concentrate.

Dialysis schedules included at least 3 weeks dialyses of 10 to 12 hours duration; some patients required one dialysis every other day. 40 to 60 l of dialysate were used for each session, with a total of 120 to 210 l/week according to the dialysis schedule. Most patients dialysed overnight. Great aseptic care was used at the beginning and the end of dialysis when the dialysate delivery circuit was connected or disconnected from the Tenckhoff catheter.

Management of diabetes

Diet

All patients had a diet with a controlled carbohydrate intake, ranging from 120 to 220 g/day according to the patients' body weight and life style. A protein intake of 1.2–1.5 g kg body weight^{-1} day^{-1} was recommended. The patients were also encouraged to limit their dietary sodium and water intake. On dialysis days, the patients were advised to reduce their carbohydrate intake to a minimum (20 g) to avoid the effects on blood glucose level of too large a carbohydrate load resulting from an excessive dietary intake and glucose diffusing from the peritoneal cavity.

Blood glucose monitoring and insulin prescription

Daily blood glucose determinations were done 3 to 4 times a day as a guide for insulin requirements. Blood glucose levels were measured with the finger prick technique using Dextrostix; the readings were made by a reflectance meter (Glucometer, Ames Corp, Elkhart, IN, USA). During the first week on dialysis, 3 daily subcutaneous injections of regular insulin were given and the insulin dosage was adjusted to maintain glucose levels between 4 and 10 mmol/l. This permitted one to determine empirically for each patient the insulin requirement on dialysis and non-dialysis days. The amount of supplemental insulin needed on dialysis days was a function of the dextrose concentration in the dialysis solutions selected for a given dialysis session; this supplemental insulin varied greatly from patient to patient and was defined on an empirical basis. After a few weeks, when satisfactory control of blood glucose was obtained, insulin injections were prescribed twice daily (semi-lente insulin) but some patients preferred to have only one daily injection of a mixture of regular and lente insulin.

For long term surveillance, daily blood glucose measurements were recommended and the following readings were suggested: fasting, before lunch, before dinner, plus extra readings in case of thirst or malaise.

Other treatments

The management of diabetes in Type II B patients was adapted according to the effects of IPD on blood glucose levels. Some patients had a satisfactory result with diet alone; others were prescribed sulphonyl urea preparations either every day or on dialysis days only; a smaller number of patients received subcutaneous injection of regular or semi-lente insulin on dialysis nights only.

Diabetes surveillance

Every 2 to 3 months, the patients were seen at the outpatient clinic. Standard biochemistry, EKG, motor nerve conduction velocity (MNCV) and telethorax X-ray were checked on this occasion; MNCV was measured on 4 nerves (median, ulnar, tibialis anterior and posterior) with a normal mean value of 49 ± 5(SD) m/s. Figures 1 to 5 present some of these data collected in patients treated for at least 6 months; the number of patients for which data were available at the start of treatment and at one, two, three, four and five years later respectively was the following: Type I diabetics: 15, 11, 9, 9, 7 and 4; Type II diabetics: 25, 18, 9, 6 and 3. Rehabilitation was assessed according to the scoring system adopted by the Registry of the European Dialysis and Transplant Association[8].

Statistics

The life table method[9] was chosen to determine patient cumulative survival rates at 6 month intervals; actuarial survival was computed separately for Type I and Type II patients. Furthermore, the same statistical approach was used to calculate the technique success rate which was computed by counting as 'dead' a patient who was transferred to another treatment modality (e.g. CAPD) except transplantation. Two patients who were temporarily transferred to another treatment modality and later received again IPD were considered as new patients in the patient survival computation.

RESULTS

Treatment duration and outcome

The cumulative treatment duration for both Types I and II patients amounted to 133.2 years of experience. The cumulative as well as the individual (mean per patient) treatment durations for Type I, Type II A and Type II B patients are shown in Table 2 which indicates also the experience acquired with cyclers versus RO machines: the latter were almost exclusively used in Type I diabetics who were more skilled at utilizing this more complex equipment.

Table 2 Total treatment duration for 3 subgroups of diabetics receiving IPD and duration of treatment according to the technique used (automatic cycler or reverse osmosis (RO) machine)

	Type I		*Type II A*		*Type II B*	
Number of patients	19		10		29	
Cumulative duration (y)						
Total	60.5		15.9		56.8	
Cycler	12.4		11.0		49.6	
R.O.	48.1		4.9		7.2	
Mean per patient (y ± SD)						
Total	3.2 ± 1.9	(15)	1.6 ± 1.8		2.0 ± 1.4	
Cycler (*n*)	2.5 ± 2.1	(5)	1.4 ± 1.8	(8)	1.9 ± 1.6	(26)
R.O. (*n*)	3.0 ± 1.7	(16)	2.4	(2)	1.8 ± 0.6	(3)

Six patients were previously treated with CAPD (1 Type I, 5 Type II) and were transferred to IPD for the following reasons: loss of the capacity of the peritoneum to ultafilter, 3; severe hypertriglyceridaemia, 1; permanent hypotension, 1; patient's preference, 1. Fifteen patients, including 9 Type I diabetics (47.4%) and 6 Type II diabetics (15.4%), were transferred from IPD to CAPD with the following indications: patient's preference, 7; pain during infusion in IPD, 2; intolerable thirst, 2; inadequate dialysis, 1; poor diabetic control, 1; unable to cope with IPD, 2. One patient was transplanted with her brother's kidney; she rejected one year later and was started again on IPD.

Overall, 22 deaths were observed, including 3 Type I (15.8%) and 19 Type II patients (48.7%). By 30 November 1982, 20 patients (6 Type I and 14 Type II) were continuing on IPD with treatment durations ranging from 4.5 months to almost 6 years.

Control of diabetes mellitus

The blood glucose level obtained in 16 Type I patients on 6 consecutive days once a year showed that the control of DM was good in 5 patients, fair in 4 and poor in 7 with mean weekly blood glucose level (in mmol/l ± SD) of 6.4 ± 0.6, 7.4 ± 1.3 and 9.8 ± 1.5 respectively.

In Type II patients, diabetes control was evaluated from daily blood glucose measurements made 3 times a day by 32 patients: control was rated good in 22 patients, fair in 8 and poor in 2.

Blood pressure control

As shown in Figure 1, the control of blood pressure was satisfactory in both Type I and Type II diabetics. However, an increasing number of Type I patients required antihypertensive therapy. In this group of patients, it should be noted that supine mean blood pressure remained in the hypertensive range, whereas standing blood pressure was normal.

Among Type II diabetics, blood pressure was more easily controlled, particularly in those patients who had the longest follow-up. It is worth noting that

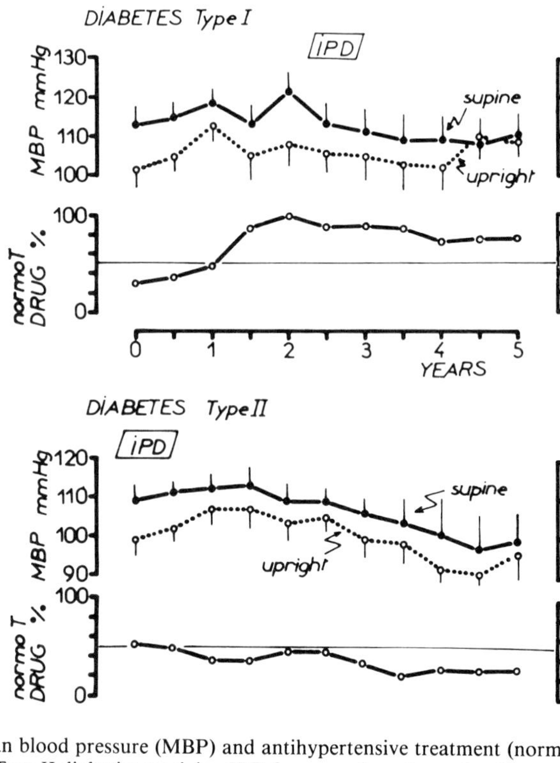

Figure 1 Mean blood pressure (MBP) and antihypertensive treatment (normoT. drugs) in 15 Type I and 25 Type II diabetics receiving IPD for more than 6 months. The number of patients on treatment at each interval is indicated in the text (page 266). Each point is a mean value for the group; the vertical bars indicate standard deviations.

the percentage of patients receiving antihypertensive treatment never exceeded 50% and decreased progressively with time.

Nutritional status and anaemia

Most patients maintained good nutritional status. As a group, Type II patients remained in the range of 10 to 20% excess body weight by reference to the calculated ideal body weight; however, as shown in Figure 2, there were wide interpatient differences.

Type I diabetics were in most cases malnourished when they were referred to us. After the initial ultrafiltration necessitated by an almost constant severe extracellular volume (ECV) excess, the mean body weight remained below the ideal body weight up to the end of the second year of treatment. Later on, the mean for the group stabilized until the 42nd month of IPD, some patients still being underweight. In the patients observed beyond the 42nd month, there was a progressive increase in weight up to + 15% ± 12%(SD) ideal body weight.

As shown in Figure 3, serum albumin levels remained in the normal range (36 ± 2 g/l) in both groups of diabetics for up to 36 months of IPD. In the fourth year of treatment, serum albumin decreased significantly to 30 g/l in Type II diabetics, whereas Type I patients were able to maintain normal levels during the whole period of follow-up.

The anaemia of renal failure was only partially corrected in both Type I and Type II patients. However, the haematocrit value remained stable without transfusion after reaching a mean value of 30.6 ± 2.3% at the end of the first year of treatment.

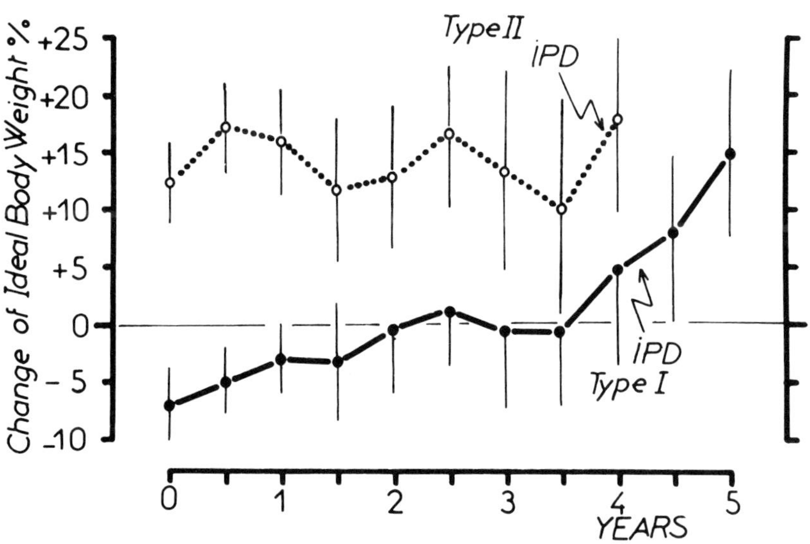

Figure 2 Changes in body weight during IPD in diabetics treated for more than 6 months (same patients as in Figure 1). Each point is a mean value for the group; vertical bars indicate standard deviations.

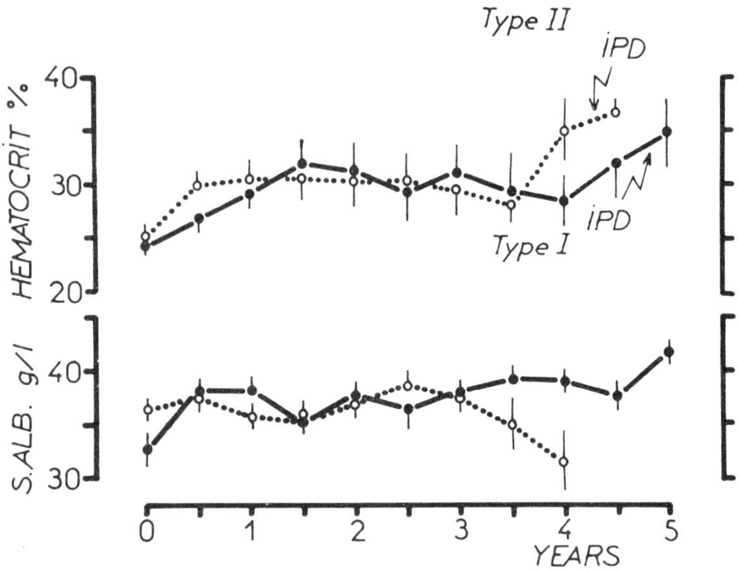

Figure 3 Serum albumin levels and haematocrit values of diabetics receiving IPD for 6 months or more (same patients as in Figures 1 and 2). Each point is a mean value for the group; vertical bars indicate standard deviations.

Residual renal function and control of uraemia

After starting IPD, a rapid decrease in creatinine clearance was observed among Type I patients from a mean intitial value of 3.8 ± 1.2 ml/min to 1.6 ± 1.1 at 6 months, and 1.1 ± 1.0 at one year. At the end of the second year, most patients were anuric (mean creatinine clearance: 0.3 ± 0.5 ml/min). This rapid decrease in residual renal function was the consequence of the considerable reduction in ECV required in the early phase of IPD to bring the patient down to his dry weight (average weight reduction during the first month: 4.2 ± 3.7 kg).

In Type II patients, there was also a progressive decline in residual renal function: however, this reduction in clearance was smaller in magnitude than in Type I patients. Mean values for creatinine clearance (in ml/min) dropped from 4.2 ± 1.7 to 1.9 ± 1.5 after one year of treatment and to 1.3 ± 1.4 at two years.

These changes in creatinine clearance as a function of time are depicted in Figure 4 where pre-dialysis serum urea and creatinine levels are also shown. Urea levels were similar in both Type I and Type II diabetics, whereas serum creatinine levels were higher among Type I patients (1200 ± 140 μmol/l) than in Type II diabetics (870 ± 120 μmol/l).

Visual status and peripheral neuropathy

Table 3 summarizes the visual status of the patients and confirms the remark-

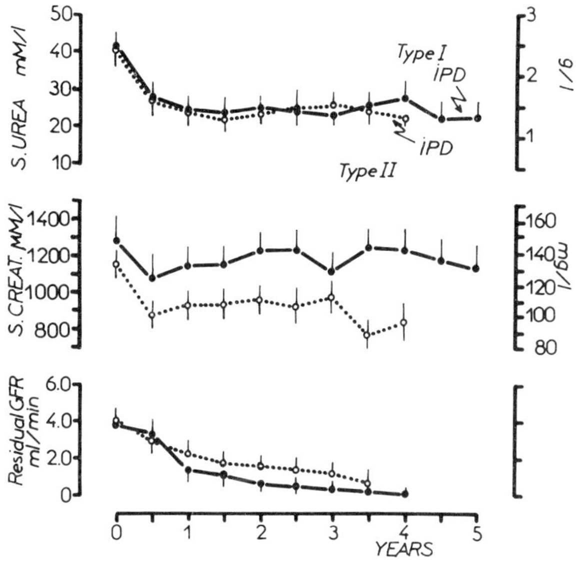

Figure 4 Serum urea and creatinine levels, and residual renal function in diabetics treated with IPD for 6 or more months (same patients as in Figures 1–3). Each point is a mean value for the group; vertical bars indicate standard deviations.

able stability of this parameter over the whole period of follow-up.

Two Type I and 2 Type II diabetics improved remarkably after phakectomy for cataract, 3 of them being able to read after the operation.

As shown in Table 4, peripheral neuropathy was stable in most patients: signs and symptoms of deterioration were observed in 4 Type I and in 12 Type II diabetics. However, the clinical manifestations were minor in most cases (e.g. disappearance of deep tendon reflexes) and were not accompanied by major difficulty in walking. One young female (Type I DM) with severe autonomic neuropathy and marked orthostatic hypotension (standing systolic blood pressure: 70–80 mmHg) improved only slightly after intensive physical therapy and remained severely handicapped after 4 years of treatment. Figure 5 depicts the outcome of MNCV. This parameter was below normal in all patients before treatment. However Type II patients had higher MNCV values

Table 3 Visual status before treatment and outcome

	19 Type I		*39 Type II*	
	Before IPD	*Last control*	*Before IPD*	*Last control*
Can read	7	8	24	26
Can see but not read	4	5	13	11
Blind	8	6	2	2

Table 4 Peripheral neuropathy: status before IPD and outcome

	Type I n	(%)	*Type II* n	(%)
Improved	10	(53)	12	(31)
Stable	5	(26)	15	(38)
Worsened	4	(21)	12	(31)
Total	19	(100)	39	(100)

than Type I diabetics; furthermore, at follow-up, the MNCV remained stable in the former while they decreased steadily in the latter.

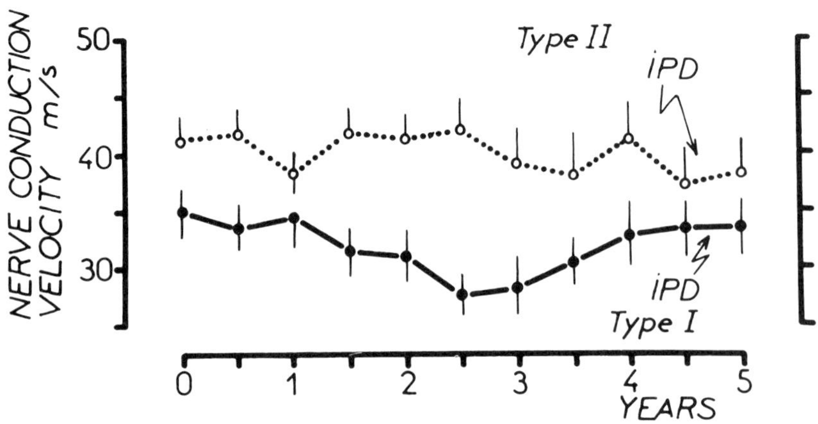

Figure 5 Mean nerve conduction velocity in 15 Type and 25 Type II diabetics treated with IPD for 6 months or more (same patients as in Figures 1–4). Each point is a mean value for the group; vertical bars indicate standard deviations.

Peritonitis

As shown in Table 5, the rate of peritoneal infection was kept at a low level among both Type I and Type II diabetics, ranging from one episode per 5.2 patient treatment years to 1 per 15.3 years. The higher rate of peritoneal infection was observed in Type II B patients, who had an incidence of peritonitis 3 times higher than Type II A patients.

Table 5 Incidence of peritonitis

	Type I	*Type II A*	*Type II B*
Number of patients	19	10	29
Patients with peritonitis	3	1	11
Cumulative treatment duration (y)	60.5	15.9	56.8
Number of PE[1]	5 (1)[2]	1	11 (4)[2]
PE incidence per patient treatment year	1/12.1	1/15.9	1/5.2

[1] PE = peritonitis episodes; [2] between parenthesis: episodes of PE secondary to acute visceral disease.

Causes of death

Among the 22 deaths observed, 3 occurred in Type I patients, 4 in Type II A and 15 in Type II B diabetics, representing 15.8, 40 and 48.3% of the patients in each subgroup. The causes of death are indicated in Table 6, showing a striking predominance of cardiovascular deaths (16 of 22 deaths or 72.7%). Three deaths occurred as a complication of infectious peritonitis, including 2 episodes secondary to appendicitis and diverticulitis.

Table 6 Causes of death

	Type I	*Type II A*	*Type II B*
Number of patients	19	10	29
Number of deaths (%)[1]	3 (16)	4 (40)	15 (51)
Causes of death			
Cardiovascular (16 deaths, 72% of deaths)			
CVA	1	2	2
Gangrene	1	—	3
Intractable CCF	—	—	2
Arrhythmias and sudden death	—	1	4
Infectious (5 deaths, 26% of deaths)			
Peritonitis	1[2]	1	1[2]
Pulmonary	—	—	2
GI bleeding	—	—	1

[1] Percentage of patients in each subgroup
[2] Peritonitis secondary to appendicitis or diverticulitis

Rehabilitation

The degree of rehabilitation was difficult to assess among this population as many patients had not been working for several months or years when IPD was initiated. The main causes of unemployment were impaired vision, severe peripheral vascular disease or retirement. At the most recent review 15 patients representing 78.9% of Type I diabetics and 25 subjects representing 64.1% of Type II patients were not able to work, as shown in Table 7. Most patients

Table 7 Rehabilitation status of 48 diabetics at most recent review (evaluated according to EDTA scale)

	Type I	*Type II*
Able to work		
Working full time	2	2
Working part time	1	1
No work available	1	—
Social security benefits greater than earning capacity	—	4
Retired	—	7
Unable to work		
Living at home	12	20
Equivalent to hospital care	3	5

living at home were able to take care of themselves without help, only 3 Type I and 5 Type II diabetics requiring assistance equivalent to hospitalization.

Survival

Figure 6 shows the actuarial survival of the patients and also the technique success rate (TSR). Among Type I diabetics, the actuarial survival was excellent (95% at one and 2 years, 83% at 3 and 4 years) but the TSR was low (65% at one year, 55% at 2 years, 48% at 3 and 4 years) as a result of transferring patients to CAPD or transplantation. As expected, the per cent actuarial survival of Type II patients was much lower, with percentages of 79, 68 and 41.2 at 1, 2 and 3 years respectively. On the other hand, the patients in this group being exclusively treated with IPD, the TSR was almost identical to the patients' survival.

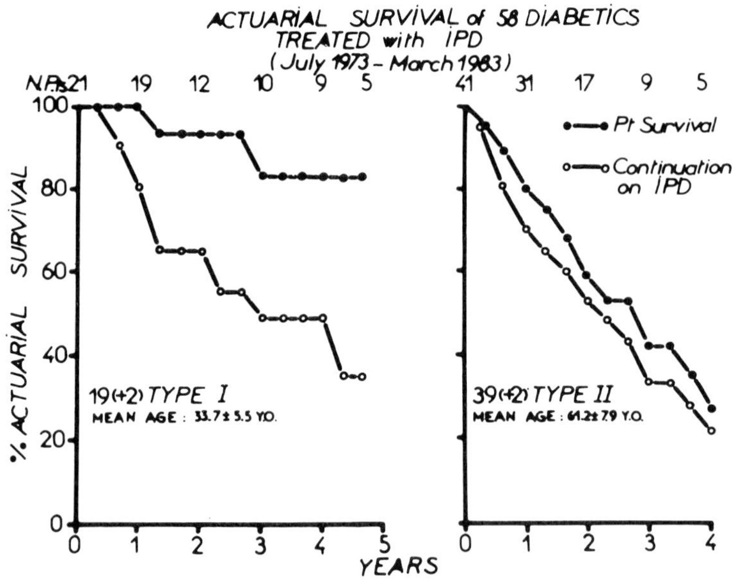

Figure 6 Actuarial survival and technique success rate of diabetic patients treated with IPD. Two patients who were temporarily transferred to another treatment modality are considered as 'new patients' when started again on IPD.

DISCUSSION

The present report confirms our previous observations concerning the satisfactory results obtained in the long term with IPD in patients with end stage diabetic nephropathy[1,2]. The per cent actuarial survival of Type I diabetics remains one of the highest ever reported and compares very favourably with those obtained by Shapiro and Comty[10] in similar patients treated with haemodialysis (HD); on the other hand, our Type II diabetics had a slightly poorer survival than that obtained with HD by the same authors.

The results presented here demonstrate the prognostic value of identifying the type of DM in diabetics with end-stage renal failure. Type I DM and Type II DM correspond to 2 distinct groups of patients differing in their age and the severity of cardiovascular complications at the time of initiating maintenance dialysis. Our Type II diabetics belonged to the age group 60 years or more so it was no surprise that their survival was much poorer than that observed among the younger Type I patients. The separation of diabetics into their two main subgroups (Type I or insulin dependent and Type II or non-insulin dependent diabetics) is therefore a necessary prerequisite to survival studies using the life-table method.

The main reasons for using IPD in our programme were: (1) the preference of our patients who dislike the constraint of CAPD with its multiple daily bag exchanges; (2) the extremely low incidence of peritonitis observed with this technique; and (3) the total dependence of some patients, making it impractical to use CAPD. The long term results obtained demonstrate that IPD may be used with success provided the dialysis schedule and the weekly volume of dialysate are adapted to the needs of the individual patient, particularly when creatinine clearance is declining. When asked to do one dialysis every other night because of persisting hypertension or deterioration in peripheral neuropathy, our patients have preferred to increase their weekly IPD duration rather than transferring to CAPD.

The main advantage of IPD was its remarkably low risk of peritoneal infection. The extremely low incidence of peritonitis among Type I diabetics was surprising in view of the well known susceptibility of diabetics to infection. Our IPD experience suggests that young diabetics fare better in that regard than non-diabetic patients using the same technique[11]. In spite of routine use of IPD as a home technique accomplished as a routine without close supervision, peritonitis was virtually eradicated from the list of PD complications. The peritoneal infection rate observed among Type II B patients was twice that of Type I diabetics, but did not differ from that of other non-diabetic patients of the same age group. Type II A diabetics had a rate of infection three times lower than Type II B: whether this difference was due to the small number of Type II A patients with a short aggregated observation period or resulted from better diabetes control and improved immune defences from insulin treatment remains uncertain.

The limitations of IPD have been recognized in recent years[12] and this dialysis method gave poor results in diabetics in the hands of Katirzoglou *et al*[13]. Our results do not support such pessimistic conclusions, although some of our data may suggest the possibility that inadequate dialysis was more frequent in Type I patients than eventually recognized.

The main difficulty encountered in our patients concerned the control of blood pressure, particularly in Type I diabetics. One year after starting IPD, 80% of them were using antihypertensive drugs. It should be stressed, however, that except in 4 Type I patients, the antihypertensive regimen was mild and used only one drug (usually acebutolol 100 to 400 mg p.o. daily). Another problem was the poor control of diabetes in about $\frac{2}{3}$ of Type I diabetics: reports stressing the superiority of administering insulin via the peritoneal route with CAPD[14,15] to normalize blood glucose were confirmed in those of our patients transferred to CAPD. Finally, the progressive decline in MNCV among Type I diabetics may indicate that these patients were inadequately dialysed; the fact that the reduction of MNCV was observed with a simultaneous decrease in creatinine clearance gives some support to this hypothesis. In one patient, transferred to CAPD because of inadequate dialysis, the peripheral neuropathy stabilized then improved, but this improvement was difficult to assign to CAPD alone, as diabetes control was simultaneously improved by intraperitoneal insulin administration.

CONCLUSION

Although we accept the theoretical advantages of CAPD in diabetics[14,15], we believe from our experience that IPD still has an important role to play in the treatment of diabetics with end-stage renal failure. This technique has enabled us to treat a large group of unselected diabetics in their homes in spite of the various handicaps observed in such patients. Furthermore, IPD permitted the continuation of maintenance peritoneal dialysis in those CAPD patients whose peritoneum had lost its capacity to ultrafilter. We propose therefore that IPD should remain available in any end-stage renal disease treatment programme, to solve some of the problems that occur in diabetics treated with CAPD (e.g. frequent peritonitis, loss of ultrafiltration capacity).

ACKNOWLEDGEMENTS

We wish to express our many thanks to Mrs M. Elie for her kind cooperation in the preparation of this manuscript.

References

1. Mion, C, Slingeneyer, A., Oulès, R., Selam, J. L., Delors, J. and Mirouze, J. (1979). Home peritoneal dialysis in diabetics with end stage renal failure. *Contrib. Nephrol.*, **17**, 120–130
2. Slingeneyer, A., Mion, C. and Selam, J. L. (1981). Home intermittent and continuous ambulatory peritoneal dialysis as a long term treatment of end stage renal failure in diabetics. In Gahl, G. M., Kessel, M., Nolph, K. D. (eds), *Advances in Peritoneal Dialysis, International Congress Series 567*, pp. 378–388. (Amsterdam: Excerpta Medica).
3. Najarian, J. S., Sutherland, D. E. R. (1982). Continuous ambulatory peritoneal dialysis in diabetics with end stage renal disease. Letter to the Editor. *N. Engl. J. Med.*, **307**, 1083
4. Anonymous (1980). World Health Organisation. *Technical Report Series, no. 646.* (Geneva, Switzerland: WHO).
5. Slingeneyer, A., Mion, C., Charpiat, A., Balmès, M. (1981). Is an alternative to the Tenckhoff catheter necessary? In Gahl, G. M., Kessel, M., Nolph, K. D. (eds), *Advances in Peritoneal Dialysis, International Congress Series 567*, pp. 179–184. (Amsterdam: Excerpta Medica)

6. Mion, C. (1975). A peritoneal dialysis programme. *Proc. Eur. Dial. Transpl. Assoc.*, **12,** 140
7. Tenckhoff, H., Meston, B. and Shilipetar, G. (1972). A simplified automatic peritoneal dialysis system. *Trans. Am. Soc. Artif. Intern. Organs*, **18,** 436
8. Jacobs, C., Brunner, F. P., Chantler, C., Donckerwolcke, R. A., Gurland, H. J., Hathway, R. A., Selwood, N. H. and Wing, A. J. (1977). Combined report on regular dialysis and transplant in Europe VII, 1976. *Proc. Eur. Dial. Transpl. Assoc*, **14,** 1
9. Kaplan, E. M. and Meier, P. (1958). Non parametric estimation from incomplete observations. *J. Am. Statis. Assoc.*, **53,** 457–481
10 Shapiro, F. L. and Comty, C. M. (1980). Hemodialysis in diabetics: 1979 update. In Friedman, E. A. and L'Esperance, F. A. (eds), *Diabetic Renal-Retinal Syndrome*, pp. 333–343. (New York: Grune and Stratton)
11. Slingeneyer, A., Mion, C., Despaux, E., Perez, C., Duport, J. and Dansette, A. M. (1981). Use of a bacteriologic filter in the prevention of peritonitis associated with peritoneal dialysis: long term clinical results in intermittent and continuous ambulatory peritoneal dialysis. In Atkins, R. C., Thompson, N. P., Farrell, P. C. (eds), *Peritoneal Dialysis*, pp. 301–312 (Edinburgh: Churchill Livingstone)
12. Ahmad, S., Gallager, N. and Shen, F. (1979). Intermittent peritoneal dialysis: status reassessed. *Trans. Am. Soc. Artif. Intern. Organs.*, **25,** 86
13. Katirzoglou, A., Izatt, S., Oreopoulos, D. G., Dombros, N., Blair, G. H., Chisholm, L., Meema, H. E., Ogilvie, R., Vas, S., Leibel, B. and McCreedy, W., (1980). Chronic peritoneal dialysis in diabetics with end stage renal failure. In Friedman, E. A., L'Esperance, F. A. (eds), *Diabetic Renal-Retinal Syndrome*, pp. 317–331. (New York: Grune and Stratton)
14. Flynn, C. T., Hibbard, J. and Dohrman, B. (1979). Advantages of continuous ambulatory peritoneal dialysis to the diabetic with renal failure. *Proc. Eur. Dial. Transpl. Assoc.*, **16,** 184–193
15. Amair, P., Khanna, P., Leibel, B., Pierratos, A., Vas, S., Meema, E., Blair, G., Chisholm, L., Vas, M., Zingg, W., Digenis, G. and Oreopoulos, D. G. (1982). Continuous ambulatory peritoneal dialysis in diabetics with end stage renal disease. *N. Engl. J. Med.*, **306,** 625–630

19.1
Further experience with CAPD in diabetics with end-stage renal disease

R. KHANNA, G. WU, L. CHISHOLM and D. G. OREOPOULOS

INTRODUCTION

Diabetes is no longer a contraindication to kidney replacement, and throughout the world the proportion of diabetics among ESRD patients is increasing[1]. In part, this increase is due to the remarkable improvement in recent years in cumulative survival following chronic dialysis (both haemo- and peritoneal) and transplantation in ESRD diabetic patients[2,3]. After the encouraging results of Katirtzoglou[4] and Flynn[5] continuous ambulatory peritoneal dialysis (CAPD) is now being used extensively in diabetic patients who require dialysis, although experience with CAPD is relatively short, compared to that with haemodialysis. Nevertheless, to date the reported cumulative survival of diabetic on CAPD[3] has been similar to, if not better than, that achieved with haemodialysis[2]. This paper describes our experience with 37 diabetic patients with ESRD who were treated with CAPD at the Toronto Western Hospital over a period of 54 months.

PATIENTS AND METHODS

Patients

Between July 1978 and December 1982, 37 unselected diabetic patients with ESRD were trained for CAPD. They had not been on any form of dialysis previously. Twenty-eight were men and nine were women; their ages ranged from 26 to 70 years (average 49.8). They received dialysis for 2–54 months for a mean of 14.5 months and a total experience of 589 patient-months. Concerning their disease, 29 had Type I (juvenile, insulin-dependent), and eight had Type II (non-insulin-dependent, maturity onset) diabetes.

Dialysis technique and laboratory determinations

In all peritoneal access was achieved through the Toronto Western Hospital catheter[6]. The details of the (CAPD) technique have been reported previously[7]. Four 2 litre bag exchanges were performed every day. Dialysis solutions (Dianeal, Baxter) were available in the following dextrose concentrations: 0.5, 1.5, 2.5 and 4.25 g/dl. The patients were taught to add insulin to the dialysate solution according to the protocol previously described[3]. Antihypertensive medications were given if hypertension persisted after the patient had reached 'dry weight' (oedema free with no cardiac failure). Vitamin D3 or 1,25-dihydroxyvitamin D3 was given in doses appropriate to maintain the serum calcium level (corrected for protein) between 10.0–10.5 mg/dl (2.5 and 2.6 mmol/l), and phosphorus binders were administered to keep the serum phosphorus below 5 mg/dl (1.6 mmol/l). A multivitamin preparation was given daily to all patients.

The patients were seen weekly during the first month after the completion of training and monthly thereafter; visual acuity was measured at 6 month intervals.

Control of blood sugar

Blood sugar was controlled by intraperitoneal administration of insulin along with the dialysis solution[3]. The aim of this treatment was to achieve a fasting blood sugar level of less than 140 mg/dl (8 mmol/l) and a level of less than 200 mg/dl (11 mmol/) 1 hour after meals.

Statistical analysis

The rates for survival and for continuation of dialysis were calculated according to the actuarial method (life-table analysis).

RESULTS

The clinical characteristics of these 37 patients are shown in Table 1.

Table 1 Clinical characteristic of diabetic patients treated with CAPD

	Type I (No.)	*Type II (No.)*
Male	25	3
Female	4	5
Mean age (years)	47	58
Age range (years)	25–69	53–70
Duration of diabetes (years)	20.5	3.5
Hypertension	28	2
Retinopathy	29	5
Residual kidney function (ml/min)	5.3	2.9

Peritonitis

Seventeen of the 37 had 29 episodes of peritonitis – an incidence of one episode every 20.3 patient months. The predominant organisms were Staphylococci (*Staph. epidermidis* and *Staph. aureus*). Two patients had peritonitis due to Candida and Mucor species.

The outcome of these episodes was uniformly good; all but one patient improved with standard treatment previously described[8]. In three patients it was deemed necessary to remove the catheter; in two, because of fungal peritonitis; and in one due to a *Staphylococcus aureus* exit-site infection. One patient died of severe staphylococcal peritonitis.

Other complications

There was a high incidence of gastrointestinal complications, such as drug-induced gastritis, oesophagitis and diabetic gastroparesis (Table 2).

Table 2 Complications other than peritonitis in diabetics on CAPD

Complication	*No. of episodes*
Exit site infection	4
Dialysis leak	4
exit site	3
abdominal wall	1
Catheter one-way obstruction	1
Cardio-cerebrovascular	
Myocardial infarction	4
Hypertension	4
CVA	2
completed stroke	1
TIA	1
Peripheral vascular disease	3
femoral bypass	1
gangrene–amputation	2 (legs)
Gastrointestinal	
Nausea – vomiting	frequent
Gastric ulcer	1
Cholecystitis	1
Perianal abscess	1
Hernia	1
Other complications	
Fluid overload	4
Pulmonary embolism	1
Pneumonia	3
Herpes zoster	1

One patient required amputation of both legs because of progressive ischaemic changes. Another patient with ischaemic changes in one leg was stabilized with a femoropopliteal bypass.

Five patients experienced various degrees of depression, secondary to the strain of chronic illness – diabetes and uraemia, and the stress of dialysis. Two patients attempted suicide and one asked that treatment be stopped, both family and medical staff agreed and eventually this patient died. In 33 patients hypertension was controlled with dialysis alone; only four required medication for control.

Visual acuity

Table 3 shows the status of visual acuity among these patients, and Figure 1 shows the progressive change during CAPD in 22 eyes. At the start of CAPD, 28 eyes had either normal visual acuity (20/20) or mild impairment (20/160), and 30 eyes were classified as legally blind (> 20/200).

Table 3 Visual acuity in 29 CAPD diabetic patients (58 eyes)

Visual acuity	*Initial no. of eyes*	*Last status no. of eyes*
20/20 - 20/60	19	21
20/70 - 20/160	9	3
> 20/200 - total blindness	30*	34

* 8 eyes started totally blind

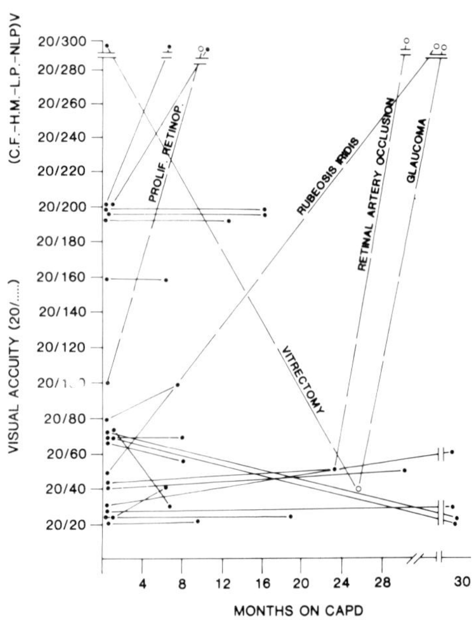

Figure 1 Changes in visual acuity in 22 eyes of diabetics on CAPD

Nineteen eyes with good vision at the start remained more or less unchanged at the end of the study. Four eyes with moderately impaired vision (20/70–20/160) deteriorated gradually to severe visual impairment: all had underlying severe opthalmological diseases such as severe proliferative retinopathy, rubeosis iritis, postvirectomy glaucoma and central retinal artery thrombosis.

Residual kidney function

In 22 patients, creatinine clearance was measured at the start and again at 3 month intervals after CAPD was begun. In these patients the mean creatinine clearance at the start was 4.2 ml/min. After at least 3 months of follow-up, the clearance had decreased to 2.3 ml/min, and the decline continued with time on CAPD. The change for individual patients are shown in Figure 2.

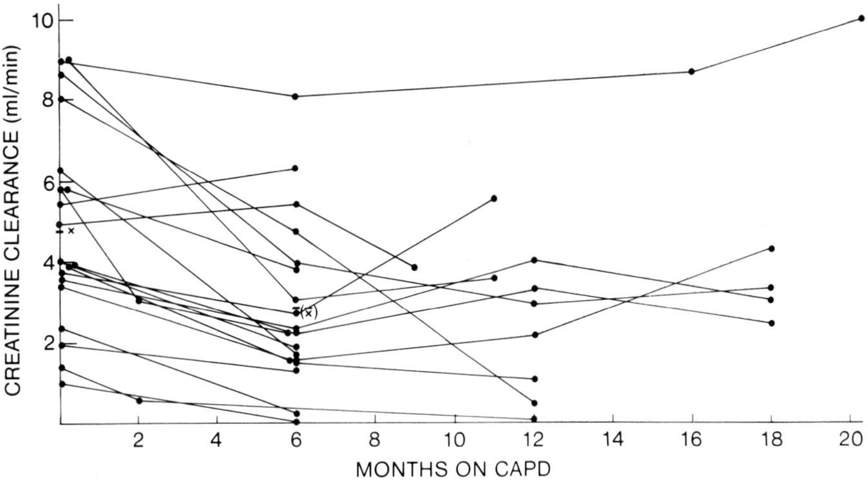

Figure 2 Change of residual kidney function with time on CAPD in 22 individual diabetics (x indicates mean)

Vascular calcifications and peripheral vascular disease

Radiologically demonstrated vascular calcification progressed in most patients. One of the 37 patients required below knee amputation of both legs because of the progressive peripheral vascular disease. Another patient required femoral popliteal bypass to one of the legs.

Hospitalization

Table 4 shows the number of hospital days for complications during CAPD in diabetics. Thirty-three days in hospital for diabetics per patient year of follow-up is almost twice the rate (16 days) for all the CAPD patients in our programme. One-half of these days (15.3 days/patient year of follow-up) was due to peritonitis-related complications. The rate of hospitalization for Type I and Type II diabetics was similar.

Table 4 Back-up hospitalization of diabetics on CAPD (days/patient treatment years)

	Year				
	1979	*1980*	*1981*	*1982*	*1979–82*
All diabetics					
All complications	72	22.5	26.9	32.1	33.1
For peritonitis only	48	0.5	3.6	9.4	—
Type I diabetics					
All complications	68	21.5	25.8	36.1	33.1
For peritonitis only	41	0.6	3.6	9.4	—

Rehabilitation

Table 5 shows the rehabilitation status of these 37 patients. Twenty-one were able to carry out normal activity and seven of these were gainfully employed full-time and three for part-time. Three housewives had normal daily activity. Six patients remained unemployed even though they could have been employed.

Table 5 Rehabilitation status of 37 CAPD diabetic patients

Occupational status	*(no.)*	*Daily activity*	*(no.)*
Fulltime	7	normal	21
Retired	8	restricted	11
Housewife	8	required care	5
Part-time	3	confined to bed	0
Sick leave	5		
Unemployed	6		
TOTAL	37		37

In Figure 3 we compared the cumulative survival for all diabetics (Type I and Type II) with that of the non-diabetics on CAPD during the same period. Despite a comparable age (49 *vs.* 51 y) the death rate of diabetics at 48 months is almost 20% higher than that for non-diabetics.

The cumulative survival of the Type I diabetic patients is shown in Figure 4. The Type I survival rate at 4 years is 62% as opposed to 27% for Type II. The numbers of patients are not large enough to make a meaningful comparison.

The cumulative technique survival for the type I diabetic is also shown in Figure 4. At 2 years with nine patients at risk, the technique survival of 62% is similar to that of non-diabetics (64%) on CAPD a the Toronto Western Hospital.

The number of patients is too small to show the influence of age on the outcome of these diabetic patients.

Among the 37 diabetics, there were four dialysis 'failures' and nine deaths (Table 6); an additional eight Type I patients received a kidney transplant.

The reason for the 'failures' (withdrawal from the programme) are shown in

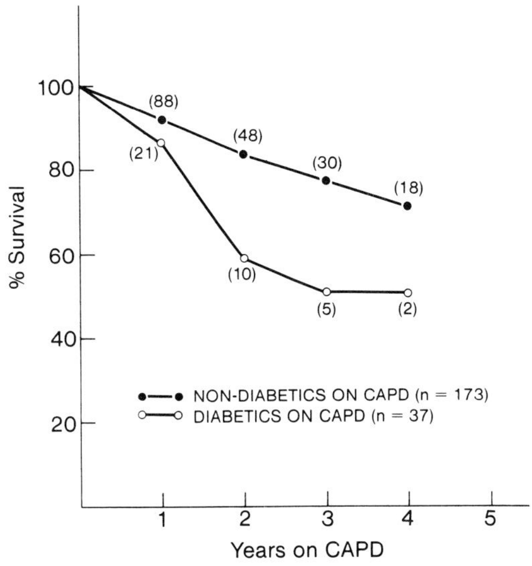

Figure 3 Cumulative survival of 37 diabetics on CAPD, compared to non-diabetics

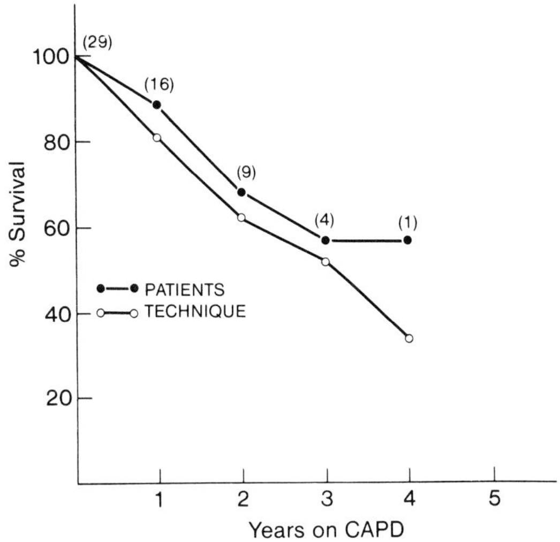

Figure 4 Cumulative patient and technique survival of 29 Type I diabetics on CAPD

Table 7. One Type II diabetic patient developed a rapidly progressive peripheral neuropathy after she had been on CAPD for 8 months. In one of the two patients who failed because of peritonitis, peritoneal access could not be re-established because of repeated profuse bleeding from the peritoneum and dialysate leak after catheter implantation.

Table 6 Outcome of 37 diabetic patients on CAPD

	Type I (n = 29)	*Type II* (*n* = 8)
Continued on CAPD	13	3
Transplanted	8	
Transferred to haemodialysis/IPD	2	2
Death	6	3

Table 7 Reasons for discontinuing CAPD in four diabetic patients

Complication	*No.*
Peritonitis	2
Progressive neuropathy	1
Backache	1

Table 8 shows the causes of death in these nine patients whose mean age was 55 years. As expected, most of the causes were cardiovascular and were associated with systemic atherosclerosis. Two patients who died suddenly had no obvious electrolyte abnormalities and we believe these deaths were also due to cardiovascular causes.

Table 8 Causes of death in nine patients (mean age 55 years)

Myocardial infarction	4
Cerebrovascular accident	1
Sudden death	2
Peritonitis	1
Withdrawal of treatment At patient request	1

DISCUSSION

At our institution CAPD has been the preferred mode of dialysis for diabetics with end-stage renal disease since mid-1978. These 37 diabetic patients comprised 18% of Toronto Western Hospital CAPD population. Twenty-nine (78%) of these 37 patients were Type I, insulin-independent diabetics.

The cumulative survival rates for all diabetics at 4 years was lower than that of the non-diabetics on CAPD, despite their lower mean age. This is not surprising because of the high incidence of cardiovascular complications in diabetics. However, the survival for the Type I diabetics at 4 years was comparable to that of non-diabetics, and to that of insulin-dependent diabetics under 61 years maintained on haemodialysis[2]. The continued good survival for Type I diabetics on CAPD may be due to several factors, such as good control of blood pressure, steady cardiovascular status without rapid fluid shifts and good control of blood sugar with insulin in the dialysis solution.

Cardiovascular disease accounted for nearly 80% of the deaths among these patients. Peritonitis was not a common cause of death; thus, in CAPD diabetic patients, it is a cause of morbidity but not of mortality. One of our patients suffered a rapid progression of peripheral neuropathy despite adequate control of blood pressure and blood sugar - an observation that casts some doubt on the importance of good blood sugar control in arresting this complication.

A most encouraging aspect in this group, was stabilization of vision in most of these patients. The four eyes in which the visual acuity deteriorated all had complicating underlying pathology. Overall, patients with good visual acuity tended to maintain good vision throughout the period of observation.

Peripheral vascular disease requiring amputation was infrequent in diabetics on CAPD as opposed to the high rate reported in transplant diabetics[9].

Our CAPD patients showed a continuous decline in residual kidney function. Some workers have suggested that liberal use of high doses of furosemide may preserve the kidney function[10], but we could not confirm this observation.

The frequency of 'back-up' hospitalization in diabetics continues to be high and exceeds that for non-diabetics. One-half of the hospitalization was related to peritonitis.

The number of people rehabilitated enough to resume their original occupations is still low (38%). Many of these patients have varying degrees of visual impairment, which may prevent them from taking gainful employment. Moreover they also have frequent medical complications, which require hospitalization care and contribute to morbidity.

In conclusion, the cumulative survival of diabetics on CAPD continues to rise. Good control of blood sugar, blood pressure, and steady state control of uraemia may be the contributing factors. Patients with good vision at the start tend to maintain good vision. Rate of hospitalization due to peritonitis and other medical complication is much higher than that of non-diabetic patients. CAPD does not preserve the residual kidney function in these patients. Because of the many advantages, and promising rate of survival, CAPD seems to be the treatment of choice for diabetics who require dialysis.

References

1. Kjellstrand, C., Comty, C. and Shapiro, F. (1982). A comparison of dialysis and transplantation in insulin dependent diabetic patients. In Friedman, E. A., L'Esperance, F. A. Jr. (eds.). *Diabetic Renal–Retinal Syndrome*, pp. 405–417. (New York: Grune & Stratton)
2. Shapiro, F. L. and Comty, C. M. (1981). Hemodialysis in diabetics. In Friedman, E. A., L'Esperance, F. A. Jr. (eds.). *Update in Diabetic Retinal Syndrome,* pp. 309–320. (New York: Grune & Stratton)
3. Amair, P., Khanna, R., Leibel, B. *et al.* (1982). Continuous ambulatory peritoneal dialysis in diabetics with end-stage renal disease. *N. Engl. J. Med.,* **306,** 625–630
4. Katirtzoglou, A., Izatt, S., Oreopoulos, D. G. *et al.* (1980). Chronic peritoneal dialysis in diabetics with end-stage renal disease. In Friedman, E. A., L'Esperance, F. A. Jr. (eds.). *Diabetic Renal–Retinal Syndrome,* pp. 317. (New York: Grune & Stratton)

5. Flynn, C.T. and Nanson, J.A. (1979). Intraperitoneal insulin with CAPD. An artificial pancreas. *Trans. Am. Soc. Artif. Intern. Organs,* **25,** 114
6. Oreopoulos, D.G., Zellerman, G., Izatt, S. *et al.* (1980). The Toronto Western Hospital permanent peritoneal catheter and continuous ambulatory peritoneal dialysis connector. In Legrain, M. (ed.). *Proceedings 1st. Symposium on CAPD.* pp. 161–166. (Amsterdam: Excerpta Medica)
7. Khanna, R., Oreopoulos, D.G., Dombros, N. *et al.* (1981). Continuous ambulatory peritoneal dialysis after three years: still a promising treatment. *Perit. Dial.* Bull., **1,** 24
8. Williams, P., Khanna, R. and Oreopoulos, D.G. (1981). Treatment of peritonitis in patients on CAPD. No longer a controversy. *Dial. Transplant.,* **10,** 272
9. Sutherland, D.E.R., Fryd, D., Peters, C. *et al* (1982). Current status of kidney transplantation in uremic diabetics at the University of Minnesota. In Friedman, G.A. and L'Esperance, F.A. (eds.). *Diabetic Renal-Retinal Syndrome,* pp. 373-383. (New York: Grune & Stratton)
10. Rottembourg, J., Shahat, Y.E., Agrafiotis, A. *et al.* (1983). Continuous ambulatory peritoneal dialysis in insulin dependent diabetics mellitus: A 40 months experience. *Kidney Int.,* **23,** 40

19.2

Experience with CAPD in diabetic patients

N. LAMEIRE, M. DHAENE, E. MATTHIJS, M. DE PAEPE,
P. VEREERSTRAETEN, M. DRATWA and S. RINGOIR

INTRODUCTION

The preferred mode of treatment for diabetic end-stage renal disease (ESRD) remains still controversial, although it becomes more and more clear that the young uraemic diabetic patient should be offered at least one chance to be transplanted, certainly when an HLA-identical donor is available[1,2]. Impressive improvement in the survival results in dialysed diabetics have been reported with either haemodialysis[1,3] or continuous ambulatory peritoneal dialysis (CAPD)[4,5]. The latter technique especially has some advantages for the older patient, since it is a form of home treatment, otherwise rarely applied in the diabetic. The results with CAPD in two relatively large series of diabetic patients have recently been published; in the experience of Toronto[4] a dramatic patient survival rate of 92% at 1 year and of 81% at 2 years was noted. Rottembourg and co-workers[5] also reported similarly excellent results with a survival rate of 84% at 1 year and of 72% at 18 months.

The present paper describes the combined experience from three Belgian renal units in treating diabetic patients with CAPD.

PATIENTS AND METHODS

Between January, 1979 and March, 1983, 19 diabetic patients (10 men and 9 women) with end-stage kidney disease were admitted in the CAPD programme of the University units of Gent and Brussels. At the start of CAPD, the mean age of the patients was 56 years (varying between 34 and 74 years) and the duration of the diabetes mellitus ranged from 9 to 31 years. Only twelve patients were on insulin therapy prior to CAPD. Their daily insulin therapy ranged from 16 to 45 units (a mean of 33 units). Fifteen patients suffered from insulin-dependent and four from non-insulin dependent diabetes (NIDD). CAPD was the primary therapy in 16 patients; three were transferred from the haemodialysis programme. They received CAPD from 2 to 15 months, for a mean of 7.3 months, representing a total experience of 139 patient months. Eight patients were followed for longer than 1 year.

All patients were performing CAPD through an indwelling double cuff Tenckhoff catheter and used three to four 21 bags of Dianeal(R) solutions (Travenol Co) per day. The following dextrose dialysate concentrations were available: 1.5, 2.5 and 4.25 g per dl. The CAPD technique has previously been described in detail[6,7].

All patients or their partners were trained to add an amount of insulin into the bags according to frequently measured blood glucose levels during the initial hospitalization. Patients were instructed to change their bags 30–60 minutes before taking each meal. All patients were advised to restrict dietary calories mainly by adhering to a low carbohydrate (125–150 g), high protein diet (1.2–1.5 g/kg). Salt restriction was only applied when hypertension persisted.

No training for self-control of glucose levels was given, except for three patients. Once on an ambulatory basis, the diabetes control in almost all patients was performed at the outpatient department. For practical reasons, this was limited to one or two blood glucose levels once a month and to a series of four blood glucose readings per day every 3 months, together with the other routine blood tests.

RESULTS

All patients presented with one or more serious extrarenal complications at the

Table 1 Extrarenal complications in 19 diabetic patients at start CAPD

Hypertension (>160/95 mmHg)	13	(68%)
Retinopathy	17	(90%)
Peripheral neuropathy (nerve conduction <35 m/s)	7	(37%)
Autonomic dysfunction	3	(16%)
Cardiac problems		
Clinical and/or e.c.g. angor	12	(84%)
Previous heart failure	4	
Peripheral vascular disease		
Clinical (claudication)	4	(21%)
Absent peripheral arterial pulsations	11	(58%)
Pre-gangrene	3	(16%)
Enteropathy	1	(5%)

start of CAPD. The most important complications are summarized in Table 1.

Table 2 Clinical and biochemical profile in 19 diabetic uraemic patients treated with CAPD (means ± SEM)

	Months			
	0 ($n=19$)	*3* ($n=16$)	*6* ($n=9$)	*12* ($n=5$)
Weight (kg)	67·5 ± 2.2	65.1 ± 1.9	65.1 ± 2.7	66.6 ± 2.9
Blood pressure (mmHg)				
systolic	165 ± 5.8	152 ± 4.5	158 ± 10.2	147 ± 10.8*
diastolic	92 ± 3.4	87 ± 2.4	84 ± 4.0	82 ± 5.2*
Daily peritoneal protein loss (g/24 h)**	10.2 ± 1.6	12.6 ± 1.5	13.6 ± 2.2	13.9 ± 3.5
Peritoneal creatinine clearance (ml/min)**	4.47 ± 0.40	4.70 ± 0.30	4.35 ± 0.50	4.80 ± 0.40
Daily ultrafiltration (ml/day)**	−975 ± 120	−877 ± 120	−995 ± 192	−1160 ± 283
Residual creatinine clearance (ml/min)	6.9 ± 0.8	4.3 ± 1.9	3.2 ± 1.3*	1.5 ($n=2$)
Urea (mg/dl)	193 ± 10.9	124 ± 11.2*	149 ± 20*	134 ± 29*
Creatinine (mg/dl)	8.05 ± 0.70	7.25 ± 0.78	7.3 ± 2.8	7.84 ± 2.6
Hgb (g/dl)	9.32 ± 0.34	10.3 ± 0.48	9.8 ± 0.87	9.02 ± 0.43
Hct (%)	27.2 ± 1.14	31.7 ± 1.50*	30.9 ± 1.60	28.4 ± 1.30
Total protein (g/l)	61.6 ± 1.80	64.0 ± 1.05	64.7 ± 2.0	58.8 ± 3.30
Albumin (g/l)	32.0 ± 1.56	33.3 ± 1.12	33.5 ± 1.90	30.3 ± 2.60
Na (mmol/l)	137 ± 1.10	138.2 ± 0.80	136 ± 1.10	137 ± 1.60
K (mmol/l)	4.5 ± 0.18	4.8 ± 0.17	4.7 ± 0.30	4.2 ± 0.20
Ca (mg/dl)	8.45 ± 0.25	8.98 ± 0.22	8.81 ± 0.28	8.44 ± 0.55
P (mg/dl)	5.83 ± 0.46	5.60 ± 0.37	4.55 ± 0.29	6.38 ± 1.60
Alk. phosph. (U/l) (96–272)	271 ± 58	268 ± 14	226 ± 37	391 ± 100 ($n=3$)
Cholesterol (mg/dl)	211.5 ± 18	264 ± 14*	243 ± 22	207 ± 13
Triglycerides (mg/dl)	188 ± 26.3	209 ± 32	282 ± 75*	347 ± 120* ($n=3$)

* $p < 0.05$
** Calculated after 1 week of CAPD

Except for two patients with NIDD, all others suffered from diabetic retinopathy. Information on visual acuity was available in 34 eyes at the start of dialysis. Only 11 (32%) eyes had a 'good' visual acuity (VA between 50/100 and 100/100).

Particularly important were the cardiovascular problems with three patients suffering from uni- or bilateral pregangrene of the foot.

The evolution of the most relevant clinical and biochemical parameters in these patients is summarized in Table 2.

After an initial drop in body weight during the first 3 months, there was a trend to gain weight at the end of the first year of CAPD.

Improvement of hypertension was noted in many patients, resulting in almost normal mean systolic and diastolic pressures at 12 months.

The proportion of the CAPD patients taking antihypertensive medication at the start and after 6 and 12 months was 11/19 (58%), 6/9 (67%) and 5/7 patients (71%), respectively.

The daily peritoneal protein loss after 1 week of dialysis varied from 2.6 to 23 g (mean 10.2 ± 1.6 g) but did not change consistently during follow-up. At 6 months the peritoneal protein losses ranged from 9 to 23.6 g (mean 13.6 ± 2.2 g) in the seven patients where data were available. The peritoneal creatinine clearances and daily ultrafiltration rates were calculated, and did not change over this first year of treatment. The residual endogenous creatinine clearance dropped from a mean of 6.9 ± 0.8 at start to 3.2 ± 1.3 ml/min after 6 months.

After an initial increase in haematocrit and haemoglobin levels after 3–6 months, the mean values of both parameters returned to base line in the five patients that were followed over 1 year. No consistent changes in serum total protein, albumin and major serum electrolytes were noted. A moderate elevation of mean serum cholesterol levels, but a sharp and continuous rise in serum triglycerides was observed throughout the follow-up period.

The data on follow-up of diabetes control are summarized in Table 3. Due to

Table 3 Daily glucose profile in diabetic CAPD patients (mg/dl). Mean ± SEM

	Months			
	0	*3*	*6*	*12*
Morning	171 ± 16	164 ± 17	232 ± 30	244 ± 26
Noon	233 ± 19	199 ± 30	194 ± 40	271 ± 48
Afternoon	190 ± 20	219 ± 42	225 ± 23	310 ± 63
Evening	201 ± 16	202 ± 33	309 ± 51	348 ± 58
Daily amounts (U) of insulin (i.p.)	20.8 ± 4.2	53.2 ± 5.3*	53.8 ± 5.5*	53.2 ± 11*

* $p < 0.05$

the fact that 7 out of the 19 patients did not need insulin therapy before the start of CAPD, the mean daily dose of intraperitoneal insulin at the start was only 20.8 ± 4.2 units, with a range from 0 to 44 units per day. From 3 months to 12 months, the mean daily dose of insulin was stabilized at a mean of 53 units per day, ranging from 24 to 92 units. As can be noted, there was a steady increase in glycaemia, not only in the fasting, but also in the postmeal blood glucose levels during the first 12 months of CAPD.

As already stated, the monitoring of the blood glucose levels was quite irregularly performed by the patient's general practioner or by the outpatient clinic at 3 months interval.

No change in the frequency of using the more concentrated glucose solutions over 1 year was noted. No follow-up data on serum glycosylated haemoglobin are available. Symptomatic hypoglycaemia occurred in two patients but no hospital admission was required because of this complication.

Table 4 gives a summary of the evolution of the visual function and status of peripheral neuropathy in the CAPD patients.

Table 4 Evolution of visual function (A) and peripheral neuropathy (B)

	Months	
	0	*6–12*
A. *Visual acuity*		
Number of eyes (*n*)	34	18
10/100	13 (38%)	10 (55%)
10–50/100	10 (30%)	6 (33%)
50–100/100	11 (32%)	2 (11%)
B. *Peripheral nerve conduction (m/s)*		
n	18	8
Mean of all patients	32.2 ± 2.46	22.4 ± 6.1
Paired observations (*n*)	27.3 ± 5.7(7)	20.8 ± 6.2(7)

mean ± SD

In the seven patients whose visual acuity was assessed both at the start and after 12 months, the visual status did not change in four of them, but deteriorated in three patients. The deterioration was due to aggravation of the diabetic retinopathy in two patients and to severe intravitreous haemorrhage, despite acceptable blood pressure control, in a third patient. When combined with the results obtained in two additional patients at 6 months, an overall deterioration in visual acuity was observed.

The mean value for nerve conduction velocity in 18 patients at the start of CAPD was 32.2 ± 2.4 m/s. In the seven patients who could be tested before and after 1 year of CAPD the nerve conduction deteriorated in four, improved in one and remained stable in two. The mean values in these seven patients were 27.3 ± 5.7 and 20.8 ± 6.2 m/s, respectively.

Despite the presence of severe peripheral vascular disease with pregangrene in three patients, only three amputations, two of a lower limb in one patient and one foot in another man were performed.

PERITONITIS AND OTHER INFECTIOUS COMPLICATIONS

The overall incidence of peritonitis was 13 episodes over 139 patient months, occurring in 9 of the 19 patients (one episode every 10.7 patient months). In the overall CAPD programme, this incidence is one episode every 13 patient months. The risk of a first episode of peritonitis by the end of the first year of CAPD was 54.5% in the diabetics.

Eleven episodes yielded a pathogen: *Staph. Aureus* in three, *Staph. Epidermidis* in five, *Corynebacterium* in two and *E. Coli* in one episode. Aseptic peritonitis occurred in two episodes. All episodes of peritonitis were treated in the hospital with intraperitoneal administration of antibiotics.

Skin catheter exit infections with *Staphylococcus Aureus* were noted in three patients, leading to peritonitis in two patients.

Other infectious complications noted were an ischiorectal abcess following peritonitis in one patient, an acute pyelonephritis requiring nephrectomy in an other patient, while two cases of severe bronchopneumonia were additionally observed.

GENERAL OUTCOME

The actuarial patient and technique survival rates were calculated by the Life Table Method and are depicted in Figure 1. The results are compared with the overall results obtained in 85 non-diabetic patients treated with CAPD over the same time interval.

In the diabetic, a patient survival of 64% at 12 months and of 43% at 15 months is noted. This is in sharp contrast with the survival rates of 81% at 12 months in the non-diabetic CAPD population. In the latter, a similar patient survival of 64% is obtained after 4 years of CAPD. After 1 year only 41% of the diabetic patients were continuing CAPD in contrast with 65% of the non-diabetics, who are maintained in the programme at the same time.

The reasons for drop out in the diabetics are death in six patients and transfer to haemodialysis in four, and to intermittent peritoneal dialysis in one patient. Three patients died from acute myocardial infarction, two from a severe cerebrovascular bleeding and one from acute pulmonary oedema.

Two young patient were transferred to haemodialysis in view of a planned pancreas and kidney transplantation; one because of recurrent peritonitis and

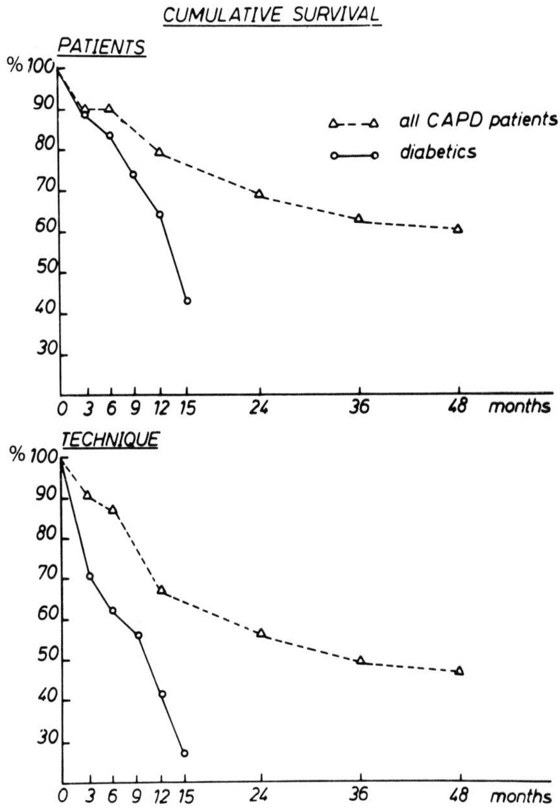

Figure 1 Actuarial patient and technique survival in 19 diabetic patients, compared to 85 non-diabetics, treated with CAPD

one because of protracted vomiting. The latter two patients and the one patient transferred to intermittent peritoneal dialysis subsequently died within a mean period of 5 months after drop out from CAPD.

The mean training time for CAPD in the diabetics was 25 ± 2.7 days/patient. The overall hospitalization rate was 63 ± 10 days per patient year. This is two times higher than the hospitalization rate in the overall CAPD programme.

DISCUSSION

Theoretically, CAPD offers several advantages over other therapeutic strategies in diabetic end-stage nephropathy. The most important are a better control of blood pressure, a more stable cardiovascular status with avoidance of the wide fluctuations in plasma- and extracellular fluid volume associated with intermittent haemo- or peritoneal dialysis, and not least, improvement in the glucose homeostasis due to the steady and continuous transperitoneal absorption of glucose and intraperitoneally administered insulin.

Many of these advantages seemed to be realized in two major CAPD programmes which recently described their short-term (2 year) experience in diabetic patients[4,5]. Unfortunately, our own experience does not seem to confirm these excellent results. Our patient survival dropped to 65% and the rate of continuation of CAPD to 40% after 1 year. These results are in marked contrast with our overall results obtained with the same mode of dialysis in the non-diabetic patients. In the latter, the 1 year patient and technique survivals in our three centres vary between 80 and 93% and 68 and 89%, respectively.

Although it is always difficult to compare directly different groups of patients, the obvious question arises why our experience is less favourable than the experience of others.

It must be stressed that no selection policy was followed and that all diabetic uraemic patients, except for three, were treated with CAPD as a first choice.

The presence of severe cardiovascular and peripheral vascular disease before CAPD in the large majority of our patients partially explains the relatively high mortality rate. All six deaths observed in this study were directly due to either myocardial infarction or to cerebrovascular catastrophes.

However, this alone cannot account for our unfavourable results, since in the two other reported series similar cardiovascular problems were encountered[4,5].

The most important factor explaining the divergent results is, in our opinion, the inadequate control of blood glucose homeostasis in our CAPD patients over time. The observed deterioration in visual acuity and nerve conduction velocity are probably directly related to the poor control of the diabetic state.

This is reflected by the progressive increase in daily blood glucose levels over the studied time interval. As has been stated before, blood glucose control was left to the policlinical check-up or to the family physician. Until now, the great majority of our diabetic patients (16 out of 19) could not be motivated to learn self-monitoring of their diabetes. Moreover, many elderly patients refused more frequent daily glucose profile determinations even at the monthly outpatient consultation. The collaboration with the family physicians was highly variable, and is in our experience not sufficiently reliable to provide adequate blood glucose monitoring.

On the other hand, it is also clear from our experience that by itself CAPD can easily be performed and is an adequate alternative dialysis technique in diabetics, provided the complications directly related to poor diabetes control can be prevented.

Problems directly related to the CAPD technique were not more frequent than in the non-diabetic patient population of a similar age.

The ultrafiltration and clearing capacity of the peritoneum remained unaltered at least over 1 year, and reasonable control of the uraemic biochemical parameters and of hypertension can be achieved. However, we have observed a steady increase in the triglyceride levels, and longterm consequences of this hypertriglyceridaemia on the cardiovascular system need to be assessed.

In contrast to other reports[4,5], the incidence of peritonitis was slighly higher than in the non-diabetic CAPD patients although the number of treated diabetic patients is too small to make any firm statement on this aspect.

In conclusion, based on these preliminary results in a relatively small number of patients, we wonder whether it would not be better to restrict CAPD therapy in diabetics only to those patients who are willing to be admitted in a diabetic self-care programme. It could also be recommended that the training for diabetic self-care should be started as soon as possible in the foliow-up of the diabetic nephropathy, and before the CAPD treatment has to start. This should eliminate at least one of the numerous medicotechnical and psychological problems present at the beginning of a CAPD treatment in the diabetics. For the other patients, not able to perform diabetic self-control, hospital haemodialysis creates, at least three times a week, the opportunity to follow more accurately their diabetic status.

References

1. Kjellstrand, C., Comty, C. and Shapiro, F. (1982). A comparison of dialysis and transplantation in insulin-dependent diabetic patients. In Friedman, E. A. and L'Esperance R. (eds.). *Diabetic Renal-Retinal Syndrome*, Vol. 2, pp. 405–417, (New York: Grune and Sratton)
2. Najarian, J.S., Sutherland, D.E.R., Simmons, R.L., Howard, R., Kjellstrand, C., Ramsay, R., Goetz, F., Fryd, D. and Sommer, B. (1979). Ten year experience with renal transplantation in juvenile onset diabetics. *Ann. Surg.*, **190**, 487
3. McCrary, R.F., Pitts, T.O. and Puschett, J.B. (1981). Diabetic nephropathy: natural couıse, survivorship and therapy. *Am. J. Nephrol.*, **1**, 206
4. Amair, P., Khanna, R., Leibel, B., Pierratos, A., Vas,S., Meema, E., Blair, G., Chisolm, L., Vas, M., Zingg, W., Digenis, G. and Oreopoulos, D. (1981). Continuous ambulatory peritoneal dialysis in diabetics with end-stage renal disease. *N. Engl. J. Med.*, **306**, 625
5. Rottembourg, J., Shahatel, Y., Agrafoitis, A., Thuillier, Y., De Groc, F., Jacobs, C. and Legrain, M. (1983). Continuous ambulatory peritoneal dialysis in insulin-dependent diabetic patients: a 40-month experience. *Kidney Int.*, **23**, 40
6. Dratwa, M., Tielemans, C., Smet, L., Gouttenegre, M.J., Kinnaert, P., Anthonis, D., Vereerstraeten, P. and Toussaint, C. (1980). Infectious complications and therapy in continuous ambulatory peritoneal dialysis (CAPD). In Lameire, N. and Ringoir, S. (eds.). *Proceedings 1st Benelux Symposium on CAPD.* pp. 34–44
7. Lameire, N.H., De Paepe, M., Vanholder, R., Verbanck, J. and Ringoir, S. (1981). Experience with CAPD in Belgium. *Perit. Dialys. Bull.*, **1**, 54

19.3
Experience with glycerol as the osmotic agent in peritoneal dialysis in diabetic and non-diabetic patients

M. DE PAEPE, E. MATTHIJS, F. PELUSO, R. DOLKART and N. LAMEIRE

INTRODUCTION

In peritoneal dialysis, the removal of excess water from the patient occurs through a process of transperitoneal ultrafiltration, by the creation of an osmotic pressure gradient. This function is achieved by adding a solute to the dialysate at adequate concentrations. Currently, the most widely used osmotic agent is glucose. The disadvantages of the use of glucose have been previously summarized[1]. The most important ones are: first, the diffusion of the intra-peritoneally injected glucose into the blood, challenging the CAPD patient with a considerable caloric load and leading to obesity and hyperlipidaemia; second, due to the heat sterilization, the glucose solutions must be acidified to prevent caramelizing the sugar. The low dialysate pH may alter and irritate the peritoneal membrane. Therefore, the search for alternative osmotic agents has led to the testing of dextran, xylitol, fructose, sorbitol and amino acid mixtures[1]. Several of these agents have been subsequently abandoned for either toxic or practical reasons. Among the small molecules that are available for substituting glucose as the osmotic agent in peritoneal dialysis, glycerol presents some advantages: first, it does not require insulin for its metabolization[2], which could make it particularly suitable in diabetic patients; second, based on theoretical calculations by the manufacturer (Travenol), the caloric load for a similar ultrafiltration could be 30% lower than with corresponding glucose solutions and third, the pH of the glycerol dialysate is substantially higher than the glucose solutions.

The present paper describes our clinical experience with a peritoneal dialysate, containing different concentrations of glycerol.

In the first part of the study, the peritoneal clearances, ultrafiltration capacity and blood and dialysate glycerol kinetics were acutely studied over a single dwell time and compared with a glucose dialysate.

In a second part, the more chronic effects of the glycerol dialysate were studied over a 1 year period in five non-diabetic and five diabetic patients.

METHODS AND MATERIALS

Three different glycerol or glucose concentrations were used: the glycerol concentrations were 0.85% (712–1), 1.40% (712–2) and 2.50%, (712–3) while the glucose solutions were 1.36%, 2.27% and 3.86% Dianeal solutions. The glycerol concentrations were chosen not on equimolar base, but on the basis of a theoretically equivalent ultrafiltration capacity.

The protocol for the acute study is outlined in Table 1. Six stable CAPD patients were hospitalized for 2 weeks in the Division of Nephrology of the University Hospital. During the first week, they continued the CAPD treatment with different concentrations of glucose dialysates; during the second week they were dialysed with different glycerol solutions.

Table 1 Acute tolerance study with glycerol (CAPD)

Protocol	: 6 stable CAPD patients, female
First week	: Glucose dialysate 3 or 4 dwells studied (biochemistry, ultrafiltration)
Second week	: Glycerol dialysate 3 or 4 dwells studied (biochemistry, ultrafiltration)
Comparison of	1.36% glucose to 0.85% glycerol 2.27% glucose to 1.4% glycerol 3.86% glucose to 2.5% glycerol

(chosen not on equimolar base but on 'equi-uf' base)

On a test day, the peritoneal ultrafiltration capacity was measured in the morning. For that purpose, the peritoneal dilution of autologous hacmoglobin was used as a volume marker. This method has been recently described by Canaud *et al*[3]. Experimental work in rabbits and patients has shown that haemoglobin is a useful and reliable volume marker when compared to albumin and dextran blue, provided the necessary corrections for recovery are made (De Paepe, M. *et al*, unpublished results).

In the afternoon, a second dwell was used for chemical analysis of dialysate and plasma.

For the analysis of the chronic effects, five non-diabetic patients, previously studied in the acute protocol, were placed continuously on four exchanges per day with glycerol-dialysate. In addition, five insulin-dependent diabetic patients were transferred from the usual CAPD protocol with glucose to a longterm study with glycerol dialysate. All patients were admitted on the renal ward and the glucose dialysate was progressively replaced by glycerol dialysate under careful clinical and biological monitoring. The concentrations of both solutes were selected on the basis of the individual ultrafiltration need.

For calculation of the transperitoneal energy uptake, the drained bags of 24 hours were collected and the glucose, respectively glycerol, concentrations were determined. These studies were performed in six patients who were on a stable schedule of exchanges with the respective dialysates. The energy-containing osmotic agents transferred across the peritoneum were calculated according to the following numerical factors: 1 g D glucose = 16.6 kJ, 1 g glycerol = 18.06 kJ[4].

All patients gave their informed consent for this study after careful explanation of its experimental nature. All results are represented as Mean ± SEM. For statistical analysis, paired and unpaired Wilcoxon tests were performed, and significance was accepted at $p < 0.05$ level.

RESULTS

Acute studies

Figure 1 depicts the evolution of dialysate to plasma mean concentration ratios of ureum and creatinine with the glycerol 2.5% and glucose 3.86% solution

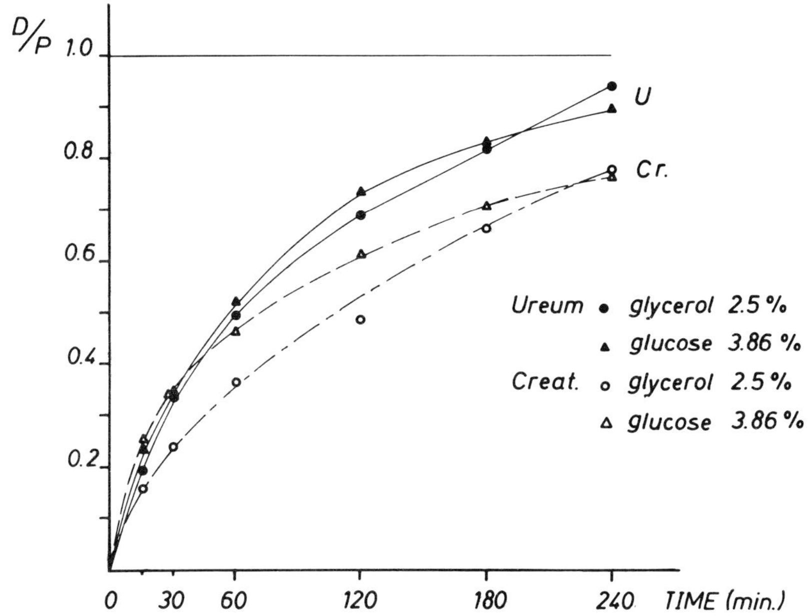

Figure 1 Evolution of dialysate to plasma ureum and creatinine ratios during a 4 h dwell time with glycerol 2.5% and glucose 3.86% dialysate (means ± SEM)

during one single 4 hour dwell in five patients. No difference in these ratios between the two different dialysate solutions was detected. Qualitatively similar results were obtained with the lower concentrations of each solute.

Figure 2 depicts the change in dialysate osmolality observed with the same solutions as in Figure 1. Up to 2 hours the dialysate osmolality remains statistically higher with the glycerol than with the glucose dialysate. The plasma osmolality did not change significantly with either solution, so that, at least during the first 2 hours of the dwell, a greater transperitoneal osmotic gradient existed during the glycerol exchange.

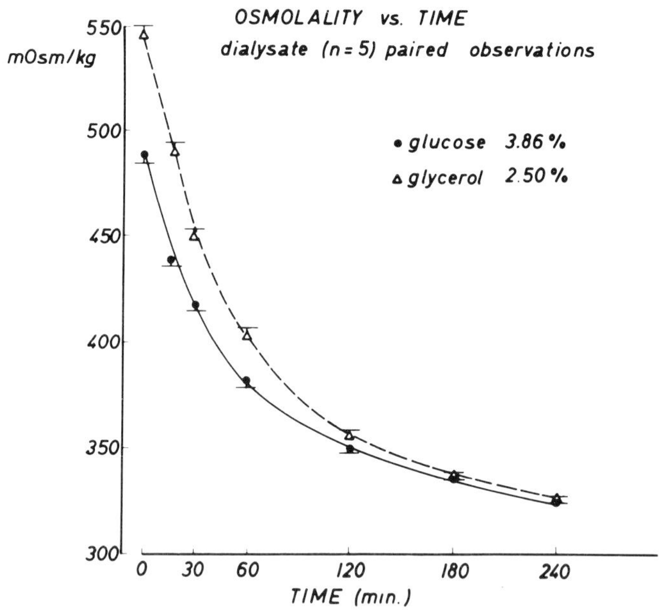

Figure 2 Changes in dialysate osmolalities (same solutions as in Figure 1)

The change in dialysate volume profile during a single 4 hour dwell with the two highest solute concentrations measured by the haemoglobin dilution technique, is depicted in Figure 3. It is clear that the volume profile with glycerol was consistently lower over the whole dwell time, except for the first 30 minutes. Again, qualitatively similar results were obtained with the two lower solute concentrations.

Table 2 summarizes the end-volumes obtained with the different solutions in seven paired studies. It is important to note that the mean volumes after a 4 h exchange were systematically lower when a given glycerol solution was compared with the corresponding glucose dialysate.

Figure 4 depicts the changes in dialysate concentrations of both solutes with the 2.5% glycerol and 3.86% glucose, respectively. Despite a more rapid fall in

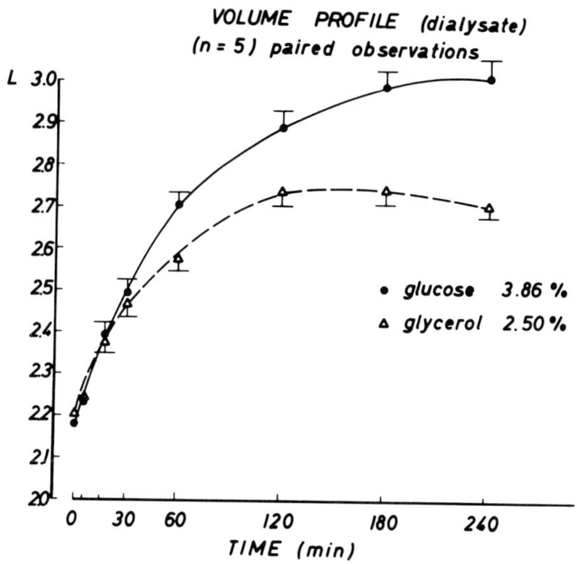

Figure 3 Changes in dialysate volume as measured by the autologous haemoglobin dilution technique, corrected for recovery (same solutions as in Figure 1)

glycerol than in glucose levels during the first 60 minutes, the glycerol concentrations over the first 60–90 minutes remain statistically higher than the glucose concentrations; it takes approximately 3–4 hours before equal osmolar concentrations are achieved.

Table 2 Volumes** (ml) (means ± SEM) after 4 h dwell, paired observations ($n = 7$)

Glucose	*Glycerol*
1.36% 2333 ± 43	0.85% 2119 ± 51*
2.27% 2574 ± 63	1.4% 2291 ± 27*
3.86% 3038 ± 70	2.5% 2729 ± 56*

* $p < 0.05$
** corrected Hb dilution curve

Figure 5 illustrates the blood glycerol levels obtained during dialysis with the three available glycerol concentrations in five acute, 4–8 hour exchanges. Where the blood glycerol level in the normal individual is around 0.1 mmol/l, substantial increases were noted, especially when the 2.5% glycerol solution

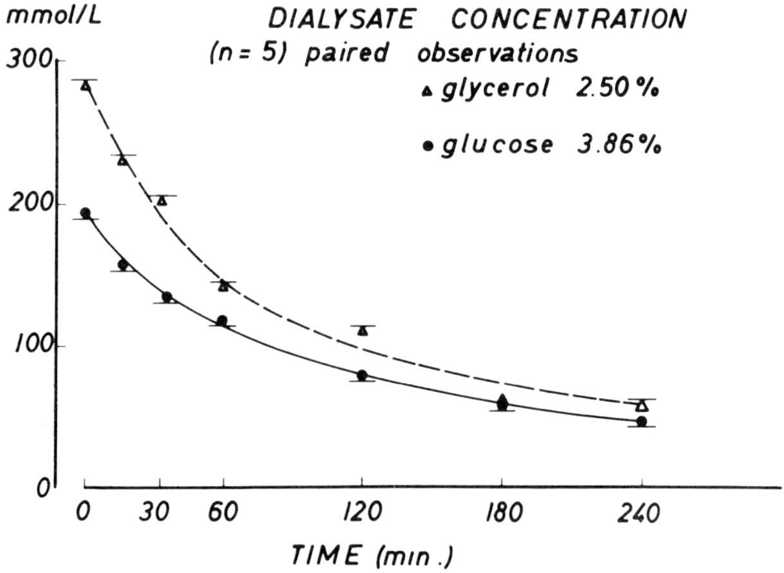

Figure 4 Changes in dialysate concentrations of glycerol and glucose (mmol/l) (same solutions as in Figure 1)

was used. In the latter situation, the mean peak blood glycerol level of 5.3 mmol/l was achieved after 4 hours of instillation and then gradually decreased, but did not normalize, after 8 hours of dwell time.

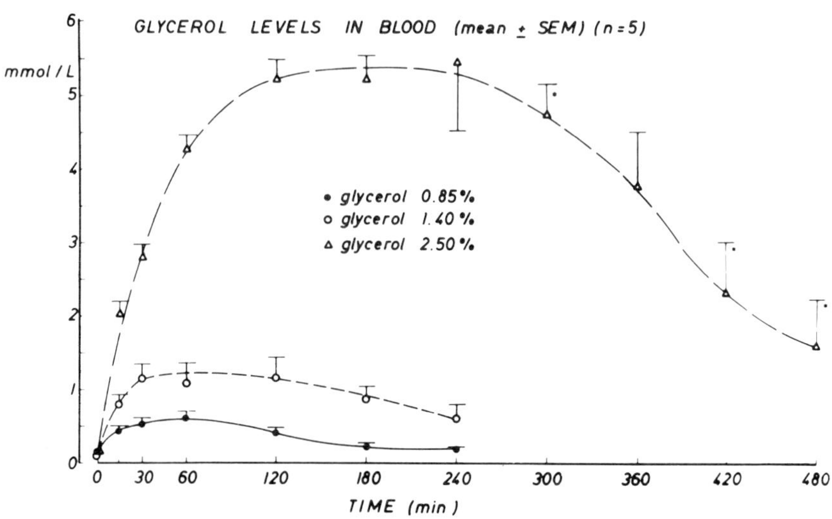

Figure 5 Evolution of blood glycerol levels (mmol/l) studied with the three available glycerol solutions over a 4–8 h exchange

The blood glucose levels achieved during a 4 hour acute exchange with the two most concentrated glycerol and glucose dialysates are shown in Figure 6. In contrast with the marked hyperglycaemia noted under glucose dialysis, no significant change in blood glucose level occurred during glycerol dialysis.

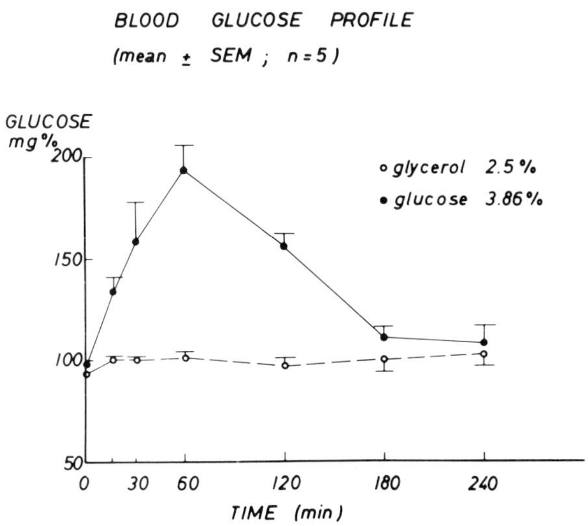

Figure 6 Changes in blood glucose levels (mg/dl) with glucose 3.86% and glycerol 2.5% during a 4 h exchange

In summary, the acute studies revealed:

(1) Glycerol peritoneal dialysis was clinically well tolerated, and no biochemical abnormalities were observed.

(2) The blood glucose levels did not increase with the glycerol dialysate which was in marked contrast with the results observed with glucose dialysis.

(3) At the proposed concentrations, glycerol seemed to be a less effective osmotic agent compared to glucose.

(4) The peritoneal transport of urea and creatinine was not different between glycerol or glucose dialysate.

Chronic studies

Ten patients were on CAPD with glycerol dialysate for a total of 81 patient months and four were followed for as long as 12 months. The glycerol dialysis was clinically well tolerated and there were certainly no more subjective complaints when compared to the patient's experience with glucose. No changes in blood pressure or intake in antihypertensive medication were noted.

Table 3 summarizes the changes in body weight, and the evolution of the

Table 3 Evolution of body weight and most relevant biochemical data (mean ± SEM)

	Months				
	0 n = 10	*2* n = 7	*6* n = 7	*9* n = 7	*12* n = 4
Body weight (kg)	66.5 ± 3.7	66.8 ± 3.8	69.5 ± 4.2	70 ± 4.2	68.9 ± 3.8
Urea mg/dl	150 ± 16	126 ± 23	121 ± 22	124 ± 25	128 ± 32
Creatinine mg/dl	9.50 ± 0.64	9.90 ± 0.93	9.91 ± 1.50	9.80 ± 1.32	10.7 ± 1.14
Uric acid mg/dl	6.67 ± 0.47	7.0 ± 0.50	—	6.3 ± 0.25	7.7 ± 1.20
Sodium mmol/l	137 ± 1.50	138 ± 1.35	139 ± 1.4	139 ± 1.3	142 ± 0.29
Potassium mmol/l	5.21 ± 0.30	5.0 ± 0.35	4.67 ± 0.15	4.47 ± 0.21	4.40 ± 0.32
Bicarbonate mmol/l	23 ± 1.33	22.2 ± 0.9	22.3 ± 1.13	22.6 ± 0.98	22 ± 1.20
Lactate mmol/l	0.95 ± 0.17	0.74 ± 0.09	0.96 ± 1.13	1.20 ± 0.98	1.39 ± 0.49
Phosphate mg/dl	4.78 ± 0.60	5.02 ± 0.64	5.13 ± 0.39	5.11 ± 0.46	5.92 ± 0.44
Haematocrit %	32 ± 1.7	31 ± 1.9	32.5 ± 1.2	32.4 ± 1.4	36.8 ± 2.9
Tot. protein g/dl	6.66 ± 0.21	6.89 ± 0.37	6.98 ± 0.37	6.50 ± 0.34	6.97 ± 0.56
Alk. phosphatase U/l (96–272)	377.5 ± 64.6	338 ± 103	—	426 ± 110	340 ± 110
Cholesterol mg/dl	265 ± 25	284 ± 33	298** ± 31	—	296** ± 17.5
Blood glycerol§ mmol/l	0.10 ± 0.004	5.90** ± 1.50	7.17** ± 1.55	—	7.47** ± 3.12
Osmolality§ mosmol/kg	310 ± 4.10	313 ± 3.12	309 ± 2.41	310 ± 4.7	319 ± 7.8
Blood glucose*§ mg/dl	86 ± 1.9	97** ± 9.4	—	97** ± 1.0	94** ± 2.3

* in 5 non-diabetics only
** $p < 0.05$, compared to start values
§ peak values 1–2 h after instillation

most relevant biological data over 12 months. The mean body weight at the start of glycerol therapy was 66.5 ± 3.7 kg, and a tendency for slight increase was noted at 9 months. In the four patients followed for 12 months the body weight at start was 67.2 ± 3.9 kg and was 68.9 ± 3.3 kg after 1 year ($p > 0.05$).

Stable values for blood urea, serum creatinine and the major serum electrolytes were noted. No significant accumulation of either uric acid or lactate was observed.

Serum phosphate concentrations remained unchanged and there was no need for change in the intake of phosphate binders.

Haemotocrit values did not change during the glycerol dialysis; the higher mean value of 36.8 ± 2.9% at 12 months was not statistically different from the initial value, due to the limited number of observations.

Total protein concentration and values for alkaline phosphatases were not altered. Other liver parameters, such as transaminases (not shown) did not change.

Correct interpretation of the routine analysis of blood triglyceride levels is impossible because of the falsely elevated values due to the presence of glycerol in the blood. All lipid analysis will further be carried out, using the more sophisticated techniques by Malmendier and co-workers (University of Brussels). Preliminary results show that glycerol dialysis does not induce hypertriglyceridaemia by itself and does not modify the levels of apoprotein B (Malmendier, personal communication). However, definite statements on this important issue cannot yet be made.

The cholesterol levels moderately increase from 265 ± 25 to 296 ± 17.5% mg/dl ($p<0,05$).

For correct interpretation of the non-fasting blood glucose, glycerol and blood osmolality values, it should be stressed that the blood samples were taken in the outpatient department, approximately 1–2 h after instillation of a fresh morning bag. Thus, they represent more or less peak values during one single dwell. Only the blood glucose levels of the five non-diabetic patients are included in Table 3. A small but significant increase in glycaemia was already noted after 2 months of glycerol dialysis. No dramatic increase in blood osmolality was found, although occasionally a value of 330 mosmol/kg was observed correlating with high blood glycerol levels.

Concerning the latter, a mean peak serum glycerol level of 7.47 ± 3.12 mmol/l was found ranging from 1.91 to 16.3 mmol/l in the four patients at 12 months. The values obtained at 2, 6 and 9 months were not statistically different from each other. No change in serum LDH and haptoglobin levels were noted over the whole follow-up period (not shown).

The effect of glycerol dialysis on glucose homeostasis, level of glycosylated haemoglobin, daily dose of intraperitoneal insulin, body weight and types of dialysate used in the 45 year old diabetic with the longest follow-up is shown in Table 4. The daily 24 hour blood glucose profiles the last 3 months on glucose dialysate were certainly far from ideal, as can be judged from both the high

Table 4 Evolution of blood glucose and fasting haemoglobin levels, need of insulin, body weight and types of dialysate in a diabetic patient.

	Blood glucose (mg/dl)				$HgbA_{1c}$	*i.p. Insulin*	*Body weight*	*Dialysate*
Months	7 h	10 h	16 h	20 h	(%)	(U/day)	(kg)	
−3	480	430	390	250	13.6	58	59	4 × 1.36
−2	200	380	350	220	—	54	57.5	2 × 1.36, 2 × 3.86
−1	310	300	160	100	—	56	59	2 × 1.36, 2 × 3.86
+1	320	310	250	300	11.6	30	59	3 × 1.4, 1 × 2.5
+2	230	150	100	130	—	50	60	2 × 1.4, 2 × 2.5
+3	110	70	60	140	8.4	62	60	2 × 1.4, 2 × 2.5
+6	130	140	150	270	8.7	67	61	2 × 1.4, 2 × 2.5
+9	140	170	230	270	8.9	60	63	3 × 2.5, 1 × 1.4

−: months on glucose
+: months on glycerol

blood glucose and elevated $HgbA_{1c}$ levels. For maintaining a relatively stable weight, more concentrated glucose solutions were used during the last 2 months on glucose dialysate and despite this, the amount of insulin was not adequately adapted on the outpatient control visit. In the first month on glycerol dialysis, the body weight remained stable with the use of three bags of 1.4% and 1 bag of 2.5% of glycerol. The blood glucose profile and $HgbA_{1c}$ level were not markedly different from the results noted under glucose dialysis, but were obtained with a drastic reduction in the amount of intraperitoneal insulin. Better glucose profiles and a sustained decrease in $HgbA_{1c}$ level were noted from the 3rd till the 9th month on glycerol when the amount of insulin was increased to 60–67 U/day. At 9 months, two bags of 2.5% glycerol were used to maintain ultrafiltration, and no oedema or hypertension developed. 'Dry' body weight increased by 4 kg over 9 months. Qualitatively similar results were obtained in the four other diabetic patients treated with glycerol dialysis. After an initial drop in the needs for insulin, an increase was necessary after 2–3 months but with better control of glucose homeostasis, at least over the short time interval that they were followed.

Table 5 summarizes the data on calculated daily energy uptakes in six paired observations with glucose and glycerol dialysis, respectively. The mean values were 2058 ± 190 kJ with glucose and 2294 ± 281 kJ/day with glycerol. This corresponded with a daily absorption of a mean of 124 ± 11 g of glucose and of

Table 5 Energy uptake (kJ/day) and daily amounts of transperitoneal solute absorption (paired observations)

	Glucose		*Glycerol*	
Patient	*Absorbed* g/day	*Energy* kJ/day	*Absorbed* g/day	*Energy* kJ/day
1	125	2076[1]	86	1544[a]
2	141	2335[2]	169	3050[b]
3	136	2259[3]	160	2887[c]
4	71	1179[4]	84	1523[d]
5	150	2496[3]	153	2749[b]
6	120	2000[3]	112	2013[e]
$\bar{m}$	124 ± 11	2058 ± 190	127 ± 16	2294 ± 128
				2126* ± 276

* corrected value

means ± SEM

Exchanges per day glucose: 1 = 2 × 2.27, 1 × 3.86; 2 = 3 × 2.27, 1 × 3.86; 3 = 3 × 1.36, 1 × 3.86; 4 = 4 × 1.36

glycerol: a = 2 × 1.40, 1 × 2.5; b = 4 × 2.5; c = 3 × 2.5, 1 × 1.4; d = 4 × 1.4; e = 3 × 1.4, 1 × 2.5

127 ± 16 g of glycerol. However, due to the loss of glucose into the glycerol dialysate (mean of 11.7 g/day) the net energy uptake for the glycerol dialysate can be calculated by subtracting this loss of 'glucose-energy' from the total amount absorbed. After correction, the mean energy uptake for the glycerol dialysate became 2126 ± 276 kJ, which is only 3% higher than with glucose dialysate; a value not statistically different. For comparison, the main daily caloric intake with the glucose dialysate was 491 ± 45 kcal and for glycerol 508 ± 66 kcal, after correction.

DISCUSSION

In a recent editorial[1], Wu nicely summarized the advantages and disadvantages of glucose as an osmotic agent in chronic peritoneal dialysis.

As the first important drawback, he mentioned the low pH of the dialysate with possible negative influence on peritoneal irritation and inhibition of polymorphonuclear phagocytosis and intracellular killing of bacteria. Another negative point is the high caloric load due to the glucose absorption, exposing the patient to hyperinsulinaemia, obesity and hyperlipidaemia.

Although the continuous and more or less constant daily absorption of glucose may theoretically facilitate the blood glucose regulation in the dialysed diabetic patient, at least our experience[5] indicates that without careful monitoring the blood glucose, in practice, glucose homeostasis in diabetic CAPD patients is far from ideally maintained. It is therefore no surprise, that quite a number of other osmotic agents have been tested as a replacement for glucose in peritoneal dialysis[1]. Many of them have been abandoned for practical reasons or for toxic side effects[1].

Actually, only amino acid mixtures[6] and xylitol[7] have been used in CAPD patients. Amino acids have many advantages, but so far no chronic experience in CAPD is available. The high cost and the presence of high chloride concentrations in many of the amino acid solutions will limit their widespread use in the near future.

Bazzato and co-workers have used xylitol, an aliphatic polyalcohol in four diabetic CAPD patients for 6 months[7]. As major advantages they noted a lower need for insulin, a better control of the diabetes, a lowering of the cholesterol and triglyceride levels and a return toward normal levels of HDL cholesterol. However, an increase in plasma uric acid and lactic acid levels was observed, and clinical side effects occurred with deterioration of liver function when the total daily amount of xylitol absorption was greater than 150 g/day. From the concentrations of xylitol used (1.5 and 3.0%), it can be derived that it will be difficult to remain below this maximum in many patients.

In the present study, glycerol, a naturally occurring trivalent alcohol with a molecular weight of 92.09, was evaluated as an osmotic agent for peritoneal dialysis in both acute and chronic clinical investigations. Although a greater osmotic potential may be expected from a small molecule like glycerol, its more rapid removal from the peritoneal cavity may partly or completely overcome this advantage. Our results indeed confirm this hypothesis. In the acute experiments it was found that a much lower ultrafiltration was achieved with glycerol, compared to glucose, despite its concentration being chosen on a 'equi-ultrafiltration' capacity basis. The latter was derived from theoretical kinetic modelling and from experimental data obtained in the dog (Travenol Laboratories, unpublished observations).

The lower ultrafiltration obtained with glycerol, in the presence of a longer preserved favourable transperitoneal osmotic gradient may be due to a lower reflection coefficient of glycerol, although a direct effect on peritoneal permeability by glycerol cannot be excluded. We are now in the process of analysing the mass transfer coefficients for both glucose and glycerol obtained during the acute exchanges to look for a possible explanation for this phenomenon.

To further evaluate the results of the acute experiments, a chronic clinical study was designed in a group of ten stable CAPD patients.

Since the acute studies revealed that the blood glucose levels did not change with the glycerol dialysate, five diabetic patients were included in the chronic study, with the hope that glycerol would facilitate their glucose homeostasis at a reduced need for insulin.

At first, chronic use of the glycerol dialysate was clinically well tolerated and no subjective or objective side effects could be directly attributed to the presence of glycerol in the blood. The peak blood glycerol levels remained at a relatively stable value for 1 year follow-up, but this value was highly variable from patient to patient, ranging from 1.91 to 16.3 mmol/l. No signs of haemolysis were seen, and the frequently monitored serum levels of LDH and haptoglobin remained unaltered; in addition, an increase in haemotocrit was noted in the four patients after 1 year. As has been previously shown by us, the high haematocrit during the second year of CAPD is the reflection of an improvement in red cell mass and decreased circulating plasma volume[8].

The amount of glycerol absorbed per day varied from 83 to 169 grams with a mean of 127 grams in six patients, corresponding to a mean of 88 mg/min or approximately 1–1.5 mg kg^{-1} min^{-1}. Based on an extensive review by Frank *et al*[2], no haemolysis must be feared when an infusion with glycerol at a rate equal or less than 6 mg kg^{-1} min^{-1} is given. As a matter of fact, rates as high as 33 mg kg^{-1} min^{-1} have been safely administered for several days. Other biological parameters that were followed in our patients to monitor safety such as uric acid, lactic acid and liver enzymes all remained within normal limits.

A remarkable finding in the diabetic patients was indeed the appearance of a lower need for insulin in the first months; however, after 3–4 months this increased again toward the insulin need observed with glucose dialysate. It cannot be denied that the regulation of the diabetes was easier in these patients with achievement of lower blood glucose and better blood levels of glycosylated haemoglobin. It should be remarked here that the absolute value of glycosylated haemoglobin in the uraemic patient should be interpreted with caution[4], although in a stable uraemic situation as under CAPD treatment, a lowering of $HgbA_{1c}$ under therapy probably reflects a better glycaemia control.

An eventual additional advantage of the use of the glycerol solution in diabetics, not yet clinically explored, is the possibility of closely monitoring the diabetic state based on the analysis of the dialysate glucose level in the drained volume. A preliminary analysis of the available data, comparing the simultaneously measured dialysate and blood glucose levels in three diabetic patients, indicated a reasonable correlation between these two parameters. However, further careful studies are needed in a greater number of patients before glucose levels in glycerol dialysate can be used in addition to glucose determinations in the self-monitoring of glucose homeostasis in the diabetic CAPD patient.

The most important reason for introducing glycerol as a substitute for glucose was the hope that a major reduction in caloric load could be realized. Based on the initial theoretical analysis, a reduction in caloric load of 30% was anticipated for the same ultrafiltration rate.

Unfortunately, due to the lower ultrafiltration capacity of the glycerol solutions, the more concentrated dialysate had to be used, resulting in a complete disappearance of the caloric advantage. In fact, when the trans-peritoneal energy uptakes for both glucose and glycerol were calculated, no difference existed in the amount of kilojoules absorbed.

The results on energy uptake obtained with glucose were highly comparable with the data obtained by Von Baeyer *et al* in a greater number of patients[9]. Thus, although the present glycerol dialysates offer no caloric advantage, they certainly do not expose the patient to a greater caloric burden than the glucose dialysates, currently used in the CAPD technique.

Preliminary analysis of the blood lipids in the glycerol treated patients reveal that, by itself, glycerol does not induce more hypertriglyceridaemia than glucose. Two remarks concerning this problem should be made: first, routine analysis of the blood triglycerides cannot be performed due to the concomitant measurement of the glycerol present in the serum; second, in patients with already elevated triglyceride levels when starting glycerol dialysis, the tendency to develop further hypertriglyceridaemia is not prevented. As already previously pointed out by us, the same observation can be made with glucose dialysate[10].

In conclusion, although the most important expectation, i.e. providing a lower caloric load with glycerol containing dialysate was not fulfilled, we believe that its use in CAPD presents some advantages, especially in the diabetic patient. An easier control of the blood glucose levels and the additional help in monitoring the diabetic state by analysis of the dialysate glucose concentration are positive points. The latter is certainly worthwhile to explore further in the future.

The clinical tolerance of the glycerol dialysate is excellent and can possibly be explained by its higher pH.

The final confirmation of these, until now preliminary, observations must await further study.

ACKNOWLEDGEMENTS

The technical expertise of Mrs C. Lambert, D. Vijt, N. De Ruyck, A. Hutse and M. Van Landschoot has been greatly appreciated.

We thank Mrs I. Verslycken, Mrs L. De Torck and Miss C. Van Den Berghe for their secretarial assistance.

References

1. Wu, G. (1982). Osmotic agents for peritoneal dialysis solutions. *Perit. Dial. Bull.,* **2,** 151
2. Frank, M.S.B., Nahata, M.C. and Hilty, M.D. (1981). Glycerol: a review of its pharmacology, pharmacokinetics, adverse reactions and clinical use. *Pharmacotherapy,* **1,** 147
3. Canaud, B., Liendo, C., Claret, G., Mion, H. and Mion, C. (1980). Etude 'in situ' de la cinétique de l'ultrafiltration en cours de dialyse péritonéale avec périodes de diffusion prolongée. *Néphrologie,* **1,** 126
4. Mayer, T.K. and Freedman, Z.R. (1983). Protein glycosylation in diabetes mellitus: a review of laboratory measurements and of their clinical utility. *Clin. Chim. Acta,* **127,** 147
5. Lameire, N., Dhaene, M., Matthijs, E., De Paepe, M., Vereerstraeten, P., Dratwa, M. and Ringoir, S. (1983). Experience with CAPD in diabetic patients. This volume, Chapter 19.2
6. Williams, P., Marliss, E.B., Anderson, G.H., Orea, A., Stein, A., Khanna, R., Petitt, J., Brandes, L., Rodella, H., Mupas, L., Dombros, N. and Oreopoulos, D. (1982). Amino acid absorption following intraperitoneal administration in CAPD patients. *Perit. Dial. Bull.,* **2,** 124
7. Bazzato, G., Coli, U., Landini, S., Fracasso, A., Morachiello, P., Righetto, F. and Scanferla, F. (1982). Xylitol and low dosages of insulin: new perspectives for diabetic uraemic patients on CAPD. *Perit. Dial. Bull.,* **2,** 161
8. De Paepe, M., Schelstraete, K., Ringoir, S. and Lameire, N. (1983). Influence of CAPD on the anemia of end-stage renal disease. *Kidney Int.,* **23,** 744
9. Von Baeyer, H., Gahl, G.M., Riedinger, H., Borowzak, R., Averdruk, R., Schurig, R. and Kessel, M. (1983). Adaptation of CAPD patients to the continuous peritoneal energy uptake. *Kidney Int.,* **23,** 29
10. Lameire, N. and Ringoir, S. (1980). An overview of peritonitis and other complications of continuous ambulatory peritoneal dialysis. In Legrain, M. (ed.). *Continuous Ambulatory Peritoneal Dialysis.* pp. 229–237. (Amsterdam: Excerpta Medica)

19.4
A year of experience of continuous ambulatory peritoneal dialysis (CAPD) in the diabetic and non-diabetic patient

F. CORONEL, P. NARANJO and D. PRATS

INTRODUCTION

In the register of the European Dialysis and Transplantation Association (EDTA) of 1980[1] of a total of 91 866 patients (dead and alive) in dialysis, only 2154 were diabetics (2.34% of the population in dialysis).

According to Ahlmen[2], the prevalence of secondary uraemia or uraemia associated with diabetics mellitus is 14% in Europe, and in USA[3] can reach 26%, the risk of renal disease in diabetics being 17 times higher than the rest of the population.

In Spain[4] there is a diabetic population of 56.81 patients per 100 000 inhabitants; according to the census of the same period there is a total of 20 889 patients. If the prevalence of diabetic nephropathy is like that of Europe, there are at least 2924 patients who must, in a short period of time, receive treatment substituting the renal function and/or renal transplant, excluding the annual increase of diabetics which is 38 patients per 100 000 inhabitants.

Between 1976 and 1980 we know that the total number of diabetic patients treated by dialysis in our country (111 = 1.54% of the total dialysis population)[5] is lower than the real need and the European average. In our hospital at present, the number of diabetic patients treated in dialysis represents 21.7% of the dialysed patients.

For us, interest in this type of patient has signified a double challenge. On the one hand, we would like to be able to offer an equal opportunity to diabetic (D) and non-diabetic (ND) patients and, on the other hand, to achieve a normalizing of the blood sugar, which would permit, at least a slowing down

Table 1 Characteristics of 15 diabetic and 11 non-diabetic patients with ESRD starting CAPD

	No	*Age (years)*	*Sex*	*Age initiation diabetes*	*Years evolution diabetes*	*Initial* C_{CR} (ml/min)	*Other dialysis Pre-CAPD*	*Months on CAPD*	*Months/patients on CAPD*
Diabetic patients	15	47.7 ± 11.7	6 Females 9 Males	27.1 ± 14.7	20.6 ± 8.4	6.9 ± 2.5	1 HF	87.25	5.81 ± 4.16
				Aetiology ESRD					
Non-diabetic patients	11	51.9 ± 16	5 Females 6 Males	6 CGN 3 CPN 1 PK 1 ?		4.4 ± 3.1	1 HPD 2 HD	86.1	7.86 ± 3.99

(HF: Haemofiltration; HD: Haemodialysis; IPD: Intermittent peritoneal dialysis)
(CGN: Chronic glomerulonephritis; CPN: Chronic interstitial pyelonephritis; PK: Polycistic kidney)

or stabilizing of the progression of the existing vascular lesions[6–9]. Some early experiences[10] of the treatment of diabetics with end-stage renal disease (ESRD) in haemodialysis (HD) and intermittent peritoneal dialysis (IPD) allowed us to begin the inclusion of D patients in the programmes of continuous ambulatory peritoneal dialysis (CAPD), thinking that with this technique we could achieve both objectives.

Here we present the results in a comparative study with ND patients given the same treatment over the same period of time.

PATIENTS

In 21 months (May 1981–February 1983) we included in CAPD 26 patients with ESRD (Figure 1). They were divided into two groups, 15 insulin-

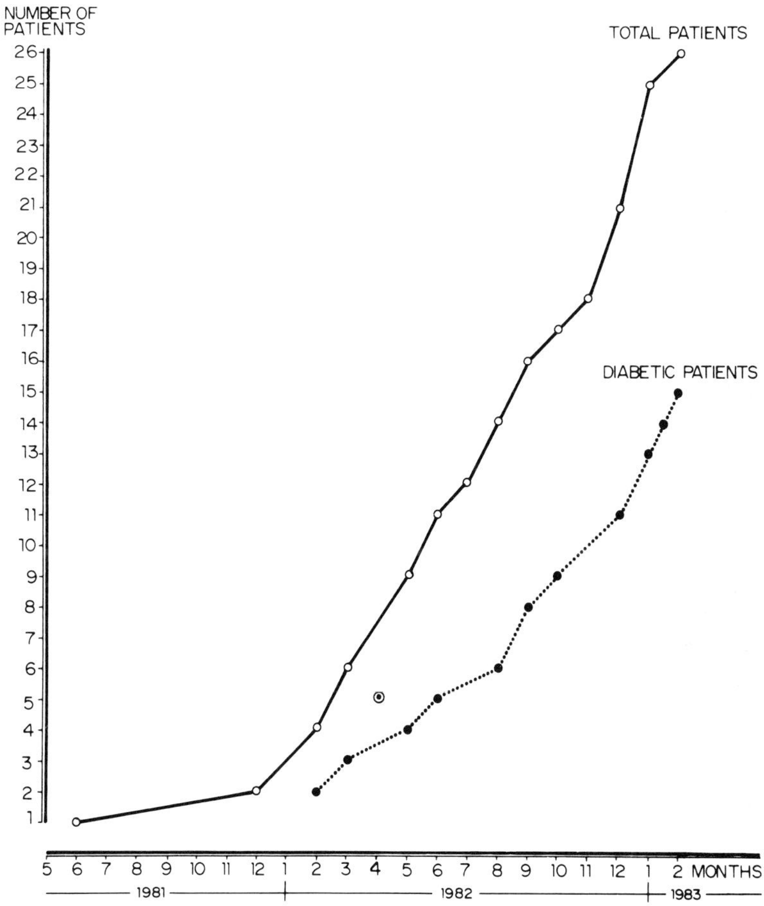

Figure 1 Patients' inclusion on CAPD

dependent diabetic patients and 11 patients who had reached renal insufficiency through chronic glomerulonephritis (CGN) 6, chronic interstitial pyelonephritis (CPN) 3, polycystic kidney (PK) 1 and one with unknown aetiology (Table 1).

The diabetics were 6 women and 9 men aged between 25 and 63 years old (mean 47.7 ± 11.7) with onset diabetes between ages 10 and 57 years (27.1 ± 14.7) with an average development time of 20.6 ± 8.4. The creatinine clearance average on being included in CAPD was 6.9 ± 2.5 ml/min. The months of treatment for this group were 87.25 which represents 5.81 ± 4.16 patient/months. Only one patient received another kind of dialysis before CAPD.

The ND patients were 5 women and 6 men aged between 20 and 70 years (51.9 ± 16), creatinine clearance at their inclusion in dialysis was 4.4 ± 3.1 ml/min with a period in CAPD of 86.5 months and 7.86 ± 3.99 patient/months. Three patients in this group had come from other dialysis techniques, one had been in IPD during the 2 previous years and the other two had to abandon HD because of loss of vascular access.

METHODS

All the patients were given the same technique of surgical implantation[11] of a permanent Tenckhoff peritoneal catheter and four exchanges of 2 litres daily. The dialysis solutions used were of 1.5 and 4.25% glucose in plastic bags (Travenol). The 4.25% was used during the night exchange. The night dwell was 8 hours and the day dwell 4–5 hours.

On stabilizing peritoneal dialysis we withdrew the subcutaneous administration of insulin to the D patients, and we used, exclusively, the intraperitoneal route, injecting into the medicine port of the bag immediately prior to infusion into the peritoneal cavity. To establish the daily dose of insulin we did not follow a general scheme but treated each case individually, depending on the previous requirements, and the blood glucose control was performed at the end of each of the exchanges of dialysis with the intention of maintaining stable levels, between 100 and 150 mg/dl. At the same time we instructed the patients in the finger-prick technique (Ames, Miles Martin) – comparing the results with those of the laboratory – to continue the same controls in their homes during the first month and diminishing them progressively in the following months, providing the patient did not show symptoms of hypoglycaemia. We followed the same study protocol for all the patients accepted into CAPD.

Pre-CAPD and every month coinciding with the set change procedure the following tests were performed:

(1) *Haematological control* – Haematocrit, red cell count, haemoglobin, leukocytes count.

(2) *Chemical constituents of blood* – Serum total proteins, albumin, serum urea, serum uric acid, creatinine, serum sodium potassium, serum bicarbonate, serum total calcium, serum inorganic phosphorus, plasma glucose, serum total cholesterol, serum triglyceride, $HgBA_{1c}$ (chromatography kit Isolab Laboratories) and iPTHc-terminal with double antibody.

(3) *Dialysate effluent* – Total protein, urea, uric acid, creatinine, sodium, potassium, calcium, inorganic phosphorus and glucose.

Additionally, every 6 months:

(1) *Cardiological study* (e.c.g. and e.c.o.). Chest and bone radiology

(2) Ocular examinations (optic fundus)

(3) Residual creatinine clearance

(4) Urine culture

(5) E.M.G.

Only in the case of cloudy effluent dialysis liquid with or without peritonitis symptoms did we do bacteriological cultures, but the treatment of the peritoneal infection was given early, if we saw a count of leukocytes higher than 200 mm^3 (Coulter count), although there was no predominance of segmented neutrophils.

During this time we did not use calcium supplements, phosphorus bindings, derivatives of vitamin D or antihypertensives.

None of the patients had blood transfusions. The NDs followed a free diet with salt, while the Ds were given diet of 1.517 kcalories with 155 g of carbohydrates, 87 g of proteins and 61 g of fats, which represents approximately 1.5–2 g prot/g. All of them received dietary additives of vitamin B complex, and in some cases protein supplements.

The results were obtained from the monthly data of all the patients taken pre-CAPD in the 1st, 3rd, 5th, 7th, 9th and the 12th months, and from the total data of the period studied.

The values obtained have been statistically analysed to determine the homogeneity of the groups following the method of comparison of variances, finding their significance in Snedecor tables as in the comparison of the averages and calculations of the Student paired *t*-test, only considering significant, values corresponding to $p \leqslant 0.05$.

RESULTS

Blood glucose control

With three exchanges at 1.5% and one at 4.25% of dextrose in 24 hours, the theoretical intake of glucose is 175 g/day, there being an absorption average in

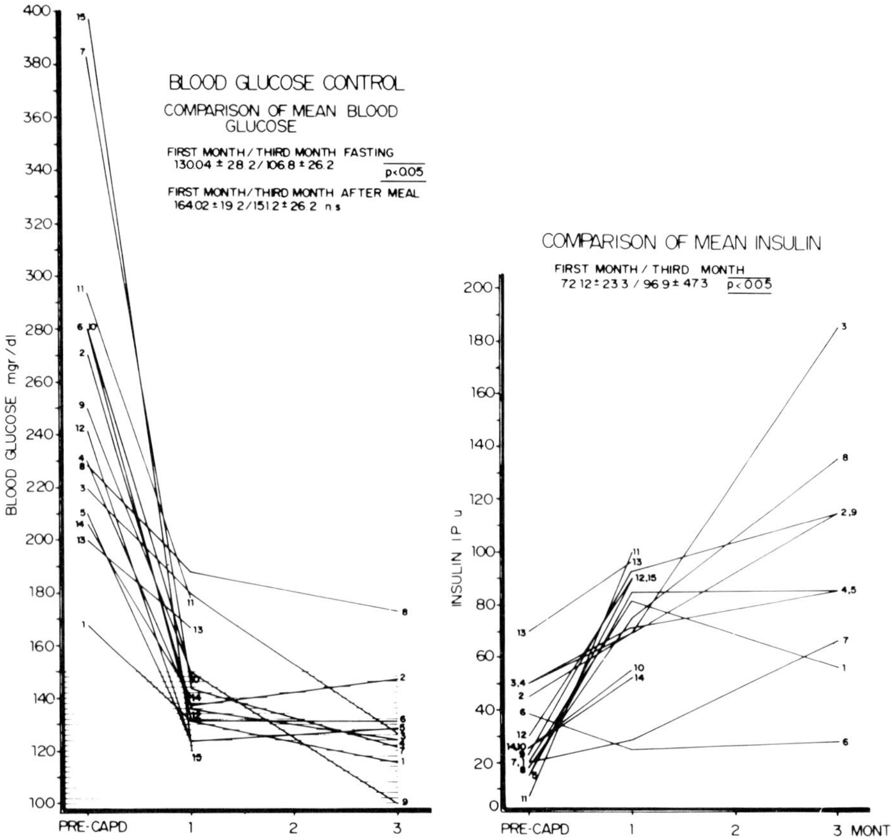

Figure 2

diabetic patients of 112.64 ± 23.63 g (68.6–145.7 g/day). With the dietary contribution of carbohydrates, these patients received approximately between 243.3–320.7 g/day, which represents 0.9734–1.2828 kcal exclusively in this manner. In Figure 2 can be seen the blood glucose levels and the intraperitoneal doses of insulin needed during the first 3 months to establish a good control. An adjustment is produced in the glycaemia levels in relation to the pre-CAPD during the first month and those near normal in the third month, with the increase of the doses of insulin. There is a significant difference ($p < 0.05$) between the average glucose data obtained in fasting subjects in the first and third month and the need for insulin in the same time ($p < 0.05$), while the after-meal levels of blood glucose, although they remain at acceptable levels, are not affected by the increase of insulin which is induced in the third month.

The average increase of insulin in the first 3 months, and maintained during

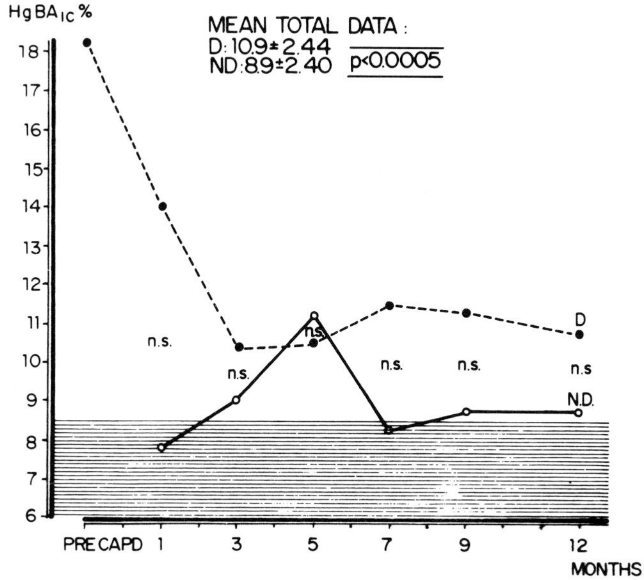

COMPARISON OF MEAN BLOOD GLUCOSE AND MEAN Hg BA_{1C} LEVELS IN INDIVIDUAL DIABETIC PRE-CAPD (r=0.80) (p n.s.)

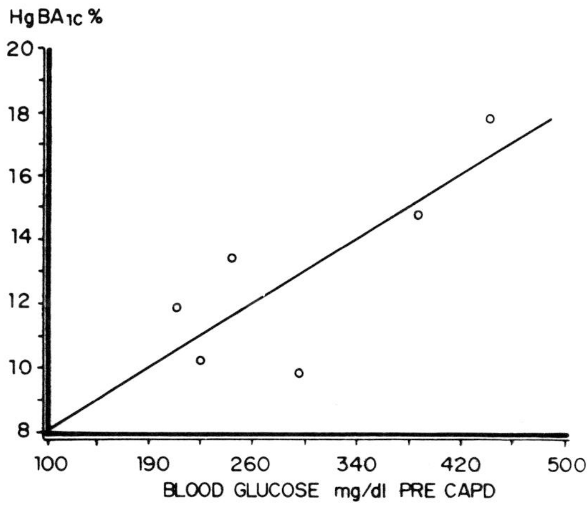

Figure 3 Mean Hg BA_{1c} levels in diabetic and non-diabetic patients during CAPD

the time studied, supposes an increase of 3.7 ± 2.2 times that necessary previous to dialysis.

In only one case was there a decrease of these needs in CAPD (case 6) with the glucose figures within normal limits.

The relationship of units of insulin to gram of glucose absorbed varies between 2.51 and 4.44 with four exchanges a day.

The control of $HgBA_{1c}$ (Figure 3) realized in both groups shows a pathological rise in the levels, significantly higher in the D patients and in the first month of treatment $p < 0.0125$.

During the study there was a drop without reaching normal in both groups, although the ND patients are closer showing a statistically significant difference $p < 0.0005$ in the entire study population. Mean random glucose determinations before initiation of CAPD were compared to $HgBA_{1c}$ predialysis; there was a correlation ($r = 0.80$), which could have been predicted, for whilst glycaemia levels remain between 100 and 140 mg% the values of $HgBA_{1c}$ will stay between 8 and 9% (Figure 3), although the statistical value isn't significant because of the little information available.

Haematological control (Figure 4)

The control of anaemia (haematocrit and haemoglobin) did not present significant differences in either group with a satisfactory evolution during the study.

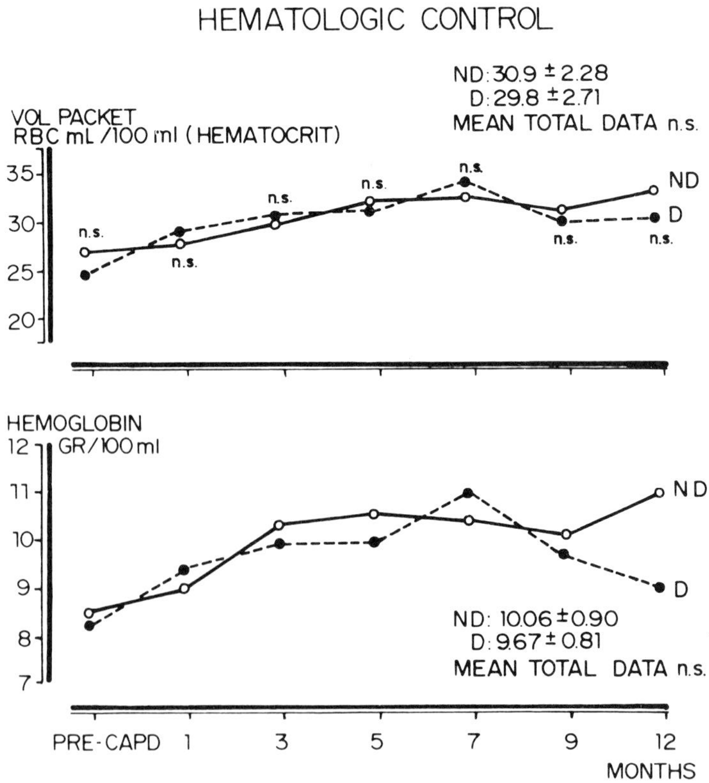

Figure 4

Biochemical control

In both the short term data and the total data there are no statistically significant differences in the serum concentrations of urea and uric acid (Figure 5), but there is a significant difference ($p \leqslant 0.0025$) in serum creatinine with higher levels in the ND patients. On comparing the initial creatinine clearance there is no difference between the two groups ($p \geqslant 0.05$). On the other hand the peritoneal creatinine clearance is slightly higher and statistically significant ($p < 0.005$) in diabetic patients although in the bi-monthly controls of the study this is not uniformly shown (Figure 6). It must be stressed that the peritoneal dialysis effluent was obtained after an overnight 8 hour dwell and always with 4.25%. In serum total proteins there is an improvement with relation to pre-dialysis, data being significantly higher in the ND patients ($p < 0.005$) (Figure 7). The average protein loss measured only in the overnight dialysate effluent is similar in both groups without significant differences.

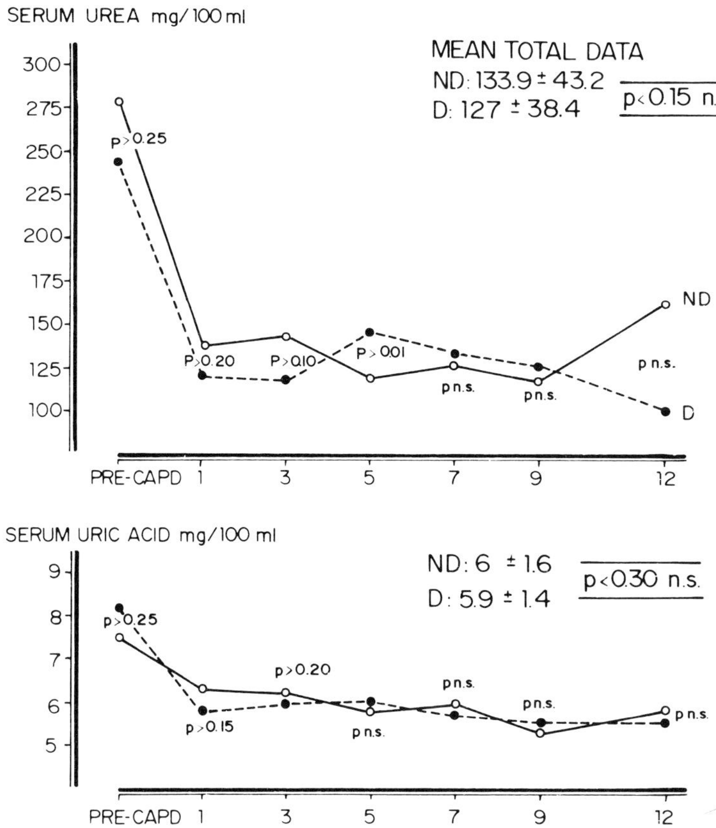

Figure 5 Serum urea and serum uric acid before and during CAPD in diabetic and non-diabetic patients

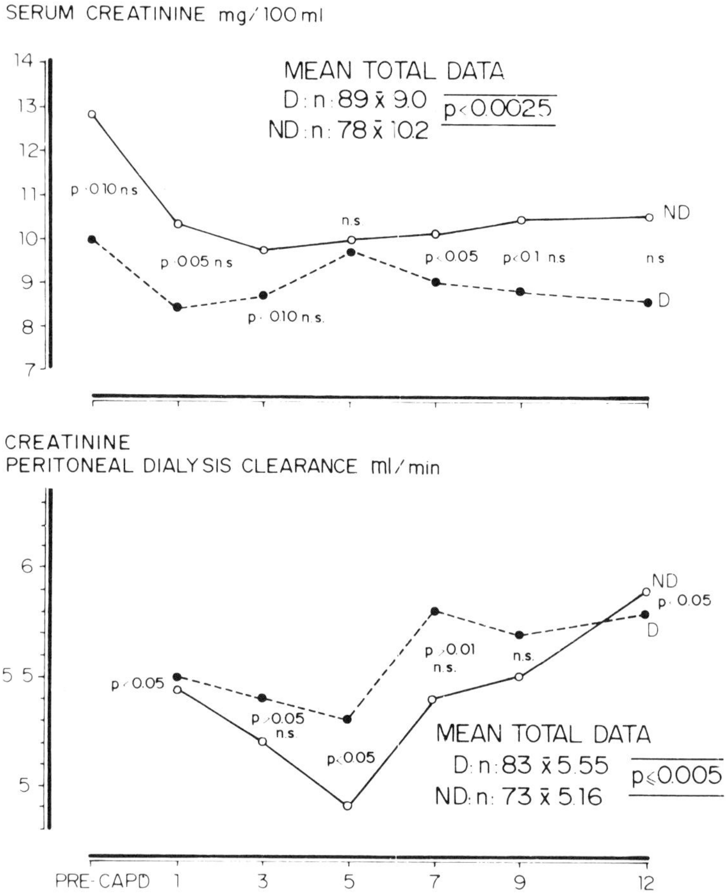

Figure 6 Serum creatinine and creatinine peritoneal dialysis clearance pre-CAPD and bimonthly during CAPD

Calcium and phosphate control, serum iPTH and alkaline phosphatase

In Figure 8 can be seen a uniform rise in serum total calcium in the two groups, previously lower than normal. The group of D patients maintain levels statistically higher ($p<0.01$).

In the phosphate control, without statistical significance, the values are reversed, the ND patients having the higher levels. High values of iPTH were found in both groups on beginning treatment with CAPD, rising higher during the time studied and being significantly higher in the ND patients ($p<0.05$), the group of patients with lower calcium and slightly higher phosphorus levels. Alkaline phosphatase is initially high in all the patients, tending to descend in the first months, and to rise again from the 7th month. There is no statistical difference between the two group of patients.

Radiologically, there is a predominance of bone pathology in the D patients

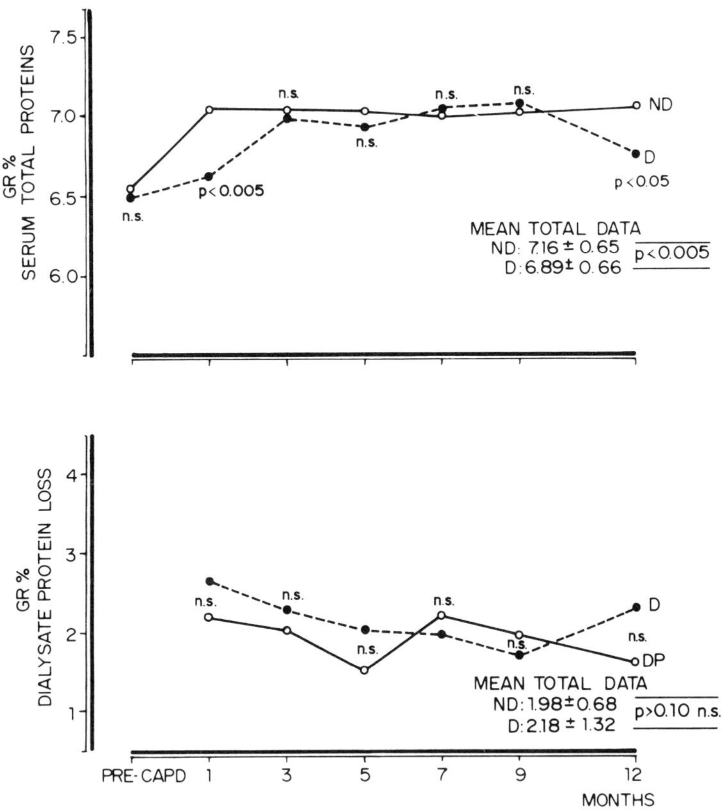

Figure 7 Serum total proteins and protein loss during CAPD

with vascular calcifications in pelvic vessels in 6 patients, 6 with osteoporosis, 2 with minimal lesions of bone reabsorptions and in 3 there are no lesions to be seen. In the ND patients 4 have no observed lesions, 2 have osteoporosis and 6 have lesions of subperiostic reabsorption.

Lipid abnormalities (Figure 9)

In our patients, during the time studied, there was a rise in total serum cholesterol with stable values in the 5th and 7th month. The total levels were statistically higher in the D patients ($p < 0.05$) though always staying in their normal limits. In the triglycerides there was a rise without significant difference. In the 12th month the scarcity of data ($n = 4$) and the disparity of such, makes their evaluation inadvisable.

Blood pressure control and weight

In the D patients group, 11 patients were hypertensive on beginning CAPD compared to 10 of the 11 ND patients. In the first month's course, the levels of

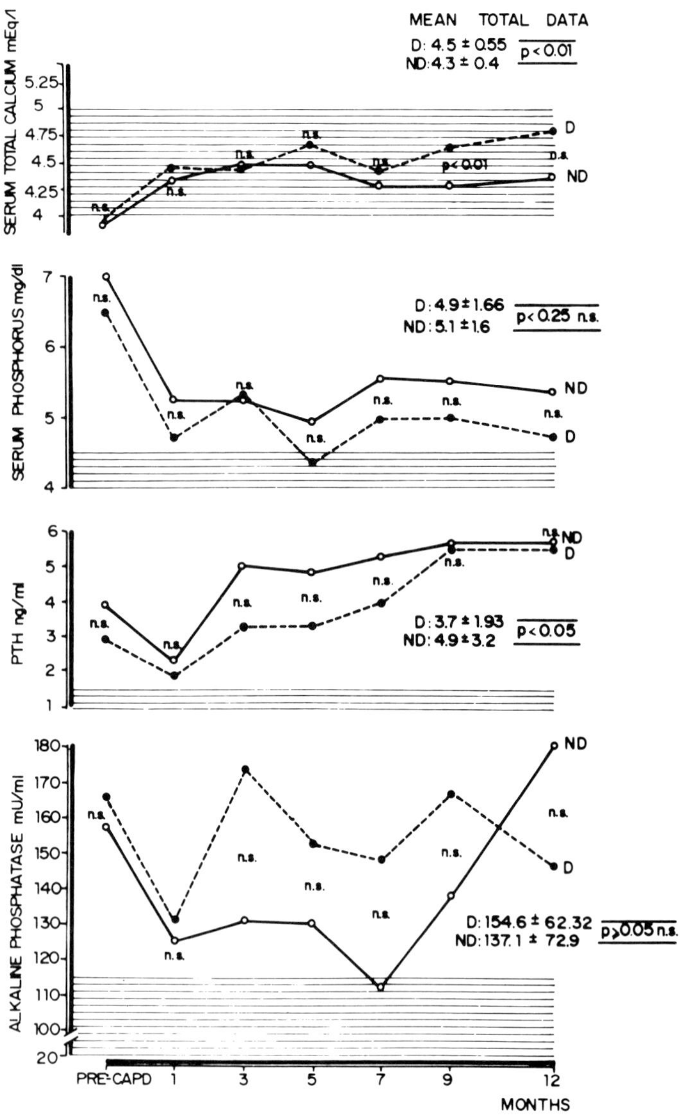

Figure 8 Serum calcium, phosphorus, PTH, and alkaline phosphatase levels prior and every 2 months subsequent to starting CAPD in diabetic and non-diabetic patients

the systolic and diastolic blood pressure normalized in the two groups, coinciding with weight loss of 1 ± 2.34 kg for the ND patients and 3.86 ± 3.72 for D patients, maintaining the stability of blood pressure. During the 12 months, there was a significant rise in weight ($p < 0.025$) for the ND patients compared with the D patients group who maintained or lost weight in the same period (Figure 10).

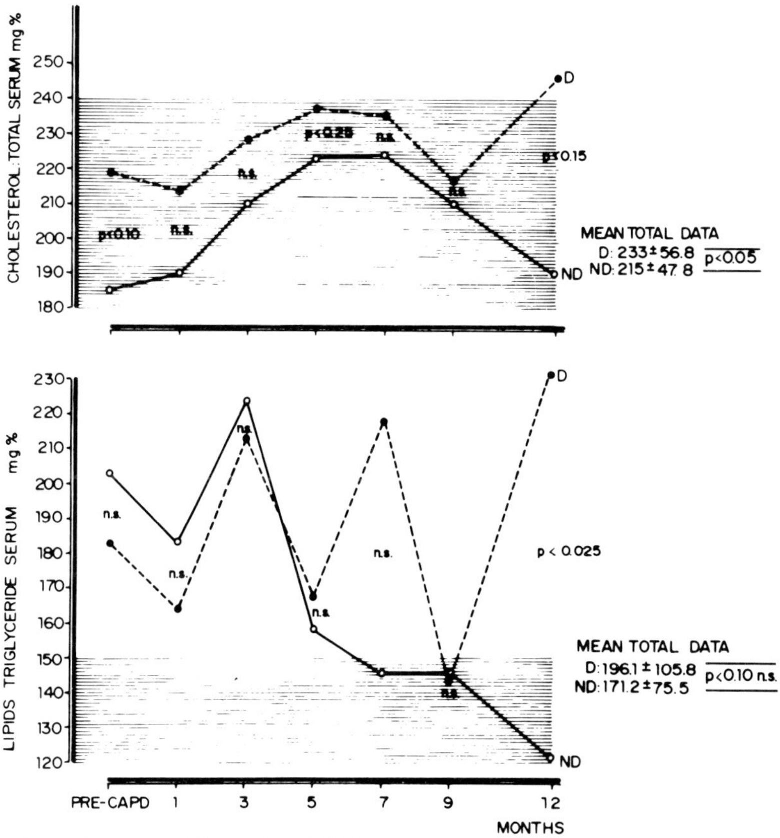

Figure 9 Lipid abnormalities during CAPD

PERITONITIS (Table 2)

The incidence of peritonitis in the group of D patients is 1 episode per 5.45 patient months, being significantly higher than that in the ND patients group, which is of 1 episode every 10.8 patient months. Of the 15 D patients, in 9 there was at least 1 episode of peritoneal infection, while of the 11 ND only in 3 was there an infection.

Table 2 Incidence of peritonitis in diabetic and non-diabetic patients on CAPD

	Diabetics	*Non-diabetics*
Number of patients	15	11
Peritonitis episodes	16	8
Total patients months	87.25	86.5
Incidence of peritonitis	1/5.45 PT.MO.	1/10.8 PT.MO.

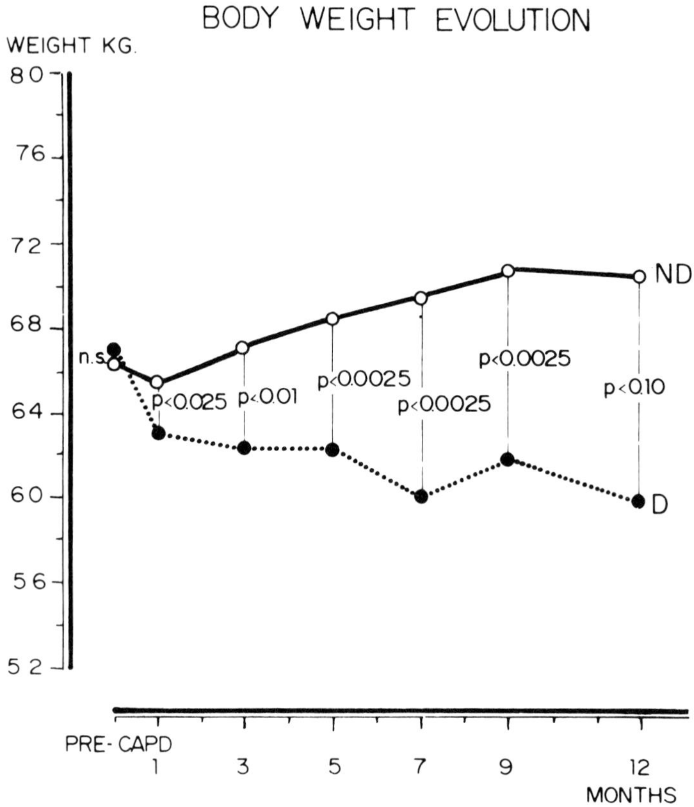

Figure 10

In both groups, the most frequent organism was *Staph. epidermidis* and on 3 occasions the bacteriological culture was negative. All the infections were rapidly cured with the treatment.

COMPLICATIONS (Table 3)

Twelve D patients arrived at dialysis with e.c.g. alterations and after 6 months evolution the same alterations persisted in 5 of them. In the ND group of the 8 who showed e.c.g. alterations this disappeared in 4 of them.

Only D patients showed pre-CAPD pericardial effusion, which after 6 months of treatment with dialysis had disappeared in 3 and diminished in the 2 others.

One patient in each group began dialysis with ischaemic heart disease, in both groups it had been corrected by the 6 month control.

Fourteen of the D patients and 7 of the ND patients had peripheral neuro-

Table 3 Complications before dialysis and evolution after 6 months CAPD

	Diabetics		*Non-diabetic*	
Complications	*Pre-CAPD* $n=15$	*After 6 months* $n=7$	*Pre-CAPD* $n=11$	*After 6 months* $n=8$
Hypertension	11	0	10	0
ECG alterations	12	5	8	4
Pericardial effusion	5	2	0	0
Ischaemic heart disease	1	0	1	0
Peripheral neuropathy (non-incapaciting)	14	6	7	4
Gastric reflux	5		0	
Hiatus hernia	6 (40%)		0	

pathy. In 6 of the first group and 4 of the second, the alteration persisted after 6 months (perineal nerve conduction less than 40 m/s). In 40% of the D patients, hiatus hernia can be detected radiologically, with symptoms of oesophagic reflux in 5 patients. None of the ND patients showed this pathology.

Opthalmological alterations (Table 4)
All the diabetic patients arrived at dialysis with retinopathy in different stages of evolution, 4 patients blind and 3 more patients with poor visual acuity. In 6 patients there were cataracts affecting 10 eyes. The lesions did not revert in any of the patients, but in those which we had enough time to observe, there was no deterioration. Of the 4 blind patients, 2 practised self-care.

In the time studied, none of the patients died and only one patient in the ND

Table 4 Diabetic retinopathy

Retinopathy		15		
Visual acuity:	Poor:	2	Self care:	0
	Blind:	4		2

group has discontinued dialysis 10 months after beginning CAPD, because of mechanical problems in the catheter (he had been 2 years in IPD). The rest of the patients still maintain the first permanent catheter.

Rehabilitation was acceptable in both groups, including the blind patients, and there is a logical difference in the periods of hospitalization between both groups due to a greater incidence of peritonitis in the D patients group.

DISCUSSION

Within the controversy of the subject there seems to exist information sufficiently valuable to establish a narrow relationship between blood glucose control and the microangiopathic and neuropathic complications related to diabetic disease.

As has been reported[13-15] the glucose control is easily performed, using the exclusively intraperitoneal access of insulin, establishing levels of glucose within near to normal limits and using the quantity necessary for each patient.

The controls of $HgBA_{1c}$ in the D group patients, including a stable control of glycaemia, were maintained during the time pathologically high, although they descended in relation to the previous levels. The $HgBA_{1c}$ value reflects the control of glucose in the 120 days previous to the determination (half life of the red cell)[12,16]. It is therefore logical to think that the levels in the first months could be high because they express the predialysis situation. Flynn[17] with serial determinations of $HgBA_{1c}$ in diabetics over more than 2 years obtains values slightly higher than normal in D patients and normal in ND patients.

The discovery of a significant difference in favour of a lesser concentration of serum creatinine in diabetic patients, on comparing all the information available in both groups, could be justified if there existed a higher residual creatinine clearance in the D group. In the initial creatinine clearance there are not statistically significant differences, and it is to be supposed that during this time the possible variations would have been minimal[18].

In patients[19,20] with severe systemic vasculitis a possible extension of the alterations to the peritoneal microcirculation (systemic lupus erythematosis, diabetes, etc) has been reported, leading to significant reduced peritoneal clearances. The changes in the capillary permeability could also explain a greater protein loss in this group of patients, that in our case does not occur. Probably our results can be explained by the use of hypertonic dialysate fluid, and they could be confirmed if similar results were obtained with dialysate fluids of different glucose concentrations.

Some reports[21,22] show the minimal bone lesions in the D patients with ESRD compared to the non-diabetic in the same situation and normal levels of iPTH in diabetic. The high incidence of vascular calcifications and osteoporosis in our D patients contrast with the lesions observed in the ND patients, as with the pathological level of iPTH since the beginning of the treatment with increases during period studied in D and ND patients.

While the number of peritoneal infections during the 12 months is similar to that described by other authors in their first experiences[23,24], the greater frequency of peritonitis in our results indicated that insulin administration in dialysate bags is a rupture in sterility and does have an influence on our environment. Introduction of some changes in the technique made in the last 4 months, have modified the incidence in both groups: 1 episode/13.3 patient months *vs.* 10.8 patient months in ND patients, and 1 episode/7.7 patient months *vs.* 5.45 patient months in D patients.

Through the studied period and the results obtained, which show minimal differences between both groups, we are encouraged to consider CAPD for the D patients as a suitable technique both for the ESRD treatment and the control of glycaemia, within stable limits near to normal; and that some of the diabetic disease sequels could be slowed in their evolution if dialysis inclusion, at least in Spain, is done before arriving at such a terminal situation as the nephrologist usually finds.

ACKNOWLEDGEMENTS

The authors would like to thank Dr A. Cruceyra, biochemist, for his help in the execution of the statistical study.

References

1. Brynger, H., Brunner, F. P., Chandler, D., Donckerwolcke, R. A., *et al.* (1980). Combined report on regular dialysis and transplantation in Europe. *Proc. Eur. Dial. Transplant. Assoc.,* **17,** 4
2. Ahlmen, J. (1975). Incidence of chronic renal insufficiency: A study of incidence and pattern of renal insufficiency in adults during 1966–1971 in Gothenburg. *Acta Med. Scand.* (Suppl.) **582,** 3
3. Ritz, E., Bommer, J. and Andrassy, K. (1981). Treatment of diabetic patients with end-stage renal failure: some clinical aspects. *Proc. 8th Int. Conf. Nephrol.* Athens
4. Instituto Nacional de Estadistica, España. (1978). Encuenta de morbilidad hospitalaria. *Ed. Ministerio. Economía y Comercia. I.N.E.* ANEXO 1, pp. 85–91, 1982
5. Garcia, G. and M. Valles, P. (1982). Informe anual del registro de pacientes en dialísis y trasplante renal en España. *Nefrología.,* **11** (Suppl. 1) 3
6. Tchobroutsky, G. (1978). Relation of diabetic control to development of microvascular complications. *Diabetologia,* **15,** 143
7. Siperstein, M. D., Foster, D. W., Knowles, H. C., Levine, R., Madison, L. L. and Roth, J. (1977). Control of blood glucose and diabetic vascular disease. *N. Engl. J. Med.,* **296,** 1060
8. Tamborlane, W. V., Sherwin, R. S., Genel, M. and Felig, P. (1978). Reduction to normal of plasma glucose in juvenile diabetes by subcutaneous administration of insulin with a portable infusion pump. *N. Engl. J. Med.,* **300,** 573
9. Viberti, G. C., Pickup, J. C., Jarret, R. J. and Keen, H. (1979). Effect of control of blood glucose on urinary excretion of albumin and β_2-microglobulin in insulin-dependent diabetics. *N. Engl. J. Med.,* **300,** 638
10. Coronel, F., Rodriguez Ibarra, R., Garcia de Lomana, M. T., Muñoz de la Paz, C., Horcajo, P., Olivan Osambele, P., Naranjo, P., Prats, D. and Docon, M. T. (1981). Dialisis en los diabéticos. *Sedyt.* III, 113
11. Horcajo, P., Prats, D., Naranjo, P., Coronel, F., Grimalt, J., Rentero, R. and Docon, M. T. (1981). Dos años de experiencia con protesis de Tenckhoff. *Sedyt,* III, 63
12. Apostolopoulus, A., Jovanovic, L. and Peterson, C. M. (1983). Current Concepts in Therapy for Diabetic Patient with Renal Disease. *Diabet. Nephrop.,* **2,** 39
13. Flynn, C. T. and Nanson, J. A. (1979). Intraperitoneal insulin with CAPD in artificial pancreas. *Trans. Am. Soc. Artif. Intern. Organs,* **25,** 114
14. Madden, M. A., Zimmerman, S. W. and Simpson, D. P. (1982). Continuous Ambulatory Peritoneal Dialysis in Diabetes Mellitus. The risks and benefits of intraperitoneal insulin. *Am. J. Nephrol.,* **2,** 133
15. Amair, P., Khanna, R., Leibel, B., Pierratos, A., Vas, S., Meema, E., Blair, G., Chisolm, L., Vas, M., Zingg, W., Digenis, G. and Oreopoulos, D. (1982). Continuous Ambulatory Peritoneal Dialysis in diabetics with end-stage renal disease. *N. Engl. J. Med.,* **306,** 625
16. Boer, J. J., Miedema, K. and Casperie, A. F. (1980). Glycoslylated hemoglobin in renal failure. *Diabetologie,* **18,** 437
17. Flynn, C. T. (1983). The diabetic patient on continuous Ambulatory Peritoneal Dialysis. *Periton. Dial. Bull.,* **3,** 16
18. Rottembourg, J., Issad, B. *et al.* (1982). Evolution of residual renal function in patient

undergoing maintenance hemodialysis or continuous Ambulatory Peritoneal Dialysis. *Proc. Eur. Dial. Transplant Assoc.*, **19**, 397

19. Nolph, K.D. and Sorkin, M.I. (1981). The peritoneal dialysis system. In Nolph, K.D. (ed.). *Peritoneal Dialysis Development in Nephrology*, Vol. II, pp. 21–41. (The Hague, Boston, London: Martinus Nijhoft Publishers)
20. Nolph, K.D., Stoltz, M. and Maher, J.F. (1973). Altered peritoneal permeability in patients with systemic vasculitis. *Ann. Intern. Med.*, **78**, 891
21. Iba, K., Ogura, F. *et al.* (1979). Rather reduced parathyroid function in chronic renal failure due to diabetic nephropathy. *Abstr., Asian Pacific Cong. Nephrol.*, **1**, 103
22. Vincenti, F., Hattner, R. (1981). Decreased secondary hyperparathyroidism in diabetic patients receiving hemodialysis. *J. Am. Med. Assoc.*, **245**, 930
23. Fenton, S., Wu, G., Cattran, D., Wadgymar, A. and Allen, A.F. (1981). Clinical aspects of peritonitis in patients on CAPD. *Dial. Bull.*, **1**, 4
24. Williams, C.C., Cattran, D., Fenton, S., Khanna, R., Manuel, A., Shiphoo, C., Oreopoulos, D.G. and Roscoe, J. (1981). Peritonitis on CAPD. Three years experience in Toronto. *Dial. Bull.*, **1**, 7

Discussant

R. TH. KREDIET

Dr Krediet (Holland): Professor Lameire was kind enough to send me his data in advance of the Symposium and I have been able to compare them with those of Dr Khanna which were published last year in *N. Engl. J. Med.* As the differences were enormous, and perhaps confusing, I thought it might be helpful, and hopefully not more confusing, to add the data of the Academic Medical Centre in Amsterdam to them.

We started our CAPD Program in August 1979, and up to December 1982 we trained 44 patients, about one-third of whom had diabetes. Our total patient experience with diabetics is about one-third of the total experience.

Our overall survival is comparable to what others have found and there is no difference between diabetics and non-diabetics. There are, however, differences in morbidity.

We can divide our patients into three groups to look at the frequency of administration after CAPD training. One is a positively selected group, that is patients who were able to choose between CAPD and other forms of treatment; the second is a group of negatively selected patients in whom CAPD was the only possibility, and the third a group of diabetic patients. It is obvious that diabetics do worst. Not one of the diabetic patients was spared re-admission.

We have studied the rehabilitation of the three groups according to EDTA criteria. 1–4 means good rehabilitation; 5 and 6 are bad rehabilitation. Diabetic patients again do worst.

Diabetic patient survival at 15 months on CAPD at the Toronto Western Hospital is 82%. Professor Lameire has suggested that different results might be due to bad control of diabetes. I have therefore compared intraperitoneal insulin requirements on CAPD. Dr Khanna showed that at the Toronto Western Hospital it currently runs at a mean of 110 units/day. Professor Caronel showed that in Spain it is about 100 units/day.

It is therefore my opinion that diabetic patients on CAPD do have higher morbidity and worse rehabilitation than other CAPD patients, but that an acceptable mortality can be achieved with close supervision of the patients and their diabetes.

Open discussion

Dr Verger (France): The dramatic hyperpermeability of the membrane in peritoneal dialysis is well known, and during these episodes we usually have to increase the rate of exchange. How can the insulin therapy be changed when insulin is being used in the bags, because the permeability may change?

Dr Khanna: At the time of training we teach every patient a sliding scale, whereby they are taught how much increment of insulin is to be added if they have to use a solution other than 1.5, either a mildly hypertonic or a severely hypertonic solution. We observe them at the time of training and check for any errors, and by the time they are ready to go home we make sure that they understand the sliding scale.

Professor M Leski (Switzerland): Could we have some new information about sclerosing peritonitis, which may represent a frightening pitfall?

Professor Mion: Among our diabetic patients we have observed only one case of sclerosing peritonitis in one young lady, a type I diabetic who had had 5.5 years of integrated IPD and CAPD. In my series she is left alive outside because she had only one year of IPD and then three or four years of CAPD. It does not seem to be a problem specific to diabetics. It is a matter of length of time on peritoneal dialysis; perhaps more on IPD than on CAPD.

I would agree that it is an upsetting problem.

Professor Shapiro: I want to answer Dr Parsons's comments about selection of patients. I believe that we probably have the most liberal selection criteria in the world for acceptance of patients. Our only criterion was that they be dying of uraemia and not require permanent nursing home care. To substantiate the difference in the patient populations that we are seeing, since 1976, 28.5% of our patients accepted into dialysis were diabetic. In the last two years that has gone up to 33% and this last year it is 38%. Of the patients accepted into the dialysis programme, 62.5% are either diabetic, and/or > 61 years old. That is skewed because of the emphasis of the University of Minnesota Transplant

Programme – which is only a mile away from us. The ideal transplant candidates are for the most part sent directly to the University and the other patients come to us.

The data I report on include all patients, and the only rejection is because they are permanent nursing home patients. That amounts to maybe five a year in an average of a 200 patient intake.

Dr Khanna: What percentage of Professor Shapiro's patients are on home dialysis?

Professor Shapiro: Right now our total programme represent about 25%; 125 out of about 450.

Dr H J Goldsmith (UK): I should like to ask Professor Shapiro some details about his heparinization regime in relation to the good effects on the patients. For example, arterial or venous, and how much?

Professor Shapiro: We use normal heparinization procedures with the usual loading dose of 1.5–2 cc and anywhere from 1–2 cc/h by infusion. We see no reason to modify at all for diabetes. The only time that we would modify is in a post vitreal haemorrhage period, which fortunately occurs relatively rarely. We handle the diabetic basically no different to the non-diabetic.

Dr Triolo (Italy): Is there any experience of haemofiltration of diabetics? The reason for my question is that within the past three years we have treated a number of diabetics – 8 of them – with a good result. The survival rate in the first year is 90%.

Professor Shapiro: We commenced a programme in May 1982. There are three diabetics in the group and all three are surviving.

If one is adequately controlling blood pressure, and particularly if one can do that without the use of antihypertensive agents, that optimizes the chance of patient survival. In that respect, haemofiltration, as it becomes more practical to apply, may offer some advantages, because fluid removal can be manipulated a little more easily.

Professor Piccoli: I agree. It is very important to gear the haemofiltration to some very sick patients who cannot continue with CAPD and who do not tolerate traditional haemodialysis.

Professor Shapiro: That is precisely our intent with the next phase of our study.

Dr J P Godon (Belgium): Surely residual renal function is decreased with glycerol? Everybody knows that experimental acute renal failure can be produced with glycerol.

Professor Lameire: Yes. But the doses that are used for producing experimental acute renal failure are a little bit higher than the amount of glycerol that was absorbed from the peritoneal cavity. The rate of endogenous creatinine clearance was exactly the same as with glucose. There was no difference in that.

Dr Coronel: When Dr Mion treats diabetic patients with IPD, does he use insulin by the intraperitoneal route when they are on dialysis?

Professor Mion: We have never done it, for practical reasons. The technique the patients are taught is to have an extra dose before they start the peritoneal dialysis session. Some very unstable patients will even monitor their blood sugar during sessions, for instance every four hours, to check whether an extra dose is needed.

It is just a matter of practicality, but it might be useful to put it through the peritoneum as well.

Dr Coronel: Does Professor Lameire find any secondary problems with glycerol?

Professor Lameire: So far as we have looked for them clinically and biologically, there are no side effects that can be attributed directly to the presence of glycerol in the plasma.

So far as the metabolism of glycerol is concerned, most of it goes to the glucose pathway, so that the slight increase in blood glucose to be observed in the non-diabetics with glycerol is due to neoglucogenesis. There is also some shift to glycogen. There may also be a little bit incorporated in the glycerides. There are also other minor metabolic pathways that we shall not discuss now.

20
Residual renal function and control of blood glucose levels in insulin-dependent diabetic patients treated by CAPD

J. ROTTEMBOURG, B. ISSAD, J. L. POIGNET, P. STRIPPOLI, A. BALDUCCI, G. SLAMA and G. M. GAHL

INTRODUCTION

Diabetic patients with end-stage renal disease (ESRD) are at a high risk for renal replacement therapy[1,2]. The choice between the different dialysis methods is largely influenced by the medical team's experience as well as the available technical facilities. Recently continuous ambulatory peritoneal dialysis (CAPD) has been considered as a satisfactory dialysis method for insulin-dependent diabetics (IDD), and very encouraging results at 2 years were reported by Amair[3] and our own group[4]. This communication will focus on residual renal function and quality of blood glucose control in IDD patients treated by CAPD.

CLINICAL MATERIAL

Between August 1978 and March 1983, 38 unselected diabetic patients with end-stage renal disease were trained in an individualized Unit of the Department of Nephrology of the Hôpital de la Pitié, in Paris. They accounted for 25% of 150 patients trained during the same period. 29 patients were exclusively treated by CAPD. Since October 1981, four patients (1 for personal convenience, three for blindness with the help of their relatives) have been treated by continuous cyclic peritoneal dialysis (CCPD) using a cycler overnight. Five patients were transferred from haemodialysis because of cardiovascular (three patients) ocular (one patient) or vascular access (one patient) complications. As of March 1983, the cumulative duration of CAPD treatment was 47 patient-years. The average time on CAPD was 14.7 months (range 1–38 months).

Age of the patients (18 males and 20 females) ranged from 22 to 76 years (mean age 52.1 ± 13 years). The mean age at start of diabetes was 30.7 ± 15.6 years. Mean duration of renal failure (time between creatinine level over 200 μmol/l and start of dialysis) was 24.5 ± 8.6 months. At start of dialysis all patients were treated with insulin, but 13 had previously been treated by oral antidiabetic agents. All patients had severe extrarenal complications: hypertension in 35 patients, a history of myocardial infarction in 16, angina pectoris in 20, peripheral vascular disease in 22, clinical peripheral neuropathy in 27. Five patients were totally blind and seven legally blind.

The actuarial survival rates were 85%, 65% and 62% at 1, 2 and 3 years, respectively. The rates of continuation on dialysis were 80% and 55% at 1 and 2 years. *Causes of drop out* were death in eleven cases and transfer to haemodialysis in seven cases. Four patients died from a vascular accident including three of myocardial infarction and one of stroke. Peripheral vascular arteritis required lower limb amputations in four cases, which was followed by sepsis and death. Two patients died from peritonitis including one case secondary to bowel perforation. Cessation of treatment was decided for a cachectic blind woman. Transfer to haemodialysis was necessary because of malnutrition in three cases, peritonitis in two patients and encapsulated sclerosing peritonitis in two other patients. On April 1st, 1983, 20 patients remained on peritoneal dialysis, 16 on CAPD and 4 treated by CAPD.

RESIDUAL RENAL FUNCTION

Residual renal function in patients with ESRD on maintenance dialysis is an important factor of the well-being of the patients and influences the dialysis schedule[5,6]. We recently reported[7] the stabilization of the residual renal function in 25 patients including four insulin-dependent diabetics treated by CAPD over an 18 month period compared to a matched group of 25 patients treated by haemodialysis. These facts led us to investigate the evolution of the glomerular filtration rate (GFR) expressed by the creatinine clearance in two diabetic groups, one treated by CAPD, the other by haemodialysis. In the CAPD group the evolution of the peritoneal clearances and protein losses were equally studied.

Patients and methods

Patients

The CAPD group included the 22 patients dialysed at least for 1 year, their clinical and biological parameters are listed on Table 1. There were 12 males and 10 females, with a mean age of 52.4 ± 12.9 years at start of CAPD. Daily dialysis was performed mainly over a schedule of four exchanges using commercial solutions with three 2l 1.5% dextrose bags and one 2l 4.5% dextrose bag.

Table 1 Evolution of clinical and biological parameters*

	Months				
	0 (n = 22)	*6* (n = 22)	*12* (n = 22)	*18* (n = 12)	*24* (n = 8)
Weight (kg)	62.7 ± 10	64.4 ± 11	66.2 ± 12	65.5 ± 9	63.1 ± 12
Blood pressure mmHg					
systolic	185 ± 26	157 ± 30	150 ± 27	142 ± 28	140 ± 22
diastolic	112 ± 16	91 ± 13	85 ± 16	85 ± 16	88 ± 20
Haematocrit %	28.9 ± 4.6	34.5 ± 6.6	32.7 ± 7.3	32 ± 8	32 ± 9
Creatinine μmol/l	854 ± 220	771 ± 247	722 ± 249	803 ± 243	810 ± 267
Bicarbonates mmol/l	220 ± 2	23.8 ± 3	25.3 ± 3.8	25.0 ± 3	26.9 ± 2.8
Potassium mmol/l	4.8 ± 0.6	4.4 ± 0.7	4.4 ± 0.6	4.4 ± 0.6	4.2 ± 0.2
Calcium mmol/l	2.2 ± 0.2	2.2 ± 0.2	2.3 ± 0.2	2.4 ± 0.2	2.4 ± 0.2
Phosphorus mmol/l	1.8 ± 0.4	1.6 ± 0.3	1.5 ± 0.3	1.4 ± 0.3	1.5 ± 0.5
Albumin g/l	32.5 ± 4.3	31.3 ± 3.5	31.8 ± 4.8	30.9 ± 3.3	28.5 ± 5.3
Cholesterol mmol/l	5.5 ± 1.3	6.3 ± 1.3	6.2 ± 1.7	5.5 ± 1.8	6.1 ± 1.8
Triglycerides mmol/l	2.1 ± 0.9	2.6 ± 1.1	2.8 ± 1.8	2.5 ± 1.9	2.0 ± 1.6

* all values are expressed as mean ± SD
n = number of patients

The haemodialysis group was composed of 56 insulin-dependent diabetic patients (37 males, 19 females) treated in the same department by haemodialysis from 1973 to 1981. Mean age at start of haemodialysis was 40.3 ± 13.3 years. Dialysis was carried out with different schedules: 24 patients were dialysed twice a week (average weekly dialysis time: 14 h) and 32 patients three times a week (average weekly dialysis time from 12 to 14 h). 45 patients were treated for at least 1 year and 34 for at least 2 years.

Methodology

The residual renal function was evaluated in each group just before dialysis therapy and every 6 months over a 2 year period using the *creatinine clearance* as a measure of the glomerular filtration rate (GFR). In the CAPD group urine was collected over a 24 h period on any day during the week and blood samples were taken at the end of urine collection period. In the haemodialysis group, during the dialysis period, a 24 h urine collection was performed on the last day of the longet period between two dialysis sessions; blood samples for serum creatinine were obtained at the end of the urine collection period at the beginning of the following dialysis session. During the same period, the *peritoneal clearance* of creatinine and phosphorus were calculated as follows: the total daily peritoneal drainage volume was measured in a graduated cylinder, divided by the time in minutes ($t = 1440$ min) multiplied by the dialysate concentration of the solute to be studied and divided by the serum concentration. Peritoneal clearance was measured at a distance from peritonitis episodes.

Results

During the first 2 years of treatment by CAPD, mean residual renal function remained stable around 4 ml/min (Table 2). There was no significant decrease in urine output volume during the same period. Nineteen out of 22 patients received high doses of furosemide (375–125 mg/d) at start of CAPD treatment. At 1 year 16 out of 22 patients continued to receive furosemide at a similar dosage. The mean peritoneal clearances of creatinine or phosphorus measured during the training period and regularly at 6 months intervals remained stable. Values were not influenced by the incidence of peritonitis. Peritoneal protein losses remained stable at around 10 g/d.

Table 2 Residual renal function and peritoneal clearances in a group of 22 IDD patients treated by CAPD*

	Period (months)				
	1 (n = 22)	*6* (n = 22)	*12* (n = 22)	*18* (n = 12)	*24* (n = 8)
GFR (ml/min)	4.07 ± 1.23	4.52 ± 2.59	3.81 ± 2.31	3.61 ± 2.25	3.42 ± 2.7
Urine output (ml/day)	1100 ± 400	900 ± 540	850 ± 380	800 ± 400	750 ± 380
Furosemide (mg/day) (number of patients)	375 ± 125 (19)	325 ± 175 (18)	325 ± 175 (16)	350 ± 125 (8)	350 ± 125 (6)
Peritoneal creat. cl. (ml/min)	4.68 ± 1.53	4.42 ± 1.18	4.40 ± 1.30	4.08 ± 1.60	3.56 ± 1.60
Peritoneal phosph. cl. (ml/min)	3.93 ± 1.58	3.69 ± 1.25	4.11 ± 1.49	3.52 ± 1.68	3.02 ± 1.57
Peritoneal protein losses (g/day)	9.2 ± 2.5	9.8 ± 2.8	9.8 ± 2.6	9.5 ± 3.2	9.8 ± 3.6

* All values are expressed as mean ± SD. The difference evaluated by Student's *t*-test between each value at first and 12th months was not statistically significant
n = number of patients

In the haemodialysis group residual renal function and urine output gradually decreased. At 2 years 20 out of 34 patients were almost anuric (Table 3).

Table 3 Residual renal function in insulin-dependent diabetics treated by haemodialysis

	Period (months)			
	0 (n = 56)	*6* (n = 53)	*12* (n = 45)	*24* (n = 34)
GFR ml/min	4.3 ± 2.6	2.5 ± 2.2	1.8 ± 1.6	0.8 ± 0.8
Urine output ml/day	1300 ± 480	670 ± 420	400 ± 240	200 ± 220
No of patients receiving furosemide	52	48	33	14

n = number of patients
values are expressed as mean ± SD

Discussion

In dialysed patients the remaining function of the existing renal mass is important. It helps to maintain a good water and electrolyte balance without too rigid diet restrictions[8]. Although very few reports recording the evolution of GFR are available, a progressive decrease of the residual renal function and urine output during the first years of treatment by haemodialysis is a common finding[5,7]. Many factors such as hypertension and evolution of the original disease can participate in the rapid destruction of the renal function[6]. In diabetics one should expect an even more rapid deterioration because of the evolution of the microangiopathy and the frequent severity of the vascular disease[1]. Indeed in our own patients a rapid predialysis deterioration of renal function was observed, if one considers the rather short time (mean 24.5 ± 8.6 months) between the occurrence of a plasma creatinine level over 200 μmol/l and the start of dialysis therapy.

Determination of GFR in haemodialysed patients is difficult: creatinine clearance has been shown to be very close to insulin clearance at the low level of GFR observed in such patients, but rigid precautions dealing with the collection of urine and timing of blood samples are required[9]. The protocol followed in this study with plasma creatinine determination being made at the end of the urine collection period underestimates the GFR of the haemodialysis group. Nevertheless, this cannot explain in a given patient the rapid decrease of renal function. Indeed 20 out of 34 haemodialysed diabetic patients were anuric at 2 years.

Very little information is available on the evolution of residual renal function of diabetic patients treated by dialysis. On intermittent peritoneal dialysis Slingeneyer reported a marked decrease in GFR which was greater in IDD patients than in NID patients[10]. At 2 years the clearance rate was almost zero in IDD patients whereas it remained stable beyond the first year value (1.9–1.5 ml/min) in the NID group. Data from Amair *et al*[3] are different from ours because their patients entered the dialysis treatment with a mean creatinine clearance of 7.9–5.0 ml/min, almost the double of our own values. These authors have observed a progressive deterioration of the residual renal function with at 1 year a creatinine clearance of 3.1 ± 3.6 ml/min.

Our results in diabetic patients treated either by haemodialysis or CAPD are in full agreement with our previously reported observation in a non-diabetic population[7]. In haemodialysed patients hypotensive episodes during dialysis sessions, cyclical variations in body weight, instability of the haemodynamic status accelerate the deterioration of the renal function. Stable GFR at least during a 2 years period in patients treated by CAPD can on the contrary be related to the constant high plasma osmolality with stable high plasma urea concentration and to the absence of acute fluid shifts. A major factor could also be the routine administration of furosemide to most of our patients. Control series are required to analyse the true efficacy of the drug. In our experience the daily prescription of furosemide in haemodialysed patients does not always prevent the reduction of urine volume. Creatinine and phosphorus peritoneal clearances and protein losses remained stable during the period of observation and were not influenced by the rate of peritonitis episodes, in agreement with data from the literature[11-13].

It is too early to predict what will be the residual renal function and the peritoneal clearances of patients after many years of treatment by CAPD. We have already observed a slow deterioration of the GFR in the eight patients treated for at least 2 years, and in the three patients treated 3 years, creatinine clearance was only 2.8 ± 1.8 ml/min.

CONTROL OF BLOOD GLUCOSE LEVELS

The main goal of the management of a diabetic patient is the normalization of blood glucose with total correction of all metabolic abnormalities. Normal insulin production is usually defined by the profile of peripheral plasma insulin concentration observed throughout the day[14]. Such peripheral venous insulin profiles reflect, however, only a fraction of the original amount secreted by the pancreas since a large proportion of the insulin is removed from the portal circulation by the liver[15]. Therefore it is apparent that it is difficult to simulate normal insulin delivery by either subcutaneous or intramuscular routes. Of all the available methods of insulin delivery the intraperitoneal route is the only one that may achieve normal portal levels of insulin, while avoiding excessive peripheral levels. The intraperitoneal insulin administration introduced by Flynn[16] to treat diabetic patients on CAPD is now routinely used in numerous centres and favoured by most patients. To evaluate the advantages and limitations of various modalities of insulin administration through the peritoneal route the following investigations were performed.

KINETICS OF RESORPTION OF INTRAPERITONEALLY ADMINISTERED INSULIN

Our purpose was to evaluate the resorption kinetics of intraperitoneally (i.p.) injected insulin in CAPD patients with respect to two parameters: the presence or absence of dialysate in the peritoneal cavity and the dextrose concentration in the dialysate[17].

Patients and protocol

Nine IDD patients treated by CAPD were investigated after informed consent of the experimental procedure. Twenty units of regular neutral insulin were injected through the line and the Tenckhoff catheter after careful drainage of the previous dialysate exchange. Three different procedures were tested in each patient and performed in random order. In the first protocol, one injection was performed in the morning, one in the afternoon of the same day and one more the following morning. Each injection was followed by only 20 ml of isotonic saline solution (enough to flush out the dead space in the tubing). The peritoneal cavity was then left empty during the 180 minute study period. In the second protocol the injection of insulin was immediately followed by the infusion of a 2 l bag with a 1.5% dextrose concentration. This solution was left i.p. for 3 hours. In the third protocol the same procedure was followed using a 2 l bag with a 4.5% dextrose concentration. Blood samples were drawn from an indwelling catheter at regular intervals for 180 min, following the i.p. insulin administration. Plasma free insulin (PFI) was measured by radio-immunossay with a talcum powder separation. Statistical analysis used the Students's *t*-test for paired data.

Results

Figure 1 shows mean PFI levels in the three protocols. Basal values were similar: 6.2 ± 2.1 μU/ml (P1), 8.2 ± 2.9 μU/ml (P2), 6.2 ± 2.5 μU/ml (P3). In protocol 1, PFI levels rose sharply and attained the maximum value (55.6 ± 18.8 μU/ml) at 45 minutes. PFI levels then fell steadily to

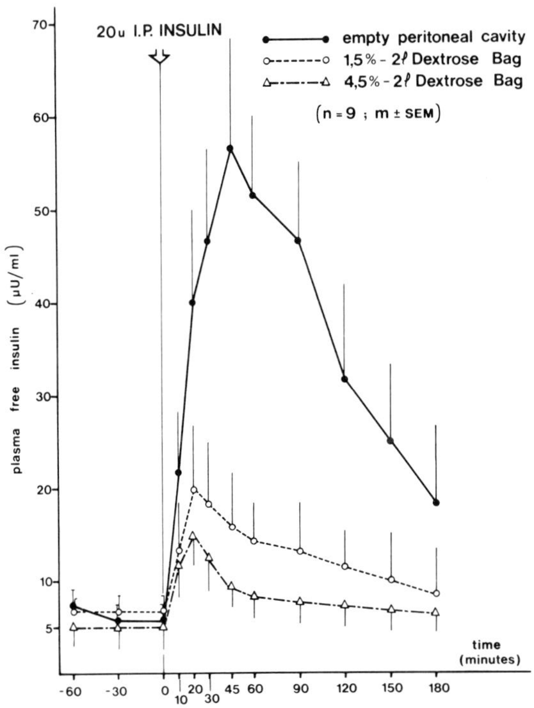

Figure 1 Mean plasma free insulin concentrations in 9 insulin-dependent diabetics receiving 20 U of insulin intraperitoneally immediately followed by instillation of either 2 l of 1.5% dextrose concentration dialysate, or 2 l of 4.5% dextrose concentration dialysate. Values are means ± SEM

17.5 ± 5.2 μU/ml at the end of 180 minutes. In protocol 2, PFI levels rose to a peak value of 20 ± 4.5 μU/ml at 20 minutes, then declined steadily to reach the end value of 9.8 ± 2.1 μU/ml. In protocol 3, a similar pattern was observed with a peak value of 15.5 ± 6.3 μU/ml. There were no statistical differences between procedures 2 and 3. Comparison between protocols 1, 2 and 3 shows significantly higher PFI in protocol 1 at 45, 60, 90 and 120 minutes ($p < 0.05$).

CONTROL OF POSTPRANDIAL BLOOD GLUCOSE LEVELS

In order to investigate the role played by the vacuity of the peritoneal cavity on the effect of i.p. administered insulin on blood glucose level a double protocol was performed in ten CAPD patients.

Patients and protocol

After careful drainage of the morning dialysate exchange two protocols were studied in a random order. The ten patients regularly treated by CAPD for a mean period of 6.2–1.7 months received the regular insulin (25 ± 8 Units) directly into the peritoneal cavity through the line. Each patient being his own control was asked to start eating after the instillation of insulin (controlled intake including carbohydrate 70 g, lipids 30 g, proteins 20 g). Study 1, 2 l of the dialysate with 1.5% dextrose concentration were introduced into the peritonal cavity immediately after the insulin injection. In study 2, the introduction of the same dialysate was performed after a delay of 30 minutes.

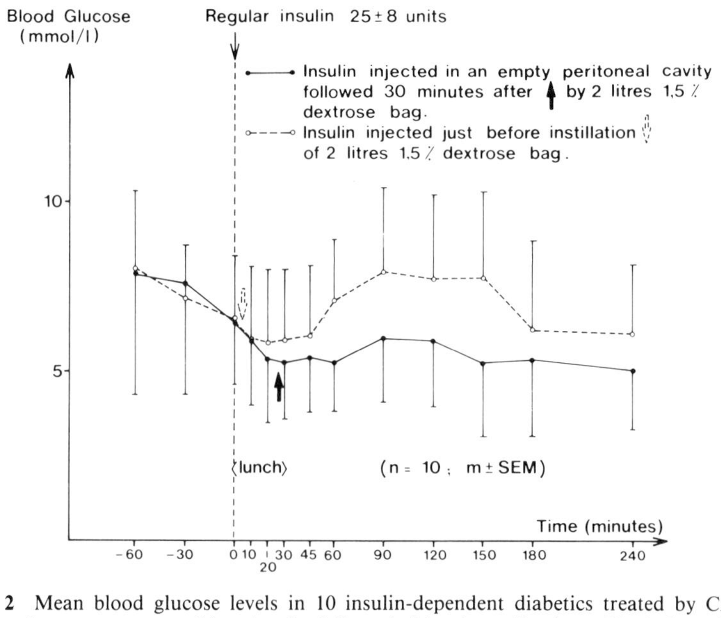

Figure 2 Mean blood glucose levels in 10 insulin-dependent diabetics treated by CAPD, receiving the same amount of i.p. insulin followed either immediately or 30 min later by the instillation of 2 l of 1.5% dextrose concentration dialysate. Values are means ± SEM

Blood samples were drawn at regular intervals for 240 minutes after the insulin administration and PFI levels were measured using the method previously described. Blood glucose levels were measured using a polarographic electrode (Yellow Spring Inst. Co, USA). Total insulin levels were also measured on two samples from the drainage fluid at the end of a 4 hours exchange.

Results

Blood glucose levels (Figure 2)

The basal values are similar in both studies (6.2 ± 2.1 mmol/l). In study 1, blood glucose levels rose progressively returning to the basal value after 240 minutes. In study 2, blood glucose levels decreased reaching the lowest value of 5.1 ± 1.4 mmol/l at 60 minutes and stabilizing around this value during the period of observation. The postprandial blood glucose levels were significantly higher at 60 minutes ($p < 0.01$), 90 minutes ($p < 0.02$), 120 minutes ($p < 0.02$)

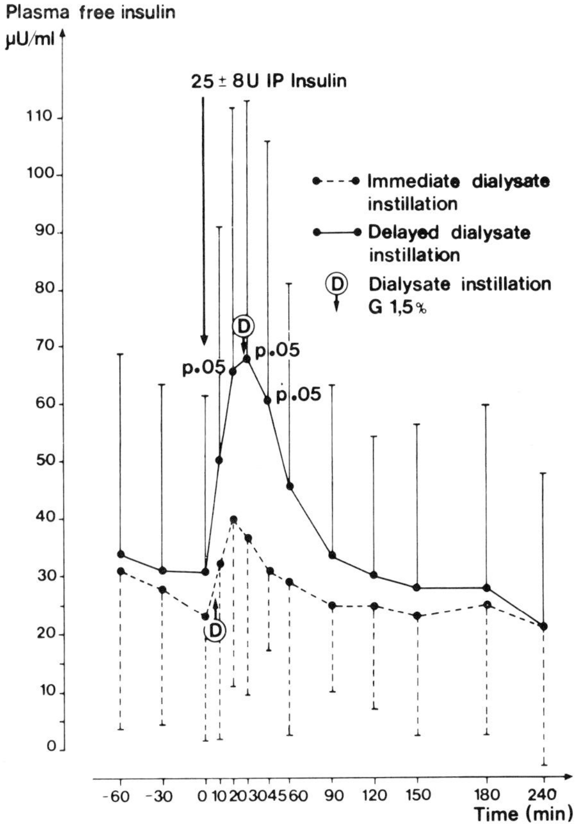

Figure 3 Mean plasma free insulin concentration of 10 insulin-dependent diabetics treated by CAPD receiving the same amount of i.p. insulin followed either immediately or 30 min later by the instillation of 2 l of 1.5% dextrose concentration dialysate. Values are means ± SEM

150 and 180 minutes ($p < 0.01$) in study 1 than in study 2. In the same manner the area under curves in study 1 (1240 ± 109 arbitrary units) was significantly higher than in study 2 (975 ± 90) ($p < 0.01$).

Plasma free insulin levels

Figure 3 shows mean plasma free levels during the 240 minutes of the study. In study 1 when the peritoneal cavity is immediately filled with the dialysate, PFI rose from the basal value of 23.5 ± 22 μU/ml to the highest value at 20 minutes of 39.5 ± 29 μU/ml and then decrease progressively. In study 2 when the peritoneal cavity was kept empty during 30 minutes, PFI rose rapidly from the basal value of 31.5 ± 35 μU/ml to the highest value of 67.8 ± 45 μU/ml at 30 minutes when the dialysate is instilled. PFI then decrease progressively. Both values in study 1 and 2 were similar at 240 minutes: 21.5 ± 27 μU/ml. PFI values were significantly higher in study 2 at 20, 30 and 45 minutes compared to the values of study 1 ($p < 0.05$).

Insulin recovery concentration in the drainage fluid

Insulin values in the bag at the end of the drainage period were measured in both studies. The total amount of insulin recovered was 6.7 ± 4 Units in study 1 and 4.2 ± 3.5 Units in study 2. We have no information on the amount of insulin adsorbed to the surface of the bag during the drainage period.

ROUTINE MODALITIES OF INSULIN ADMINISTRATION AND BLOOD GLUCOSE CONTROLS

Patients were advised to take a diet containing per day 1.2–1.5 g of protein and 2.8–3 g of carbohydrate intake per kg body weight. This diet was divided into three meals and an afternoon snack. Bags were exchanged just before each meal. Patients used routinely three 2 l bags with 1.5% dextrose concentration during the day and one 2 l bag with a 4.5% dextrose concentration overnight. Estimation of mean daily dextrose absorption through the peritoneal membrane was around 125 g and mean total daily carbohydrate intake including the oral and peritoneal route was around 285 g (Table 4). Mean daily caloric intake, all routes of administration included, was around 35 to 40 kcal per kg of body weight, half of which came from carbohydrate intake.

During training, patients' blood sugar was measured four times per day before changing the bag and occasionally 2 h after a meal. At home two controls were performed daily, one in the morning during fasting and the second before supper. Once a month a series of six readings were obtained. All controls are performed through fingerprick monitoring, the measures being made with a reflectance meter (Glucometer, Ames). Our goal was to obtain a fasting blood glucose level of less than 6 mmol/l and a postprandial blood glucose level of less than 10 mmol/l.

Insulin was administered exclusively through the intraperitoneal route

Table 4 Estimation of daily insulin requirement and daily carbohydrate intakes from food and dialysate in insulin-dependent diabetic patients treated by CAPD

	Timing of bag exchange and meals				
	7 am	12 am	4 pm	8 pm	*Total*
Dextrose concentration of the 2 l bag (%)	1.5	1.5	1.5	4.5	—
Routine dextrose absorption per 2 l bag (g)	25	20	20	60	125
Routine carbohydrate intake per meal (g)	30	70	20	40	160
Regular insulin routinely injected (U)	18	26	14	30	88

according to the following procedure: (1) drainage of the previous bag, (2) fingerprick control, (3) adjustment of the regular insulin dose, taking into account the dextrose concentration of the bag and the expected dextrose absorption, the carbohydrate intake of the meal, the value of the three last blood glucose controls performed at the same time, (4) setting of the new bag whose infusion line is kept clamped, (5) injection of the insulin through the injection site of the line followed by a 5 second flush with the dialysate to wash out the dead space of the tubing, (6) meal intake, the bag remaining clamped and (7) instillation of the dialysis at the end of the meal.

Timing and evaluation of the mean dose of insulin required daily is indicated in Table 4. The mean daily dose of insulin administered i.p. in the 20 patients treated at least 1 year was 87 ± 34 Units of regular insulin (*r.* 45–160 Units). This dose is 2.5 times higher than the subcutaneous dose of insulin used in the same patients before starting CAPD (mean daily dose 34 ± 12 Units).

Fasting blood glucose levels decreased during treatment with CAPD and at 1 year the mean values of all fasting measures performed in 9 patients treated by the protocol previously described were 5.8 ± 0.7 mmol/l.

The mean of 54 serial blood glucose determinations performed at home by ten patients was 7.32 ± 3.4 mmol/l at 8 am, 8.58 ± 3.4 mmol/l at 11 am, 8.38 ± 2.56 mmol/l at 2 pm, 8.47 ± 3.40 mmol/l at 6 pm, 7.41 ± 2.16 mmol/l at 8 pm, and 8.97 ± 2.84 mmol/l at 10 pm. The mean serum glycosylated haemoglobin ($HgbA_1$) in 22 patients dialysed for at least a year did not change significantly: 10.3 ± 2% at start of treatment and 9.6 ± 1.4% at 1 year (mean values in non-diabetic on CAPD is 8.6 ± 1.2% and 6.4 ± 0.8% in non-diabetic on HD).

DISCUSSION

Introduced by Flynn[16] the intraperitoneal administration of insulin during CAPD treatment is now routinely used in many contents, and considered as a form of artificial pancreas; some similarities exist between physiological insulin secretion and intraperitoneal insulin administration. In the non-diabetic, insulin is believed to be secreted into the portal vein in response to various secretogogues[15]. The peak blood insulin level is attained approximately 40 min after a carbohydrate load. Fifty per cent of the insulin secreted into the portal vein is removed as the blood flows through the liver. Because a large percentage of the i.p. administered insulin is in the portal vein, this route of administration mimics the physiological events.

Intraperitoneal administration of insulin is well favoured by the patients because it avoids subcutaneous injection. A potential risk of intraperitoneal insulin administration could be an increase of the incidence of peritonitis amongst diabetics but in our group[4] and in many others[3,16] the infection rates were similar or inferior to those observed in a non-diabetic population. Most dialysis units administer insulin directly into the dialysate bag and obtain excellent results[3]. This technique carries the risk that insulin could be partly adsorbed to the surface of polyvinyl chloride containers[18,19]. Nevertheless, recent studies by Twardowsky suggest that if the bag is vigorously agitated, adsorption of insulin to the surface of the bag does not exceed 5%[20].

The kinetics of i.p. injected insulin in diabetic patients treated by CAPD are in agreement with the experimental data from Shapiro[21] and Poulsen[22] and the clinical trial from Schade[23]. Our preliminary results suggest that the administration of the insulin, at least before meals, into an empty peritoneal cavity offers the highest PFI levels, and allows the best control of blood glucose level during the postprandial period. Such a procedure requires an injection site on the line and forces the patient to eat while the bag is being hung. The evaluation of the true advantages of injecting the insulin into an empty peritoneal cavity requires further controlled studies over a longterm period.

Good blood glucose control with intraperitoneal administration of insulin in diabetics on CAPD was reported in numerous recent studies[3,4,16,24–27]. The data strongly suggest that control of diabetes is actually better than that observed prior to dialysis. It should be noted that this improved control is possible only because the patient agrees to comply with frequent blood sugar monitoring.

The moderately high stable values of around 10% serum glycosylated haemoglobin ($HgbA_1$) should be interpreted with caution in uraemic patients. Elevated as well as low values of $HgbA_1$ fraction have been reported[28,29]. A significant fraction of $HgbA_1$ in chronically uraemic individuals may not be glycosylated haemoglobin but rather carbamylated, as a result of chronically elevated blood urea nitrogen levels[30]. This may be a factor involved among patients on CAPD, since these patients have high steady state values of blood urea nitrogen. In our department mean values of $HgbA_1$ in a non-diabetic population was 8 ± 1.2 in patients treated by CAPD and only 6.4 ± 0.8 in patients treated by haemodialysis. Mean value for non-diabetic and non-uraemic patients for our laboratory was $6.2 \pm 0.3\%$.

The clinical and biological status of most IDD patients treated by CAPD can be judged to be satisfactory. CAPD offers to these patients at high risk a unique opportunity to be dialysed at home. The success rate of CAPD technique within a period of 2 years compares favourably with any other replacement therapy if groups of the same age are compared. In our experience a persisting residual renal function of a few ml per minute at least at 2 years was a major contributing factor to the well-being of the patients. Intraperitoneal administration of insulin achieved good control of blood glucose levels. Administration of insulin in an empty peritoneal cavity 30 minutes before instillation of the dialysate seems to offer IDD patients treated by CAPD the most physiological route of intermittent insulin administration.

References

1. MacCrary, R.F., Pitts, T.O. and Puschett, J.B. (1981). Diabetic nephropathy natural course. Survivorship and therapy. *Am. J. Nephrol.,* **1,** 206
2. Jacobs, C., Rottembourg, J., Frantz, P., Slama, G. and Legrain, M. (1979). Treatment of end-stage renal failure in the insulin dependent diabetic patients. In Hamburger, J. *et al* (eds.). *Advances in Nephrology,* Vol. 8, p. 101 (Chicago: Year Book Medical Publishers)
3. Amair, P., Khanna, R., Leibel, B., Pierratos, A., Vas, S., Meema, E., Blair, G., Chisolm, L., Vas, M., Zingg, W., Digenis, G. and Oreopoulos, D.G. (1982). Continuous ambulatory peritoneal dialysis in diabetics with end-stage renal disease. *N. Engl. J. Med.,* **306,** 625
4. Rottembourg, J., El Shahat, Y., Agrafiotis, A., Thullier, Y., de Groc, F., Jacobs, C. and Legrain, M. (1983). Continuous ambulatory peritoneal dialysis in insulin dependent diabetic patients, a 40 months experience. *Kidney Int.,* **23,** 40
5. Milutinovic, J., Strand, M., Casaretto, A., Follette, W., Babb, A.L. and Scribner, B.H. (1974). Clinical impact of residual glomerular filtration rate (GFR) on dialysis time. A preliminary report. *Trans. Am. Soc. Artif. Intern. Organs,* **20,** 410
6. Milutinovic, J., Cutler, R.E., Hoover, P., Meijsen, B. and Scribner, B.H. (1975). Measurement of residual glomerular filtration rate in the patient receiving repetitive hemodialysis. *Kidney Int.,* **8,** 185
7. Rottembourg, J., Issad, B., Gallego, J.L., Degoulet, P., Aime, F., Gueffaf, B. and Legrain, M. (1982). Evolution of residual renal function in patients undergoing maintenance hemodialysis or continuous ambulatory peritoneal dialysis. *Proc. Eur. Dial. Transpl. Assoc.,* **19,** 397 (London: Pitman Medical)
8. Babb, A.L., Farrell, P.C., Strand, M.J., Uvelli, D.A., Milutinovic, J. and Scribner, B.H. (1972). Residual renal function and chronic hemodialysis therapy. *Proc. Dial. Transplant. Forum,* **2,** 142
9. Lubowitz, H., Slatopolsky, E., Shankel, S., Rieselbach, R.E. and Bricker, N.S. (1967). Glomerular filtration rate. Determination in patients with chronic renal disease. *J. Am. Med. Assoc.,* **199,** 252
10. Slingeneyer, A., Mion, C. and Selam, J.L. (1981). Home intermittent (IPD) and continuous ambulatory peritoneal dialysis (CAPD) as a long term treatment of end-stage renal failure in diabetics. In Gahl, G.M., Kessel, M. and Nolph, K.D. (eds.). *Advances in Peritoneal Dialysis,* pp. 378–388 (Amsterdam: Excerpta Medica)
11. Brown, E.A., Kliger, A.S. and Finkelstein, F.O. (1978). Peritoneal dialysis clearances. *Nephron,* **21,** 310

12. Rubin, J., Arfania, D., Nolph, K.D., Prowant, B., Fruto, L., Brown, P. and Moore, H. (1979). Peritoneal clearances after 6–12 months on continuous ambulatory peritoneal dialysis. *Trans. Am. Soc. Artif. Intern. Organs,* **25,** 104
13. Rubin, J., Nolph, K.D., Arfania, D., Brown, P. and Prowant, B. (1979). Follow up peritoneal clearances in patients undergoing continuous ambulatory peritoneal dialysis. *Kidney Int.,* **16,** 619
14. Porte, D. Jr. and Bagdade, J.D. (1970). Human insulin secretion. An integrated approach. *Annu. Rev. Med.,* **21,** 219
15. Eaton, R.P. and Schade, D.S. (1982). Normal human insulin secretion: the goal of management of the diabetic patient. In Peterson, C.M. (ed.). *Diabetes Management in the 80s,* p. 160. (New York: Praeger)
16. Flynn, C.T. and Nanson, J.A. (1979). Intraperitoneal insulin with CAPD. An artificial pancreas. *Trans. Am. Soc. Artif. Intern. Organs,* **25,** 104
17. Balducci, A., Slama, G., Rottembourg, J. Baumelou, A. and Delage, A. (1981). Intraperitoneal insulin in uraemic diabetics undergoing continuous ambulatory peritoneal dialysis. *Br. Med. J.,* **382,** 1021
18. Amidon, G., Reicher, J., Crutis, S.M. and Johnson, A. (1980). Absorption of insulin to the surface of polyvinyl chloride CAPD solution containers. *Proc. Dial. Transplant Forum,* **10,** 296
19. Widerboe, T.E., Smeby, L.C., Berg, K.J., Jopstag, S. and Svartas, T.M. (1981). Intraperitoneal (I 125) insulin absorption during intermittent and continuous peritoneal dialysis. In Gahl, G.M., Kessel, M. and Nolph, K.D. (eds.). *Advances in Peritoneal Dialysis,* pp. 369–370 (Amsterdam: Excerpta Medica)
20. Twardowsky, Z.J., Nolph, K.D., MacGary, T.J., Moore, H.L., Collin, P., Ausman, R.K. and Slimack, W.S. (1983). Insulin binding to plastic bags: methodological study. *Kidney Int.* (In press)
21. Shapiro, D.J., Blumenkrantz, M.J., Levin, S.R. and Coburn, J.M. (1979). Absorption and action of insulin added to peritoneal dialysate in dogs. *Nephron,* **23,** 174
22. Poulsen, J.S.D., Smith, M., Deckert, M. and Deckert, T. (1980). Comparison of intraperitoneal intraportal and intravenous insulin infusion. *Acta Endocrinol.,* **95,** 500
23. Schade, D.S., Eaton, P., Friedman, N. and Spencer, W. (1979). The intravenous intraperitoneal and subcutaneous routes of insulin delivery in diabetic man. *Diabetes,* **28,** 1069
24. Rottembourg, J., de Groc, F., Poignet, J.L. and Legrain, M. (1982). Is continuous ambulatory peritoneal dialysis the best dialysis choice for insulin dependent diabetics? *Proc. Eur. Dial. Transpl. Assoc.,* **19,** 215 (London: Pitman Medical)
25. Roscoe, J.M. (1982). Practices of insulin administration in CAPD. *Periton. Dial. Bull.,* **2,** (Suppl. 2), 27
26. Madden, M.A., Zimmerman, S.W. and Simpson, D.P. (1982). Continuous ambulatory peritoneal dialysis in diabetes mellitus, the risks and benefits of intraperitoneal insulin. *Am. J. Nephrol.,* **2,** 133
27. Flynn, C.T. (1983). The diabetic patient on CAPD. *Periton. Dial. Bull.,* (Suppl. 3), 16
28. de Baer, M.J., Miedema, K. and Casparie, A.F. (1980). Glycosylated hemoglobin in chronic renal failure. *Diabetology,* **18,** 437
29. Dandona, P., Freedman, D. and Moorhead, J.F. (1979). Glycosylated haemoglobin in chronic renal failure. *Br. Med. J.,* **1,** 1183
30. Fluckiger, R., Hamon, W., Meter, W., Loo, S. and Gabbay, K.H. (1981). Hemoglobin carbamylation in uremia. *N. Engl. J. Med.,* **304,** 823

21
Hormonal and metabolic adaptation to the glucose load of CAPD in non-diabetic patients

B. LINDHOLM, S. G. KARLANDER, H. E. NORBECK and J. BERGSTRÖM

ABSTRACT

During treatment with CAPD, 100–200 g of glucose per day are absorbed from the dialysate. This provides a substrate for increased production of triglycerides, stimulates insulin secretion and promotes anabolism. Prospective oral glucose tolerance tests indicate no further deterioration of (the uraemic) glucose intolerance, and insulin secretory capacity seems to remain unchanged during the first year of CAPD-treatment. The uraemic hyperlipidaemia and dyslipoproteinaemia is worsened during the initial 6–12 months, and is partly related to the peritoneal glucose load. However, the observed changes are transient in most of the patients. A decreased dietary intake of protein and calories is observed in many patients after 6–12 months. A possible explanation is that the continuous absorption of glucose affects the appetite of the patients. The decreased dietary intake of protein, together with the continuous losses of proteins (about 8 g per day) and amino acids (about 3 g/d) in the dialysate, may increase the risk for protein malnutrition in CAPD-patients after longterm treatment.

INTRODUCTION

The peritoneal dialysis solutions used in CAPD contain from 13.6 to 38.6 g/l of glucose. During CAPD large quantities of glucose are absorbed from the dialysate each day. This may provide a valuable source of energy to malnourished patients, but it may also cause further disturbances in the already abnormal uraemic metabolism of lipids, carbohydrates, proteins and amino acids.

In this paper we present results from a continuing prospective study of the metabolic effects of CAPD in non-diabetic patients with special regard to effects of the glucose load of CAPD.

GLUCOSE ABSORPTION FROM THE DIALYSATE

Glucose absorption from the dialysate was studied in 13 non-diabetic patients undergoing metabolic studies[1]. All patients exchanged 21 of dialysate four times per day. An average of 121 ± 40 g of glucose per day was absorbed each day representing an uptake of 71 ± 10% of the glucose instilled in the peritoneal cavity.

Grodstein *et al*[2] found that an average of 182 ± 61 g of glucose was absorbed each day. Most of their patients used five exchanges of dialysates per day. The percentage of the instilled glucose which was absorbed was almost the same as in our patients (72%). Baeyer *et al*[3] found that the mean daily absorption of glucose was 117 ± 14 g/d (four exchanges per day), while Keusch *et al*[4] have reported an uptake of 104 ± 8 g/d, and Splendiani *et al*[5] an average uptake of 156 g/d. Finally, De Santo *et al*[6] have reported an average uptake of 271 ± 5 g glucose per day (five exchanges per day).

In conclusion, these data show that under normal conditions most patients on CAPD absorb between 100 and 200 g glucose/day, depending on the number of exchanges per day, the number of hypertonic solutions and the rate of absorption in the individual patient.

GLUCOSE TOLERANCE DURING CAPD

Oral glucose tolerance tests with determination of radioimmune insulin and glucagon were performed in 18 non-diabetic patients before and after about 4 months on CAPD[7]. Glucose tolerance and insulin and glucagon response to the glucose load remained essentially unchanged after 4 months on CAPD. The glucose levels in the patients (areas under the glucose curve) were significantly higher in the patients as compared to healthy controls. Serum insulin and insulin response did not differ between patients and controls, whereas glucagon levels were significantly higher in the patients.

Glucose intolerance is common in uraemic patients and is mainly due to an impaired peripheral sensitivity to the action of insulin[8]. Glucose intolerance was also present in most of our patients. One potential hazard with CAPD is that the peritoneal glucose load could lead to a depletion of the pancreatic β-cells. This could create a diabetic state, which would add to the already impaired glucose tolerance in uraemia.

Our results, however, do not indicate any change in β-cell response after 4 months on CAPD, and when the investigations were repeated after 1 year on CAPD in 13 patients (unpublished observations) there was still no change. These results are in accordance with those of Baeyer *et al*[3], but in another study by Armstrong *et al*[9] a further deterioration in glucose tolerance as well as a decreased rate of insulin secretion was observed.

There are few reports concerning the effects of dialysate glucose load on plasma glucose and insulin levels in CAPD patients. Armstrong *et al*[10] have studied the effects of an exchange with 1.5% and 4.25% dialysate, respectively, and they found that plasma glucose and insulin levels increased above basal values only in the case of the 4.25% solutions. The authors concluded that if the use of hypertonic solutions is restricted there will be no continual stimulation of the pancreatic β-cells due to the dialysate glucose alone during CAPD. De Santo *et al*[6] and Splendiani *et al*[5] have found similar results, and also that glucagon levels decrease during a dwell with the 4.25% solution.

In conclusion, short term treatment with CAPD does not seem to lead to any further disturbances of the already abnormal glucose metabolism in uraemia, but the longterm effects are as yet unknown.

SERUM LIPID AND LIPOPROTEIN ABNORMALITIES

Serum lipids and lipoproteins were determined in 16 non-diabetic patients before CAPD, after about 4 months and after about 1 year on CAPD[11]. The determinations were performed after oral fast and with no exchanges of the dialysate 10–14 hours prior to the test. Intravenous fat tolerance tests (Intralipid®) and adipose tissue biopsies were performed before CAPD and after 1 year on CAPD. During the first 4 months the concentrations of serum and very low density lipoproteins (VLDL) triglycerides and cholesterol increased, but after 1 year the concentrations had returned to pretreatment levels in most of the patients. However, in four of the patients the triglyceride concentrations continued to rise. The increases in triglyceride concentrations were correlated to the daily amount of glucose in the instilled dialysate. High density lipoprotein (HDL)-cholesterol tended to increase during the initial 4 months, but after 1 year the levels returned to pretreatment levels, or even lower. There was a significant negative correlation between HDL cholesterol and VLDL triglyceride levels after 1 year. The fractional removal rate of Intralipid, expressed as $k2$%/min, was subnormal but did not change during the treatment. The mean diameter of adipose tissue cells increased during the treatment.

In our patients we found a significant negative correlation between changes in $k2$ values and changes in VLDL triglycerides before *vs.* after 1 year on CAPD. The findings that increases in the fractional removal rate of triglycerides are correlated to the changes in VLDL triglycerides may indicate that there was an increase of $k2$ in patients with stable or low triglyceride levels.

With the same interpretation some patients 'failed' to increase the fractional removal rate of exogenous triglycerides, and in these patients VLDL triglycerides remained high. This possible mechanism for adaptation, or lack of adaptation, may partly explain the large interindividual variations in triglyceride levels in patients with the same peritoneal glucose supply.

Uraemia is associated both with an increased prevalence of hypertriglyceridaemia and with several abnormalities in the lipoproteins: increased contents of triglycerides in the VLDL and LDL fractions, increased cholesterol in the VLDL fraction, and a decrease of cholesterol in the HDL fraction. This lipoprotein pattern, the uraemic dyslipoprotinaemia[12], has several features in common with both the Type IV and Type III phenotype according to Fredericksons's classification[13]. These abnormalities, which occur already at an early stage of the impairment of renal function, seem to persist in spite of haemodialysis treatment or treatment with protein restricted diets[12,14].

Our results indicate that the uraemic dyslipoproteinaemia persists, and in some respects (increased concentrations of serum and VLDL triglycerides and cholesterol) deteriorates during the initial 4 months of CAPD. These changes are partly related to the continuous glucose load. However, the changes seem to be transitory since the serum lipid levels return to pretreatment levels in most of the patients after 1 year on CAPD. Furthermore, investigations in six of the patients reveal that the mean lipid levels are essentially unchanged as compared with pretreatment levels, also after 2 years on CAPD.

In our patients the increases in serum cholesterol were even more marked than the increases in serum triglycerides although only a few of the patients developed hypercholesterolaemia. These changes may be due to an improved nutritional status of the patients with a normalization of previously low cholesterol levels. It has also been speculated whether the protein losses in the dialysis fluid may induce a hypercholesterolaemia, similar to that in the nephrotic syndrome[15]. However, Breckenridge *et al*[16] found little indication that the loss of lipoproteins or apolipoproteins could account for any changes in plasma lipoproteins.

Breckenridge *et al* also found an increase in HDL cholesterol levels in previously normolipidaemic patients, and Chan *et al*[17] have reported higher levels of HDL cholesterol in CAPD patients than in patients treated with haemodialysis. We have also compared HDL cholesterol levels in haemodialysis patients (after 1 year on dialysis) and CAPD patients (after 1 year) and we found no difference.

Khanna *et al* have[18] recently reported results which agree with our data, namely that serum triglycerides as well as cholesterol in all lipoprotein fractions tended to increase during the first 4–6 months. After 1 year these levels decreased again. Baeyer *et al*[3] found increased cholesterol levels and unchanged triglyceride levels after more than 6 months treatment. Keusch *et al*[4] found increases in both serum triglycerides, serum cholesterol and HDL cholesterol after 9 months on CAPD. Turgan *et al*[19] found increases in serum cholesterol levels but unchanged serum triglycerides in patients with restrictions of oral carbohydrate intake and a limited use of hypertonic solutions.

In conclusion, the hyperlipidaemic effects of CAPD seem to be transitory in most of the patients, which indicates metabolic adaptation to the glucose load and/or changes in energy intake, as discussed below.

CHANGES IN PROTEIN AND CALORIC INTAKE DURING CAPD

The dietary intake of protein, fat and carbohydrates in nine patients was assessed by our dietitian after about 4 and 12 months, respectively, on CAPD. Based on these assessments individualized balance diets were provided during metabolic balance studies[1]. The dietary intake of energy decreased from 34.6 ± 5.0 to $28.7\,kcal\,kg^{-1}\,day^{-1}$, and energy from glucose absorbed from dialysate decreased from 8.5 ± 2.9 to $6.4 \pm 1.9\,kcal\,kg^{-1}day^{-1}$. Dietary protein intake decreased from 1.46 ± 0.38 to $1.24 \pm 31\,g\,kg^{-1}\,day^{-1}$. $43.6 \pm 8.5\%$ and $42.7 \pm 5.1\%$, respectively, of the dietary energy intake was derived from carbohydrates. The corresponding figures for carbohydrates, when glucose absorbed from the dialysate was included, was $55.0 \pm 5.3\%$ and $53.2 \pm 3.5\%$, respectively.

These findings are similar to those reported by Williams *et al*[20] and by Baeyer *et al*[3]. Baeyer *et al* have suggested that the total carbohydrate intake in CAPD patients is regulated by a spontaneous decrease of the oral carbohydrate fraction in their nutrition, which could compensate for the peritoneal glucose absorption. This suggestion is supported by the relative low fraction of dietary energy derived from carbohydrates. A possible explanation is that the continuous absorption of glucose affects the appetite of the patients. The decrease in both dietary and total energy intake is probably one important factor behind the decrease in serum lipids after 2–6 months.

The decreased dietary intake of protein, together with the continuous losses of proteins (about 8 g/d) and amino acids (about 3 g/d) in the dialysate may increase the risk for protein malnutrition in CAPD patients after longterm treatment. In order to overcome this potential problem Oreopoulos *et al*[21,22] and Williams *et al*[23] from the Toronto group are performing clinical trials with substitution of amino acids for glucose as osmotic agent in peritoneal dialysis solutions.

ACKNOWLEDGEMENT

Part of this work was supported by a grant from the US National Institutes of Health (Grant No. 1R01 AM 27519-01A1).

References

1. Lindholm, B., Karlander, S.G., Norbeck, H.-E., Fürst, P. and Bergström, J. (1981). Efficacy and clinical experience of CAPD. In Atkins, R., Thomson, N. and Farrell, P. (eds.). *Peritoneal Dialysis,* pp. 147–161. (Edinburgh, London, Melbourne, New York: Churchill Livingstone)
2. Grodstein, G.P., Blumenkrantz, M.J., Kopple, J.D., Moran, J.K. and Coburn, J.W. (1981). Glucose absorption during continuous ambulatory peritoneal dialysis. *Kidney Int.,* **19,** 564
3. von Baeyer, H., Gahl, G.M., Riedinger, H., Borowzak, R., Rüdiger, A., Schurig, R. and Kessel, M. (1983). Adaptation of CAPD patients to the continuous peritoneal uptake. *Kidney Int.,* **23,** 29
4. Keusch, G., Bammatter, F., Mordasini, R. and Binswanger, U. (1981). Serum lipoprotein concentrations during continuous ambulatory peritoneal dialysis (CAPD). In Gahl, G.M., Kessel, M. and Nolph, K.D. (eds.). *Advances in Peritoneal Dialysis,* pp. 421–423. (Amsterdam, Oxford and Princeton: Excerpta Medica)
5. Splendiani, G., Acitelli, S., Albano, V., Gianforte, A. and Tancredi, M. (1981). Metabolic aspects of CAPD. In Gahl, G.M., Kessel, M. and Nolph, K.D. (eds.). *Advances in Peritoneal Dialysis,* pp. 449–451. (Amsterdam, Oxford and Princeton: Excerpta Medica)
6. De Santo, N.G., Capodicasa, G., Senatore, R., Cicchetti, T., Cirillo, D., Damiano, M., Torella, R., Gingliano, D., Improta, L. and Giordano, C. (1979). Glucose utilization from dialysate in patients on continuous ambulatory peritoneal dialysis (CAPD). *Int. J. Artif. Organs,* **2,** 119
7. Lindholm, B., Bergström, J. and Karlander, S.G. (1981). Glucose metabolism in patients on continuous ambulatory peritoneal dialysis (CAPD). In Gahl, G.M., Kessel, M. and Nolph, K.D. (eds.). *Advances in Peritoneal Dialysis,* pp. 413–416. (Amsterdam, Oxford and Princeton: Excerpta Medica)
8. DeFronzo, R.A. and Alvestrand, A. (1980). Glucose intolerance in uremia: site and mechanism. *Am. J. Clin. Nutr.,* **33,** 1438
9. Armstrong, V.W., Buschmann, E.R., Fuchs, C., Rieger, J. and Scheler, F. (1980). Biochemical investigations of CAPD: plasma levels of trace elements and amino acids and impaired glucose tolerance during the course of treatment. *Int. J. Artif. Organs,* **3,** 237
10. Armstrong, V.W., Fuchs, C. and Schelder, F. (1981). Effect of dialysate glucose load on plasma glucose and insulin levels in CAPD patients. In Gahl, G.M., Kessel, M. and Nolph, K.D. (eds.). *Advances in Peritoneal Dialysis,* pp. 421–423. (Amsterdam, Oxford and Princeton: Excerpta Medica)
11. Lindholm, B., Karlander, S.G., Norbeck, H.-E. and Bergström, J. (1982). Glucose and lipid metabolism in peritoneal dialysis. In la Greca, G., Biasioli, S. and Ronco, C. (eds.). *Peritoneal Dialysis,* pp. 217–230. (Milano: Wichtig Editore)
12. Norbeck, H.E. and Carlson, L.A. (1981). The uremic dyslipoproteinemia: Its characteristics and relations to clinical factors. *Acta Med. Scand.,* **209,** 489
13. Norbeck, H.E. (1982). Lipoprotein metabolism in chronic renal failure. In Noseda, G., Fragiacomo, C., Fumagalli, R. and Paoletti, R. (eds.). *Lipoproteins and Coronary Atherosclerosis,* pp. 337–342. (Amsterdam: Elsevier Biomedical Press B.V.)
14. Norbeck, H.E., Orö, L. and Carlson, L.A. (1976). Serum lipid and lipoprotein concentrations in chronic uremia. *Acta Med. Scand.,* **200,** 487
15. Gokal, R., Ramos, J.M., McGurk, J.G., Ward, M.K. and Kerr, D.N.S. (1981). Hyperlipidaemia in patients on continuous ambulatory peritoneal dialysis. In Gahl, G.M., Kessel, M. and Nolph, K.D. (eds.). *Advances in Peritoneal Dialysis,* pp. 430–433. (Amsterdam, Oxford and Princeton: Excerpta Medica)
16. Breckenridge, W.C., Roncari, D.A.K., Khanna, R. and Oreopoulos, D.G. (1982). The influence of continuous ambulatory peritoneal dialysis on plasma lipoproteins. *Atherosclerosis,* **45,** 249
17. Chan, M.K., Chuah, P., Raftery, M.J., Baillod, R.A., Sweny, P., Varghese, Z. and Moorhead, J.F. (1981). Three years' experience of continuous ambulatory peritoneal dialysis. *Lancet,* **ii,** 1409
18. Khanna, R., Breckenridge, C., Roncari, D., Digenis, G. and Oreopoulos, D.G. (1983). Lipid abnormalities in patients undergoing continuous ambulatory peritoneal dialysis. *Perit. Dial. Bull.,* (Suppl.), **3,** 13

19. Turgan, C., Feehally, J., Bennet, S., Davies, T. J. and Walls, J. (1981). Accelerated hypertriglyceridemia in patients on continuous ambulatory peritoneal dialysis - A preventable abnormality. *Int. J. Artif. Organs,* **4,** 158
20. Williams, P., Kay, R., Harrison, J., McNeil, K., Petitt, J., Kelman, B., Mendez, M., Ogilvie, R., Khanna, R., Carmichael, D. and Oreopoulos, D. G. (1981). Nutritional and anthropometric assessment of patients on CAPD over one year: contrasting changes in total body nitrogen and potassium. *Perit. Dial. Bull.,* **1,** 82
21. Oreopoulos, D. G., Grassweller, P., Katitzoglou, A., Ogilvie, R., Zellerman, G., Rodella, H. and Vas, S. I. (1980). Amino acids as an osmotic agent (instead of glucose) in continuous ambulatory peritoneal dialysis. In Legrain, M. (ed.). *Continuous Ambulatory Peritoneal Dialysis,* pp. 335–340. (Amsterdam, Oxford, Princeton: Excerpta Medica)
22. Oreopoulos, D. G., Marliss, E., Anderson, G. H., Oren, A., Dombros, N., Williams, P., Khanna, R., Rodella, H. and Brandes, L. (1983). Nutritonal aspects of CAPD and the potential use of amino acid containing dialysis solutions. *Perit. Dial. Bull.,* (Suppl.), **3,** 10
23. Williams, P. F., Marliss, E. B., Anderson, G. H., Oren, A., Stein, A. N., Khanna, R., Petitt, J., Brandes, L., Rodella, H., Mupas, L., Dombros, N. and Oreopoulos, D. G. (1982). Amino acid absorption following intraperitoneal administration in CAPD patients. *Perit. Dial. Bull.,* **2,** 124

22
The treatment of renal failure in diabetic patients – the best buy

M. LEGRAIN, J. ROTTEMBOURG, G. M. GAHL, A. BENTCHIKOU and P. STRIPPOLI

ABSTRACT

A recent explosion in the acceptance of diabetic patients with end-stage renal diseases (ESRD) for dialysis and transplantation is observed in all of the industrialized countries. Results of treatment are improving but diabetic patients remain at a high risk.

A critical appraisal of the literature and of data collected amongst the 108 insulin-dependent diabetics with ESRD treated in La Pitié Hospital between 1973 and 1983, including 67 treated by haemodialysis (HD) of whom 11 were transplanted and 38 treated by continuous ambulatory peritoneal dialysis (CAPD), illustrates the advantages and shortcoming of all modes of kidney replacement therapy to be offered to diabetics within an integrated programme of treatment of end-stage renal failure.

In Europe, because of the shortage of cadaver donor and the few living donor transplantations performed, most of the diabetics with ESRD are offered dialysis methods, at least for a while. Centre haemodialysis remains too often the sole form of therapy available. CAPD with intraperitoneal delivery of insulin offers excellent control of hyperglycaemia, but the dropout rate remains high. Prevention of severe infections, vascular and eye complications rely partly on better control of hyperglycaemia and hypertension before and after renal replacement therapy, and require close collaboration between the diabetologist, nephrologist and practitioner to offer the patient the best buy.

INTRODUCTION

Diabetic nephropathy is the only significant growing cause of end-stage renal disease (ESRD) in all of the industrialized countries. Recent data from the literature[1–4] and those presented in this Symposium clearly demonstrate that the exclusion of diabetic patients from renal function replacement therapy is no longer acceptable when treatment facilities are available. Indeed there has recently been an explosion in the acceptance of such patients for treatment. Currently in some regions of the United States 25% of all patients treated with dialysis or transplantation are diabetics[5,6]. In Europe the most recent data coming from the European Dialysis and Transplantation Association (EDTA) registry show the same trend[7]. In 1981 close to 1200 new diabetic patients were put on either a dialysis or a transplantation programme in Europe[8]. In France during 1982 more than 6% of all patients with ESRD on treatment were diabetic. A steady improvement of results of treatment of diabetic patients with ESRD has been observed with all methods of treatment during the last 10 years[9–13]. Nevertheless, if one considers patients of the same age group over a period of 4 years, diabetics are at a higher risk for any therapy compared to non-diabetics because of an increased frequency of septic, vascular and metabolic complications.

More diabetic patients to treat and trying to offer them longer survival, decreased morbidity and better rehabilitation are the difficult and stimulating challenges offered to the nephrology community in the coming years until the full prevention of the nephropathy in most diabetics becomes a reality.

What are the facts and the trends of the treatment of renal failure in diabetic patients in early 1983?

APPRAISAL OF THE RESULTS OF THE LITERATURE

A valid comparison of results obtained in a diabetic population with the different treatments available remains difficult because of the great heterogeneity of the populations studied[3,11,12].

Until recently in most countries, diabetic patients with ESRD were excluded from treatment. This explains that the series reported are sometimes small with too short a follow-up. The steady improvement of results for the last 15 years[1,10,11] calls for the comparison of data collected during the same period.

The choice of mode of renal replacement therapy is largely influenced by the medical team's experience and preference, as well as by the technical facilities available in a given country or even region. Both the lack of cadaver transplant and adequate centre haemodialysis facilities can lead to the restriction of transplantation to younger candidates, a positive selection and the proposal of CAPD to the desperate causes, a negative selection.

For obvious reasons the patients of different groups are often different as far as age, type of diabetes, severity of ocular or vascular lesions and social conditions are concerned.

Despite these difficulties a rational approach to what each technique or renal replacement can offer to a given patient is already possible.

Transplantation

After a 10 year experience of renal transplantation with diabetics, Bryngér and Larsson do not hesitate to consider that patients with diabetes 'constitute one of the largest group of patients in need of kidney transplantation'[9]. The recent report of Sutherland *et al*[14] on the current status of kidney transplantation in uraemic diabetics at the University of Minnesota illustrates the remarkable improvement of both patient survival and graft survival observed from 1968 to 1981 in a very large experience dealing with 425 uraemic diabetics who received a primarily renal allograft. If one considers the late era (1979–81), excellent results are obtained not only among young diabetics receiving grafts from a related donor. A graft survival at 2 years of around 80% is even observed in diabetics over 40 years old as well as in those receiving transplants from cadaver donors. The authors concluded in the following manner: 'Our recent results indicate that the diabetic should no longer be considered a high risk patient for transplantation by any definition either in relation to alternative therapy or in relation to non diabetics'. A similar opinion is shared by F. Belzer *et al*[15] reviewing their large experience in Madison despite the fact that if graft survival rate at 2 years is around 80% when the transplant comes from a related donor the rate drops to 40% when the graft comes from a cadaver!

Quality of life with a functioning graft is usually considered by all groups to be superior to that of other forms of treatment for most patients. Nevertheless, if vision is often improved, morbidity remains high. Complications, mainly of vascular origin, are more frequent than in a non-diabetic population. A high rate of amputation, between 15 and 20% of the patients, was reported after transplantation by different groups[13,15].

The encouraging results observed with transplantation should not make one forget that the shortage of donors is a major handicap for transplanting all candidates within a short time. This situation is particularly critical in Europe where for ethical reasons living donor transplantation remains exceptional and where the number of patients on the waiting list for cadaver kidney transplantation is regularly increasing. Whatever the quality of the results after transplantation, the majority of diabetic patients with ESRD will be treated by a dialysis method for many more years.

Haemodialysis

Many physicians remain impressed by the disillusioned paper of Ghavanian *et al* published in 1972[16] commenting 'on the sad truth about haemodialysis in diabetic nephropathy' and the gloomy experience of more recent reports[17]. However, survival rates have improved progressively during the past 15 years as shown in the 1981 update of haemodialysis in diabetics by Shapiro and Comty[13]. A comparison of dialysis and transplantation in insulin-dependent diabetic patients made by the same group, based on data collected from American and European registries[18] shows that the third year patient survival of a large series of patients with insulin-dependent diabetes is around 60% with a functioning transplant from a cadaver and around 50% for patients treated by haemodialysis. The trends of the recently published survival rates allows one to hope for an 80% survival at 2 years for insulin-dependent diabetics of less than 50 years of age treated by haemodialysis.

Improvements also concern the quality of life. If vascular problems including severe and frequent hypotension during dialysis, malnutrition with gastrointestinal disorders, hyperkalaemia, sometimes lethal, are still encountered, blindness is no longer inevitable in haemodialysed patients and vision can improve markedly mainly because of satisfactory control of metabolism and blood pressure[19,20].

If one wants to treat all diabetic patients with ESRD, large centre haemodialysis facilities are required. Haemodialysis will be used as a first choice treatment for some patients, for others as a temporary treatment while waiting for a transplant and as the only readily available mode of therapy when peritoneal dialysis, either intermittent or continuous, fails.

Continuous ambulatory peritoneal dialysis (CAPD)

This technique introduced by Popovitch, Moncrief and Nolph[21] was proposed in recent years as a valuable alternative to haemodialysis for insulin-dependent diabetics. Very encouraging results have been reported and authors have underlined[22-25] the high survival rate, the good quality of life at least for a majority of patients, the achievement of an excellent control of blood glucose using the intraperitoneal route for administration of insulin as proposed by Flynn[26]. Stabilization or even improvement of the visual status has been reported[22,25]. In some units a special training programme can offer, to motivated blind patients, the opportunity to take care of themselves[27]. Finally the peritonitis rate is not superior and sometimes inferior[22,24,25] to what is observed in a non-diabetic population.

Nevertheless, one should be careful before making valid comparisons between CAPD and other modes of therapy used to treat diabetics. All series published dealing with insulin-dependent diabetics are small with, excluding the collaborative study of Toronto[28], a total number of patients always below 30 and often less than 10. Either a positive selection or a negative selection makes comparison of published results very difficult. In some cases a large proportion of the patients on the CAPD programme are young juvenile diabetics waiting for a transplant, while in other programmes CAPD is offered to older diabetics in whom home dialysis seems indicated or to patients transferred if not excluded from haemodialysis because of severe vascular disease.

If advantages of the method are emphasized the shortcomings should not be forgotten. Some of the older patients as well as most of the cases with partial or total blindness will never handle the technique properly, and the burden of the daily exchange is difficult to impose on relatives. Protein malnutrition favoured by protein losses through the drainage fluid, and or excessive weight-gain due to high glucose absorption from the dialysate can require the transfer to another form of therapy in order to avoid lethal complications. On a long-term range a decreasing ultrafiltration rate already observed in a few cases can lead to oedema and overuse of 4.25 dextrose concentration bags.

For the moment CAPD has proved to offer to some diabetic patients excellent treatment, perhaps the best, but cannot be considered as the exclusive technique for this high risk population, nor should it be the ultimate solution for obviously desperate situations.

Improvement of this new method is still expected, for example, in the field of prevention of peritonitis and loss of ultrafiltration. The definite evaluation of CAPD in diabetic as in non-diabetic patients requires a longer period of follow-up.

Other forms of peritoneal dialysis

Intermittent peritoneal dialysis

IPD has major limitations such as the duration of dialysis time, between 30–40 hours per week, much longer than with HD, and the high cost of the reverse osmosis machine. Nevertheless, encouraging results have been reported in the treatment of both juvenile diabetes and non-insulin-dependent diabetes using either an automatic cycler or a reverse osmosis machine[29-31]. The results, to our knowledge, of the largest series of the literature reported by Slingeneyer *et al*[31] are quite encouraging. They stress the possibility of using the technique at home even in diabetics with physical disabilities resulting from visual impairement, cardiovascular complication, or diabetic neuropathy. The actuarial survival rate at 3 years was 89% among the insulin-dependent juvenile diabetics but only 40% in the older group of non-insulin-dependent diabetics associated with their high death rate from cardiovascular complications.

At home, IPD can be a valuable alternative to HD, the sessions being performed during the night. IPD should be considered in centres if HD is either impossible or at very high risk because of vascular access or vascular instability during session.

Cycling continuous peritoneal dialysis

CCPD using an automatic cycler has developed recently[32,33], and to our knowledge even small series of diabetic patients treated by CCPD have not yet been reported. Preliminary results indicate that the technique offers adequate ultrafiltration and is comparable to IPD and CCPD in maintaining biological values within an acceptable range. The potential advantages, besides a decreased peritonitis rate, are the reduced number of connections and the possibility of pursuing normal activities during the day, the cycler doing the exchanges overnight.

We consider that CCPD could be an excellent alternative to CAPD for diabetic patients who for different reasons, mainly visual impairement, cannot handle the technique themselves. CCPD can offer adequate care to the patient without overtaxing the dialysis partner, and this has been our positive experience with three diabetic patients treated by CCPD as a first choice.

THE EXPERIENCE OF THE HOPITAL DE LA PITIE

Patients and methods of treatment

Between January 1973 and March 1983, a total of 108 insulin-dependent diabetic (IDD) patients with a mean age of 46 ± 13.5 years have been treated by dialysis methods and/or kidney transplantation in the Hôpital de La Pitié (Table 1). Sixty seven patients with a mean age of 41 years (range 20–66) have been treated by haemodialysis. The cumulative duration of HD treatment was 167 patient-years. HD was the first choice treatment in 64 patients. Thirty eight patients with a mean age of 52 years (range 22–76) have been on CAPD since August 1978[25]. We include in this group four patients on CCPD. The cumulative duration of treatment was 47 patient-years. Seven patients were transferred to HD because of abdominal complication in four and chronic malnutrition with a decrease of ultrafiltration in three. One case was transferred from CAPD because of personal convenience. Three cases were treated by CCPD as a first choice. Since July 1978, CAPD has been the first choice treatment for a majority of our IDD patients treated by dialysis.

Table 1 Hôpital de la Pitié, Paris – 108 insulin dependent diabetics with ESRD choice of dialysis method

	HD	*IPD*	*CAPD*	*CCPD*	*TOTAL*
1973	9	—	—	—	9
1975–76	13	1	—	—	14
1977–78	16	2	1	—	19
1979–80	19	—	13	—	32
1981–82	9	—	18	4	31
1983	1	—	2	—	3
Total	67	3	34	4	108

HD = haemodialysis, IPD = intraperitoneal dialysis, CAPD = continuous ambulatory peritoneal dialysis, CCPD = cycling continuous peritoneal dialysis

Three patients, aged 55, 63, 73, were *treated by intermittent peritoneal dialysis* during a cumulative period of 4.3 patient years between 1975–1978.

Thirteen patients have received a *transplant*, in three cases from a related donor and in 10 cases from a cadaveric donor. The cumulative duration of treatment was 27 patient-years. Two patients died of infection. One patient was back to HD after rejection.

Survival rate

The actuarial survival rate of the 108 IDD patients, all methods of treatment included, is 80% at 1 year, 65% at 2 years and 50% at 4 years (Figure 1). Such results are quite encouraging if one takes into consideration the period under study (1973–1983) and the mean age, 46 years.

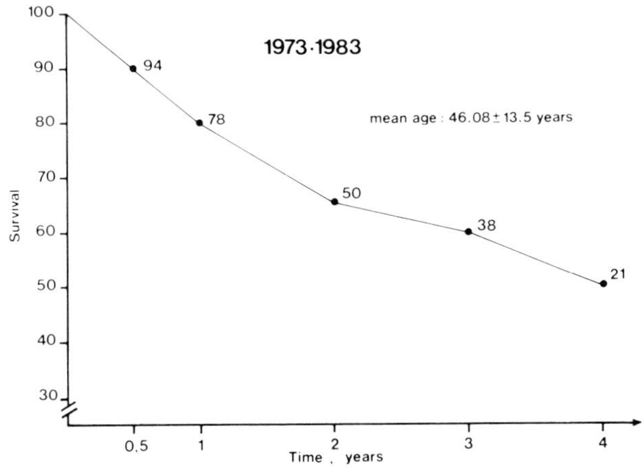

Figure 1 Actuarial survival rate of the 108 IDD patients with ESRD treated by dialysis (all methods included) and transplantation between January 1973 and March 1983

The influence of age and of the period considered on the survival rate of IDD patients treated by dialysis methods in this series is obvious. In Figure 2 one can see that the actuarial survival rate at 2 years is 72% in the group of 63 patients treated by HD and CAPD with an age under 50 y and a mean age of

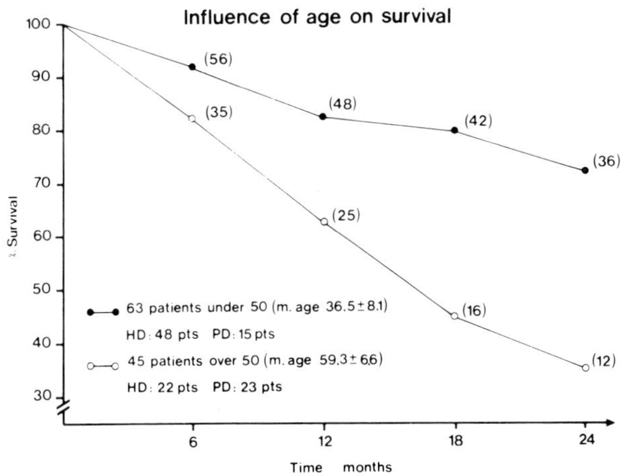

Figure 2 Actuarial survival rate of patients treated by haemodialysis and peritoneal dialysis in relation with age

36.5 ± 8.1 and only 35% in the group of 45 patients over 50 y and a mean age of 59.3 ± 6.6. If one considers the era of treatment, Figure 3 illustrates that the actuarial survival rate at 2 years of patients exclusively treated by HD increased from 56% to 68% for patients respectively dialysed between 1973–1978 and 1978–1983, despite a similar mean age, respectively 43 and 42 years.

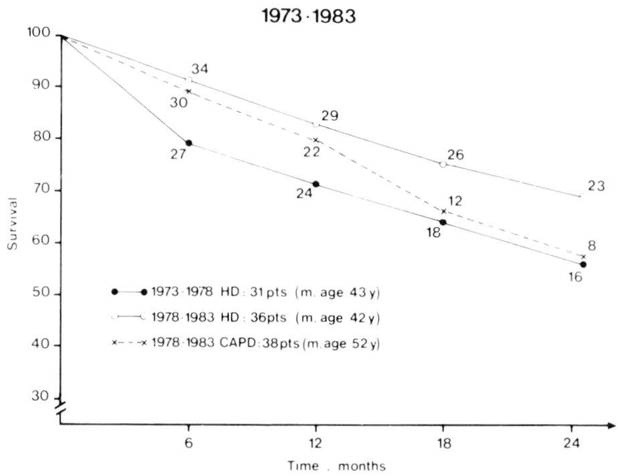

Figure 3 Actuarial survival rate with maintenance on either haemodialysis or CAPD and CCPD. Relation with the era of treatment for patients treated by haemodialysis

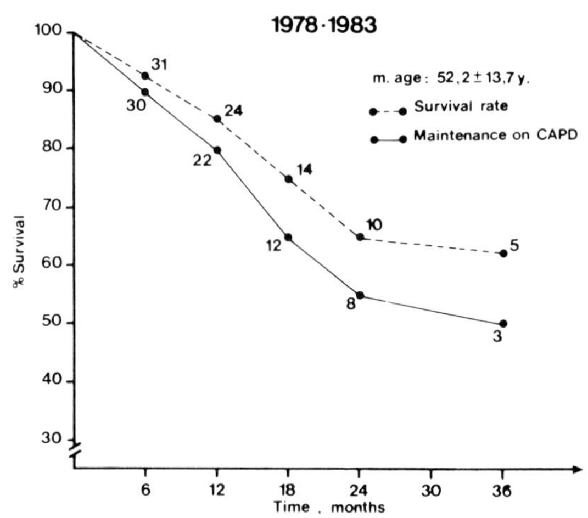

Figure 4 Actuarial rates in 38 diabetics treated by peritoneal dialysis, 34 on CAPD and 4 on CCPD

The actuarial survival maintenance rates on CAPD are respectively 85 and 80% at 1 year and 65 and 55% at 2 years (Figure 4). In this one centre experienced in offering the patients all forms of therapy the results of treatment by CAPD at 1 and 2 years compare favourably with treatment by HD during the same period (Figure 3) if one considers a mean age of 52 years for patients on CAPD and only 41 years for patients on HD. After 2 years the number of patients treated by CAPD is too small to draw any conclusion.

Causes of death

They are summarized in relation to the method of treatment in Table 2. Vascular complications including cerebral accident, myocardial infarction and arteritis appear as the main cause of death, 25 cases out of 51. One should underline the high rate of deaths observed both among patients treated by HD and CAPD related to severe arteritis leading to gangrene of the extremities and septicaemia. Twice the complications occurred in a superior limb following an attempt to create a vascular access. Patients on HD are at a higher risk of hyperkalaemia because of acute variation of blood glucose level and blood pH favoured by intermittent dialysis. Peritonitis, once in relation to a perforated bowel, was the cause of death among patients on CAPD in four cases.

Table 2 Hôpital de la Pitié, Paris - causes of death in IDD patients January 1973–March 1983 - 108 new cases

	HD	*PD*	*TRANS.*	*TOTAL*
Cer. vas. acc.	4	2	—	6
Myoc. infarction	4	4	—	8
Arteritis + sepsis	7	4	—	11
Sepsis	6	1	2	9
Peritonitis	—	4	—	4
Hyperkalaemia	3	—	—	3
Malnutrition	3	—	—	3
Cessation of treat.	4	1	—	5
Other causes	4	1	—	5
Total/Patients treated	35/67	17/41	2/13	54/108

HD = haemodialysis, PD = peritoneal dialysis, trans. = transplantation

From data of the literature and our own experience we are convinced that the encouraging results already obtained in a large group of IDD patients at high risk because of the age and the severity of the vascular disease can be progressively improved in the coming years if a careful strategy is developed.

STRATEGY FOR THE BEST BUY

To offer each patient the best buy requires a careful and adequate strategy based on a close collaboration between the practitioner and the specialists. For all diabetics as for patients with ESRD, good medical care relies on the successful education of the patient as well as on the confidence between the patient, his relatives, the nurses and the medical team. In some situations, psychological advice can be helpful to the patients and to the physicians.

The growing number of diabetic patients to be treated demands that many dialysis and transplantation units, if not all, accept the care of insulin or non-insulin-dependent diabetics. If experience can indeed contribute to the better care, this experience should be transferred through training programmes to a larger number of units so that diabetic patients could find adequate facilities within a reasonable distance of their home.

The predialysis and transplantation medical care

This is essential if one wants to avoid the severe complications, mainly ocular and vascular, which will jeopardize the future results. This delicate period requires close collaboration between all specialists and the general practitioner in charge of the patient. A medical 'task force' is required to offer the patient the best medical care concerning blood glucose and blood pressure control, treatment of eye lesions, correction of metabolic and electrolyte disturbances. Great attention should be paid to explain to the patients that progression of renal insufficiency imposes modifications of the treatment including insulin dosage and routine controls. One can expect from preliminary data[34] that such medical care will slow down the decreasing rate of the renal function and prevent some serious vascular and ocular complications.

The predialysis and transplantation check up

The purpose is to decide which mode of replacement therapy will be considered as the first choice, and to prepare the patient for the treatment selected. Because of the rapid progression of the kidney disease and of the difficulties frequently encountered with vascular access in diabetic patients, we believe that the investigations should take place when the creatinine clearance is between 15 and 10 ml/min. We prefer to rely on the creatinine clearance rather than on plasma creatinine because of large variations of the muscle mass in diabetic patients.

The best buy policy requires that all modes of replacement therapy be available within an integrated programme of treatment of ESRD either in the same unit or in close collaboration with other departments.

Numerous specialized investigations dealing with the vascular status, the gastrointestinal and urinary tract and the eye lesions all can be required to help make the decision. The advantages and shortcomings of all methods with their medical, psychological and social consequences should be carefully discussed with the patient and his relatives.

If haemodialysis is selected as the first choice treatment, vascular access should be performed as early as possible, while taking adequate precautions[11,13].

Transplantation

Because excellent results, as far as survival rate and quality of life are concerned, were reported in the most recent years, transplantation should be considered as the treatment of choice at least in the juvenile diabetics less than 40 years old. Such patients should be investigated early for transplantation, if possible before overt peripheral vascular complication and advanced neuropathy. Blindness is not considered a contra-indication for transplantation[9,12].

If a related living donor, for example one of the parents or adult HLA identical siblings wished to donate and is accepted after careful medical and psychological investigation, transplantation should be performed as soon as the creatinine clearance is around 10 ml/min, to avoid dialysis treatment. Such a situation is seldom encountered in Europe where transplantation from relatives raises many ethical problems.

Transplantation from a cadaver donor, despite less favourable results than those from a living related donor remains in most cases the only choice. The shortage of cadaveric donors, the time devoted to performing numerous investigations and treatment including the pretransplantation transfusion protocols will require in many cases that the dialysis treatment is started while the patient waits for a transplant. If home dialysis is considered suitable, CAPD can be selected as a first choice. This technique does not eliminate the chance of a successful transplantation[22,27] and can later be used to control uraemia in case of rejection. In some patients IPD can be a reasonable alternative. If on the other hand, the patient must be dialysed in a centre, haemodialysis should be considered as the first choice.

In patients over 40 years or with many invalidating complications including peripheral arteritis one should be very cautious before proposing transplantation instead of the dialysis methods. As long as the shortage of cadaveric transplants persist one must pay great attention in offering the best to every one and thus not waste a potential graft by giving a transplant to patients presenting too high a risk.

The choice of the dialysis method

Once transplantation has been excluded as the first choice, the main question to discuss is where should the patient be dialysed, taking into account his medical problems as well as his psychological, familial and social environment. The appropriate decision requires a careful investigation, including long conversations with the patient and the relatives.

To offer greater independence at lower costs *home dialysis* should be routinely evaluated and all such methods considered. If the patient is able to handle the technique of the CAPD himself we select this method as a first choice because of its efficacy and simplicity. The CAPD technique does not require any machinery and offers full independence from relatives.

However, such potential benefits are sometimes challenged because for various reasons, including impaired vision, the patient is unable to master the technique, and furthermore we do not think that the burden of the daily exchange should necessarily be imposed on the relatives. In these circumstances CCPD handled by the patient himself or by other persons from the family or even aid nurses can offer excellent clinical care.

Appropriate evaluation of daily CCPD compared to home peritoneal dialysis is not yet available. Indications for home haemodialysis remain exceptional among diabetic patients.

If centre dialysis is the only possibility, *haemodialysis* should be considered as the first choice and particular attention paid to vascular access. If for various reasons haemodialysis is considered too high a risk, *centre intermittent peritoneal dialysis* can be a satisfactory answer to the clinical problem for a few patients.

The challenging questions

Early dialysis when the creatinine clearance is still between 15–10 ml/min has been considered for both non-diabetic patients and diabetics to be the right choice for preventing the late complications of end-stage renal failure as well as decreasing the morbidity and mortality rates with better rehabilitation during the dialysis phase[1,2,10]. Diabetics should be excellent candidates for early dialysis, especially when one takes into account the severity and high rate of vascular complications which often jeopardize the later results. Nevertheless, the valid evaluation of the true benefit of early dialysis has always been difficult. The detriment to the patient and the community of a too early dialysis compared to the true potential benefit remains very difficult to evaluate[34]. We believe that early dialysis should not be considered for all diabetics, but only for those who present malnutrition and/or severe refractory hypertension despite multitherapy. In such patients the frequency of ocular and vascular complications, as well as rapid renal function deterioration make early dialysis using either haemo- or peritoneal dialysis necessary, and by the same token the best way of controlling their blood pressure. For diabetic patients with easily controlled blood pressure deferring the start of dialysis to when the creatinine clearance reaches around 7–5 ml/min seems acceptable. Unfortunately, patients are still often referred too late to dialysis units when the plasma creatinine is already greater than 1000 μmol/l.

Exclusion of a given patient from therapy when therapeutic facilities are available is always a very difficult choice. Casual good courses following adequate treatment, despite initial desperate situations make these decisions even more problematic. Nevertheless, treatments will induce more pain for the patient along with an intolerable burden for the relatives and a terrible cost for the community. Exclusion from treatment must not be a single man's decision, but should instead be the choice of a team including the relatives, nurses and physicians.

Cessation of treatment raises similar problems. The policy in our unit has been not to stop dialysis because of the severity of debilitating disorders like blindness, painful arteritis or multiple amputations, but only when cerebral lesions have led to unconsciousness or irreversible dementia.

Decisions such as exclusion from therapy or cessation of treatment should not only be discussed with all persons concerned in the medical unit, but should be, if not yet so in most centres, studied by an ethics committee so that the entire community be aware of some sad but unescapable consequences of what, nevertheless, remains a major therapeutic success.

CONCLUSION

The treatment of end-stage renal failure in diabetic patients requires close collaboration between the diabetologist, nephrologist and practitioner to offer the patient the best buy. If transplantation is a reasonable first choice for treating young juvenile diabetics, a majority of diabetic patients with ESRD will still be treated by dialysis methods for many more years. All methods including haemodialysis, continuous ambulatory peritoneal dialysis and other forms of peritoneal dialysis should be available in order to offer the best to each patient either at home or in the hospital. The most recent results obtained with all of these methods are very encouraging and still improving, nevertheless, diabetics remain at a high risk. Adequate dietary measures, excellent control of blood glucose level, vigorous control of hypertension are the best means to prevent the development of micro- and macroangiopathy, as well as slowing down the process of a progressive and often rapidly decreasing renal function. Treatment of end-stage renal failure is today's necessity, yet prevention is already a realistic objective.

References

1. Avram, M.M. (1982). Diabetic renal failure. *Nephron.*, **31**, 285
2. Jacobs, C., Rottembourg, J., Frantz, Ph., Slama, G. and Legrain, M. (1979). Treatment of end-stage renal failure in the insulin dependent diabetic patient. *Adv. Nephrol.*, **8**, 101 (Chicago: Year Book Med)
3. McCrary, R.F., Pitts, T.O. and Puschet, J.B. (1981). Diabetic nephropathy: Natural course, survivorship and therapy. *Am. J. Nephrol.*, **1**, 206
4. Polla-Imhoff, B., Pirson, Y., Lafontaine, J.J., Vandenbroucke, J.M., Costyns, J.P., Squifflet, J.P., Alexandre, G.P.F., van Ypersele de Strihou, C. (1982). Résultats de l'hémodialyse chronique et de la transplantation rénale dans le traitement de l'urémie terminale. *Nephrologie*, **3**, 80
5. Rao, T.K.S. and Friedman, E.A. (1982). Diabetic nephropathy. In Friedman, E. and L'Esperance, F. (eds.). *Diabetic Renal–Retinal Syndrome*, Vol. 2 pp. 3–7 (New York: Grune and Stratton)
6. Rostand, S.G., Kirk, K.A. and Rutsky, E.A. (1982). Racial differences in the incidence of treatment for end-stage renal disease. *N. Engl. J. Med.*, **306**, 1276
7. Jacobs, C., Broyer, M., Brunner, F.P., Brynger, H., Donckervolcke, R.A., Kramer, P., Selwood, H.H., Wing, A.J. and Bkake, R.H. (1980). Combined report on regular dialysis and transplantation in Europe 1980. In Robinson, B., Hawkins, J. and Davison, A. (eds.). *Proc. Eur. Dial. Transplant Assoc.*, Vol. 18, pp. 4–57 (Bath: Pitman)

8. Jacobs, C., Brunner, F.P., Brynger, H., Challah, S., Kramer, P., Selwood, N.H. and Wing, A.J. (1983). The changing scene in the treatment of diabetic patients with terminal uraemia in Europe. This volume, Chapter 2
9. Brynger, N. and Larsson, O. (1982). Ten years experience of renal transplantation in diabetic patients. In Kuss, R. and Legrain, M. (eds.). *Seminaires d'uronéphrologie Pitié Salpétrière.*, Vol. 8, p. 127 (Paris: Masson)
10. Friedman, E.A. (1980). Diabetic renal retinal syndrome. The prognosis improves. *Arch. Intern. Med.*, **140**, 1149
11. Kjellstrand, C., Whitley, K., Comty, C. and Shapiro, F. (1983). Dialysis in patients with diabetes mellitus. *Diabet. Nephrop.*, **2**, 5
12. Najarian, J.S., Sutherland, D.E.R., Simmons, R.L., Howard, R., Kjellstrand, C., Ramsay, R., Goetz, F., Fryd, D. and Sommer, B. (1979). Ten years experience with renal transplantation in juvenile onset diabetics. *Ann. Surg.*, **190**, 487
13. Shapiro, F. and Comty, C.M. (1982). Hemodialysis in diabetics 1981 update. In Friedman, E. and L'Esperance, F.L. (eds.). *Diabetic Renal-Retinal Syndrome,* Vol 2, pp. 309–320 (New York: Grune and Stratton)
14. Sutherland, D.E.R., Fryd, D.S., Peters, C., Ferguson, R.M., Najarian, J.S. (1982). Current status of kidney transplant in uremic diabetics at the University of Minnesota. In Friedman, E. and L'Esperance, F. (eds.). *Diabetic Renal-Retinal Syndrome,* Vol. 2, pp. 373–384 (New York: Grune and Stratton)
15. Belzer, F., Glass, N., Sollinger, H., Miller, D. (1982). Functional survival of juvenile diabetic patients after renal transplantation. In Friedman, E. and L'Esperance, F. (eds.). *Diabetic Renal-Retinal Syndrome,* Vol. 2, pp. 385–396. (New York: Grune and Stratton)
16. Ghavanian, M., Gutch, C.F., Kopp, K.F., Kilff, W.J. (1972). The sad truth about hemodialysis in diabetic nephropathy. *J. Am. Med. Assoc.*, **222**, 1386
17. Hosten, A., Cruz, I.A., Rao, M.S. (1981). Dialysis in diabetic patients with chronic renal failure. *Dial. Transplant.*, **10**, 206
18. Kjellstrand, C., Comty, C., Shapiro, F. (1982). A comparison of dialysis and transplantation in insulin-dependent diabetic patients. In Friedman, E. and L'Esperance, F. (eds.). *Diabetic Renal-Retinal Syndrome,* Vol. 2, pp. 405–417. (New York: Grune and Stratton)
19. Ramsay, R.C., Knobloch, W.H., Cantrill, H.L., Comty, C.M., Najarian, J.S. and Goetz, F.C. (1982). Visual status in transplanted and dialysed diabetic patients. *Diabetic Renal-Retinal Syndrome,* Vol 2, pp. 427–435 (New York: Grune and Stratton)
20. Steno Study Group (1982). Effect of 6 months of strict metabolic control on eye and kidney function in insulin-dependent diabetics with background retinopathy. *Lancet,* **i**, 121
21. Popovich, R.P., Moncrief, J.W., Nolph, K.D., Ghods, A.J., Twardowski, Z.J. and Pyle, W.K. (1978). Continuous ambulatory peritoneal dialysis. *Ann. Intern. Med.*, **88**, 449
22. Amair, A., Khanna, R., Leibel, B., Pierratos, A., Vas, S., Meema, E., Blair, G., Chisholm, L., Vas, M., Zingg, W., Digenis, G. and Oreopoulos, D. (1982). Continuous ambulatory peritoneal dialysis in diabetics with end-stage renal disease. *N. Engl. J. Med.*, **306**, 625
23. Katirtzoglou, A., Elzatt, S., Oreopoulos, D., Dombros, N., Blair, G., Chisholm, L., Meema, H., Ogilvie, R., Vas, S., Lieber, B. and McCreedy, W. (1980). Chronic peritoneal dialysis in diabetics with end-stage renal failure. In Friedman, E. and L'Esperance, F. (eds.). *Diabetic Retinal-Renal Syndrome,* pp. 317–331 (New York: Grune and Stratton)
24. Madden, M., Zimmerman, S., Simpson, D. (1982). Continuous ambulatory peritoneal dialysis in diabetes mellitus. The risk and benefit of intraperitoneal insulin. *Am. J. Nephrol.*, **2**, 133
25. Rottembourg, J., El Shahat, Y., Agrafiotis, A., Thuillier, Y., De Groc, F., Jacobs, C., Legrain, M. (1983). Continuous ambulatory peritoneal dialysis in insulin dependent diabetic patients: A 40 month experience. *Kidney Int.*, **23**, 40
26. Flynn, C.T. and Nanson, J. (1979). Intraperitoneal insulin with CAPD: An artificial pancreas. *Trans. Am. Soc. Artif. Intern. Organs,* **25**, 114
27. Flynn, Ç.T. (1981). The diabetic on CAPD. In Friedman, E. and L'Esperance, F. (eds.). *Diabetic Renal-Retinal Syndrome,* Vol. 2, pp. 321–330 (New York: Grune and Stratton)
28. Williams, C., Belvedere, D., Cattran, D., Clayton, S., Cole, E., Fenton, S., Gutman, K., Khanna, R., Knight, S., Manuel, A., Oreopoulos, D., Pierratos, A., Roscoe, J., Saiphoo, C., Vas, S. (1982). Experience with CAPD in diabetic patients in Toronto. *Perit. Dial. Bull.*, **2**, (Suppl.) S12

29. Hood, S. A., Frohnert, P. P., Mitchell, J. L. and Kurtz, S. B. (1980). Home peritoneal dialysis: dialysis therapy of choice in chronic renal failure of juvenile onset diabetes mellitus. *Dial. Transplant*, **9**, 843
30. Karanicolas, S. and Thompson, D. (1982). Intermittent peritoneal dialysis in the treatment of diabetics with end-stage renal disease. In CAPD in diabetics. *Perit. Dial. Bull.*, **2**, (Suppl.) S15
31. Slingeneyer, A., Mion, C., Selam, J. L. (1981). Home intermittent (IPD) and continuous ambulatory peritoneal dialysis (CAPD) as a long term treatment of end-stage renal failure in diabetics. In Gahl, G. M., Kessel, M. and Nolph, K. D. (eds.). *Advances in Peritoneal Dialysis*, pp. 378–388. (Amsterdam: Excerpta Medica)
32. Diaz Buxo, J. A., Walker, J., Farmer, C. D., Chandler, J. T., Holt, K. L. and Cox, P. (1981). Continuous cyclic peritoneal dialysis. *Trans. Am. Soc. Artif. Intern. Organs*, **27**, 51
33. Nakagawa, D., Price, C., Stinebaugh, B. and Suki, W. (1981). Continuous cycling peritoneal dialysis: a viable option in the treatment of chronic renal failure. *Trans. Am. Soc. Artif. Intern. Organs*, **27**, 55
34. Mogensen, C. E. (1982). Long term antihypertensive treatment inhibiting progression of diabetic nephroathy. *Br. Med. J.*, **285**, 685
35. Neff, M. S., Slifkin, R. F. and Eiser, A. R. (1982). Continuous ambulatory peritoneal dialysis in diabetics with end-stage renal disease. *N. Engl. J. Med.*, **37**, 1082

Closing remarks

H. KEEN and M. LEGRAIN

At the end of these two hard-working days we would congratulate our speakers and our audience on their effort and diligence. The success of the meeting has two main reasons. First, the presentations have been excellent. Second, the clear concern with the importance of the subject itself. And the catalytic activity of this splendid ambience should not be underestimated.

This first major conference of nephrologists and diabetologists in Europe marks an important stage in evolution of attitudes to the renal disease of diabetes. For the diabetologist, the appearance of persistent clinical proteinuria in a patient for whom he has been caring perhaps for decades has come to be an ominous portent that the patient's years are numbered. There has been little to do but helplessly observe the progressive decline of renal function, often increasingly complicated by visual, circulatory and neurological disabilities. Little wonder that the nephrologist, hard pressed for resources and struggling still with his own technological problems of dialysis and transplantation, was likely to counsel, albeit with compassion and regret, that his interventions would only prolong, perhaps even intensify, the patient's misery. In many cases, diabetics in renal failure were not even submitted for a nephrologist's opinion.

But now, the scene has changed and we must think again. Improvements and innovations in the care of diabetes and in the management of renal failure have significantly improved the prospect of a worthwhile extension of life for the patient with diabetic nephropathy. We must recognize the contribution made by the indefatigable workers who laboured on through the unpromising years, who refused and still refuse to admit defeat. For those standing on the sidelines it sometimes takes fine judgement to distinguish valorous from valueless activity and it is gratifying to begin to see a positive outcome from all that early effort. But as the last two days have shown, we have really just made a start in the conquest of this problem. On the diabetic side, retinal photocoagulation, adequately applied, can clearly conserve vision, and improved patient care can reduce the risk of chronic foot ulceration. But there are still the major problems of arterial disease, hypertension, autonomic and somatic neuropathy which complicate the picture. On the renal side, few problems met with in providing renal support for the non-diabetic are not magnified or more complicated in the diabetic patient. It seems clear that the intensive dialogue between the two disciplines in which we have been participating must continue, as we now go home, back to our clinics and hospitals where we must confront the patients and tackle the problems that we have been talking about.

A most hopeful view to emerge from this occasion is perhaps the growing conviction that renal failure in diabetes is preventable. As understanding of the pathogenic process grows so too will the opportunity of intervening rationally at an early stage. Present indications are that, for the first few years at any rate, the initiating abnormalities lie in the diabetic domain and that their arrest or reversal is largely a question of appropriate metabolic manipulation. In the later phases, the process has become essentially a self-generating renal one, common perhaps to many other later stage renal diseases. We are still ignorant of the point of transition from one phase to the other in diabetic nephropathy – and uncertain why some patients never seem to make that transition. All these considerations inspire us to hope and to hard work, above all to take home the memory of unanswered questions, the unfinished business of this meeting. It is only curiosity combined with enthusiasm and determination that will bring us the answers to these questions and improve the lot of our patients.

So thank you for coming, and thank you Travenol for organizing this valuable symposium. Goodbye.

Index